Obstetrics and Gynecology with Case Studies

Obstetrics and Gynecology with Case Studies

Editor: Adriana Taylor

AMERICAN
MEDICAL PUBLISHERS
www.americanmedicalpublishers.com

AMERICAN
MEDICAL PUBLISHERS
www.americanmedicalpublishers.com

Cataloging-in-Publication Data

Obstetrics and gynecology with case studies / edited by Adriana Taylor.
p. cm.
Includes bibliographical references and index.
ISBN 979-8-88740-648-0
1. Obstetrics. 2. Gynecology. 3. Generative organs, Female--Diseases.
I. Taylor, Adriana.
RG524 .H36 2023
618.2--dc23

American Medical Publishers,
41 Flatbush Avenue,
1st Floor, New York,
NY 11217, USA

ISBN 979-8-88740-648-0 (Hardback)

Contents

Preface

Obstetrics and gynecology is a medical specialty that seeks to provide medical care and support to women throughout the different stages of their reproductive lives. It focuses on two primary areas, obstetrics and gynecology. Obstetrics deals with pregnancy, childbirth, and postpartum issues. It encompasses prenatal care, monitoring the health of the mother and the developing fetus, managing and addressing any complications that may arise during pregnancy. It also provides support during labor and delivery. Gynecology focuses on the health of the female reproductive system outside of pregnancy. It deals with the diagnosis, treatment and prevention of conditions related to the female reproductive system, such as menstrual disorders, fertility issues, sexually transmitted infections (STIs), uterine fibroids, ovarian cysts, endometriosis, and gynecological cancers. This book strives to provide a fair idea about this discipline and to help develop a better understanding of the latest advances within this field. Those in search of information to further their knowledge will be greatly assisted by it.

After months of intensive research and writing, this book is the end result of all who devoted their time and efforts in the initiation and progress of this book. It will surely be a source of reference in enhancing the required knowledge of the new developments in the area. During the course of developing this book, certain measures such as accuracy, authenticity and research focused analytical studies were given preference in order to produce a comprehensive book in the area of study.

This book would not have been possible without the efforts of the authors and the publisher. I extend my sincere thanks to them. Secondly, I express my gratitude to my family and well-wishers. And most importantly, I thank my students for constantly expressing their willingness and curiosity in enhancing their knowledge in the field, which encourages me to take up further research projects for the advancement of the area.

Editor

1

A Case of Ruptured Decidualized Ovarian Endometrioma: Usefulness of Serial MRI for Determining Adequate Management

Saki Yamamoto,[1] Tomohiro Kikuchi,[1] Hiroyuki Fujii,[1] Yuko Otake,[1] Mitsuru Matsuki,[1] Risa Narumi,[2] Masashi Endo,[1] Hiroyuki Fujiwara,[2] and Harushi Mori[1]

[1]*Department of Radiology, Jichi Medical University School of Medicine, Tochigi, Japan*
[2]*Department of Obstetrics and Gynecology, Jichi Medical University School of Medicine, Tochigi, Japan*

Correspondence should be addressed to Saki Yamamoto; r1837ms@jichi.ac.jp

Academic Editor: Maria Grazia Porpora

Decidualization can originate in ovarian endometrioma by elevated serum progesterone levels during pregnancy, which mimics malignancy on ultrasonography. Moreover, decidualized ovarian endometrioma may rupture and cause acute abdominal pain during pregnancy. Magnetic resonance imaging (MRI) is reportedly useful in differentiating decidualized ovarian endometriomas from malignancies. However, to our knowledge, serial MRI of decidualized ovarian endometrioma before and after rupture has not been reported. Herein, we report the case of a 39-year-old woman with a ruptured decidualized ovarian endometrioma in which serial MRI was useful for adequate management. She had a history of right ovarian endometrioma. Transvaginal ultrasonography at 20 weeks of gestation showed the known right ovarian endometrioma with mural nodules that were not evident before pregnancy. MRI for further evaluation showed ovarian endometrioma with mural nodules with signals similar to those of the placenta. Based on the MRI findings, we diagnosed a decidualized ovarian endometrioma. At 27 weeks of gestation, she complained of sudden abdominal pain, for which MRI was performed. MRI showed disappearance of the ovarian endometrioma and bloody ascites, based on which we diagnosed a ruptured ovarian endometrioma. The abdominal pain subsided immediately, and a conservative observational treatment approach was taken. At 37 weeks of gestation, right ovarian cystectomy was performed simultaneously with an elective cesarean section, which revealed a ruptured decidualized ovarian endometrioma. Our findings demonstrate that the accurate diagnosis of a ruptured decidualized ovarian endometrioma on serial MRI can contribute to its management.

1. Introduction

Ovarian endometrioma occurs in 17–44% of patients with endometriosis and accounts for 35% of all benign ovarian cysts [1]. During pregnancy, increased progesterone levels may cause the decidualization of ovarian endometriomas, which mimics malignancies on imaging [2]. Recently, magnetic resonance imaging (MRI) has been reported to be useful in differentiating decidualized tissue from malignancies [3]. Moreover, decidualization can increase the risk of rupture of ovarian endometrioma [4]. Therefore, accurate diagnosis of a ruptured decidualized ovarian endometrioma during pregnancy is important for its adequate management.

Herein, we report a case of ruptured decidualized ovarian endometrioma in which serial MRI findings before and after the rupture were useful for determining the appropriate management.

2. Case Presentation

A 39-year-old woman (gravida 0, para 0) presented to our hospital for infertility treatment. She had a history of a 30 mm diameter right ovarian endometrioma. She became pregnant by oral clomiphene-intrauterine artificial insemination. At 20 weeks of gestation, transvaginal ultrasonography revealed that the ovarian endometrioma had enlarged

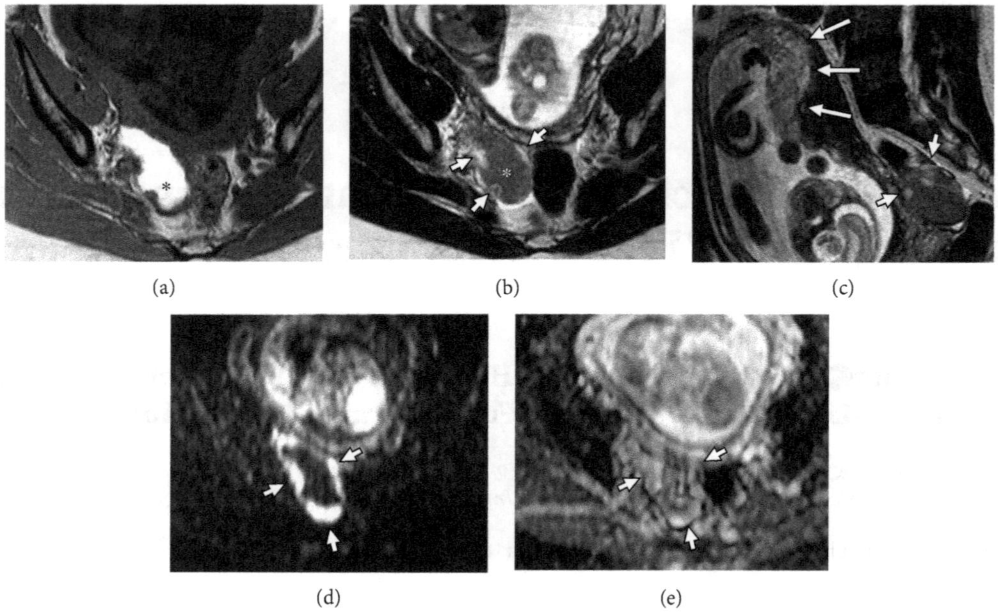

FIGURE 1: Magnetic resonance imaging (MRI) of the pelvis performed at 21 weeks of gestation. (a) Axial T1-weighted image. (b) Axial T2-weighted image. (c) Sagittal T2-weighted image. (d) Axial diffusion-weighted image (b factor: 1000 s/mm^2). (e) Apparent diffusion coefficient (ADC) map. MRI shows a well-circumscribed teardrop-shaped cystic lesion with mural nodules measuring $68 \times 45 \times 35$ mm in the right ovary. The cystic lesion shows uniformly marked high signal intensity on the T1-weighted image (a, asterisk) and intermediate signal intensity (b, asterisk) on T2-weighted images consistent with ovarian endometrioma. The mural nodules show intermediate to high signal intensity on T2-weighted images (b, c; short arrows) similar to the placenta (c, long arrows). Diffusion-weighted image (d, short arrows) and ADC map (e, short arrows) show the mural nodules with a high ADC value (1.6×10^{-3} mm^2/s). Based on these imaging findings, we diagnosed a decidualized ovarian endometrioma.

to 50 mm in diameter with mural nodules. The patient's serum cancer antigen-125 levels were slightly elevated (37 U/mL; normal, <35 U/mL), and carbohydrate antigen 19-9 levels were within normal limits (16 U/mL; normal, <37 U/mL). MRI for further evaluation showed a well-circumscribed, teardrop-shaped cystic lesion with mural nodules measuring $68 \times 45 \times 35$ mm in the right ovary (Figure 1). The cystic lesion showed uniformly marked high signal intensity on T1-weighted images and intermediate signal intensity on T2-weighted images, consistent with an ovarian endometrioma. The mural nodules showed intermediate to high signal intensity on T2-weighted images, high signal intensity on diffusion-weighted images, and a high apparent diffusion coefficient (ADC) value (1.6×10^{-3} mm^2/s) on the ADC map, which were similar to those of the placenta. Based on these imaging findings, we diagnosed a decidualized ovarian endometrioma. Further, we planned to perform MRI 6 weeks later.

At 27 weeks of gestation, the patient complained of sudden abdominal pain. Emergent MRI was performed. The decidualized ovarian endometrioma had disappeared; however, bloody ascites were found (Figure 2). Based on serial MRI findings, rupture of the decidualized ovarian endometrioma was suspected. The abdominal pain subsided immediately after injection of pentazocine 15 mg, and conservative observational management was chosen.

At 37 weeks of gestation, the patient underwent an elective cesarean section and right ovarian cystectomy simultaneously. Ruptured ovarian cystic lesions were confirmed during the surgery. The cystic lesion contained chocolate-like bloody fluid. Histopathological findings revealed decidual reaction of the ovarian endometrioma and no evidence of malignancy (Figure 3). The final diagnosis was a ruptured decidualized ovarian endometrioma. The postoperative course was uneventful, and the patient was discharged 7 days later.

3. Discussion

We have reported the case of a ruptured decidualized endometrioma during pregnancy, which was useful to diagnose accurately by serial MRI and determine the patient's treatment options. In the present case, we diagnosed a decidualized ovarian endometrioma upon the first MRI examination during pregnancy. Further, we suspected rupture of the endometrioma, due to its disappearance and bloody ascites found on serial MRI at the onset of sudden abdominal pain. We further employed a conservative observational management approach, and elective cesarean section and right ovarian cystectomy were simultaneously performed at full term. Intraoperative and histologic examination demonstrated a ruptured decidualized endometrioma.

Endometriosis is a common disease occurring in 5–10% of women of reproductive age [2]. It is one of the main causes of infertility due to mechanical factors, including adhesions, tubal blockage, and ovulation disorders [5]. The number of pregnancies with endometriosis has been increasing due to the progression of assisted reproductive technologies [2]. Decidualization can also originate in ovarian

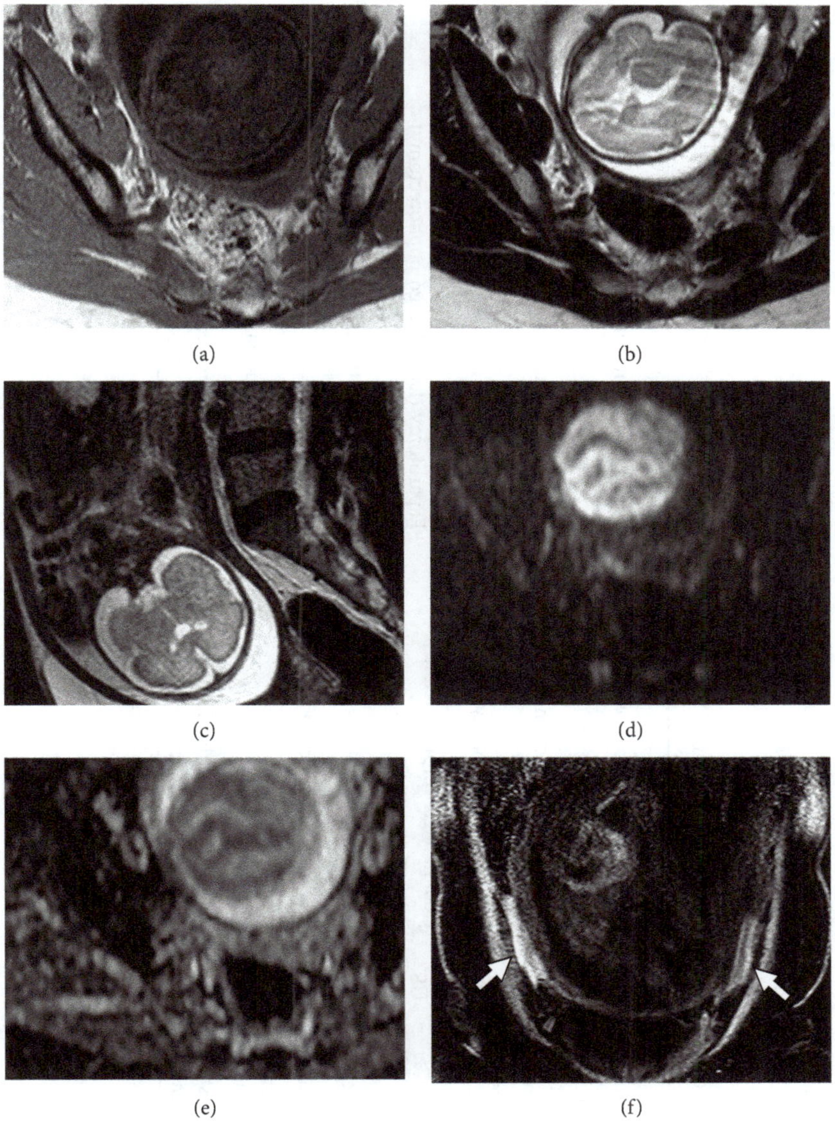

FIGURE 2: Magnetic resonance imaging (MRI) of the pelvis performed at 27 weeks of gestation. (a) Axial T1-weighted image. (b) Axial T2-weighted image. (c) Sagittal T2-weighted image. (d) Axial diffusion-weighted image (b factor: 1000 s/mm^2). (e) ADC map. (f) Coronal T1-weighted image with fat saturation. The cystic lesion disappears (a–e). Ascites around the uterus shows high signal intensity on fat-suppressed T1-weighted images, which is consistent with bloody ascites (f, arrows). Based on serial MRI findings, rupture of the decidualized ovarian endometrioma is suspected.

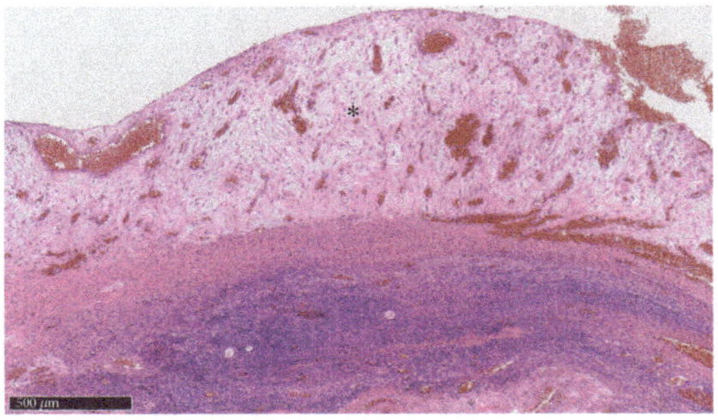

FIGURE 3: Microscopic view of a mural nodule (hematoxylin and eosin staining, magnification: 100x). Edematous tissue with abundant stromal cells' cytoplasm is visible (asterisk). These findings are consistent with decidualization.

endometrioma by elevating serum progesterone levels during pregnancy [2]. Previous reports revealed that approximately 12% of ovarian endometriomas have decidual reactions during pregnancy [2]. Decidualization primarily occurs in the second trimester and regresses during the third trimester or postpartum period [2].

Ovarian endometriomas can rupture for various reasons, including adhesions, tissue fragility, increased external pressure, or increased internal pressure due to mass enlargement. During pregnancy, increased levels of progesterone tend to shrink ovarian endometrioma [2]. However, decidualization is expected to increase ovarian endometrioma rupture due to enlargement and wall softening caused by a severe inflammatory response [2, 6]. To date, there have been six case reports of ruptured decidualized ovarian

Table 1: Summary of seven cases of ruptured decidualized endometriotic cysts.

Authors (year)	Patient age (years)	Size (mm)	Time of rupture	Imaging	Preoperative diagnosis	Treatment during pregnancy
Vercellini et al. (1992) [11]	29	80	Third trimester (35 weeks pregnant)	US	Bowel obstruction	Laparotomy (cyst enucleation and a cesarean section)
Loh et al. (1998) [9]	25	40	First trimester (6 weeks pregnant)	US	Ectopic pregnancy	Laparoscopic ovarian cystectomy
Garcia-Velasco et al. (1998) [7]	25	83×54	First trimester (9 weeks pregnant)	US	Hemorrhagic corpus luteum or endometrioma	Laparotomy (left salpingo-oophorectomy)
Gregora et al. (1998) [8]	44	60	Second trimester (17 weeks pregnant)	US	Endometriomas*	Laparotomy (opening the cyst and stripping the lining)
Ueda et al. (2010) [2]	33	61	Second trimester	US	Ovarian endometriosis*	Peritoneal washing and drainage
Reif et al. (2011) [10]	25	NA (after rupture)	Second trimester (27 weeks pregnant)	US	NA	Laparotomy (operative hemostasis and preterm cesarean section)
Present study	39	$68 \times 45 \times 35$	Second trimester (27 weeks pregnant)	US MRI	Rupture of decidualized endometriotic cyst	Conservative treatment, an elective cesarean section, and right ovarian cystectomy at 37-week pregnancy

NA: not applicable; US: ultrasonography; MRI: magnetic resonance imaging. *The preoperative diagnosis of the ruptured tumor was not described.

endometrioma (Table 1) [2, 7–11]. Among the six cases, rupture occurred during the first trimester in two cases, second trimester in three cases, and third trimester in one case.

Ultrasonography is the first choice for the screening of decidualized ovarian endometrioma. However, decidualized tissues appear as mural nodules in the cyst mimicking malignant tumors, such as endometrioid carcinoma and clear cell carcinoma arising from ovarian endometrioma [12]. Moreover, no previously reported cases (Table 1) were accurately diagnosed preoperatively with ruptured decidualized ovarian endometrioma. It is considered that ultrasonography may be limited of the visual field during pregnancy.

MRI is reported to be useful in the diagnosis of decidualized tissue, which has a thin broad structure and shows intermediate to high signal intensities on T2-weighted images, similar to the placenta. Morisawa et al. reported that the ADC values of the decidualized regions were significantly higher than those of the mural nodules of endometrioid carcinoma or clear cell carcinoma (1.77×10^{-3} mm^2/s vs. 1.13×10^{-3} mm^2/s) on diffusion-weighted images [3]. In the present case, the patient's MRI findings were similar, and we diagnosed a decidualized ovarian endometrioma. Additionally, MRI of a ruptured endometrioma can identify shrinkage or disappearance of the cyst and bloody ascites, as in the present case [13].

To our knowledge, serial MRI before and after the rupture of decidualized ovarian endometrioma during pregnancy has not been reported. In the present case, serial MRI findings before and after rupture showed disappearance of the cyst with MRI findings characteristic of decidualized ovarian endometrioma, which contributed to the accurate diagnosis.

There is no definite management for ruptured benign ovarian cystic lesions during pregnancy. All of the six patients mentioned in Table 1 underwent surgery. However, the risk of miscarriage associated with abdominal surgery during pregnancy increases in the first trimester. In addition, the risk of adverse outcomes such as miscarriage, preterm delivery, and intrauterine fetal death is increased in surgeries performed after 23 weeks of gestation [14]. Therefore, we believe that conservative treatment can be a management option in cases without torsion or malignancy and with stable hemodynamics or pain.

In conclusion, here we accurately diagnosed a ruptured decidualized ovarian endometrioma by serial MRI and chose conservative observation. In the future, the indications for conservative treatment of benign ovarian cystic lesions during pregnancy should be considered with the addition of MRI findings.

References

[1] M. Busacca and M. Vignali, "Ovarian endometriosis," *Current Opinion in Obstetrics & Gynecology*, vol. 15, no. 4, pp. 321–326, 2003.

[2] Y. Ueda, T. Enomoto, T. Miyatake et al., "A retrospective analysis of ovarian endometriosis during pregnancy," *Fertility and Sterility*, vol. 94, no. 1, pp. 78–84, 2010.

[3] N. Morisawa, A. Kido, M. Kataoka, S. Minamiguchi, I. Konishi, and K. Togashi, "Magnetic resonance imaging manifestations of decidualized endometriotic cysts: comparative study with ovarian cancers associated with endometriotic cysts," *Journal of Computer Assisted Tomography*, vol. 38, no. 6, pp. 879–884, 2014.

[4] L. R. U. Maggiore, S. Ferrero, G. Mangili et al., "A systematic review on endometriosis during pregnancy: diagnosis, misdiagnosis, complications and outcomes," *Human Reproduction Update*, vol. 22, no. 1, pp. 70–103, 2016.

[5] T. Tanbo and P. Fedorcsak, "Endometriosis-associated infertility: aspects of pathophysiological mechanisms and treatment options," *Acta Obstetricia et Gynecologica Scandinavica*, vol. 96, no. 6, pp. 659–667, 2017.

[6] A. Pisanu, D. Deplano, S. Angioni, R. Ambu, and A. Uccheddu, "Rectal perforation from endometriosis in pregnancy: case report and literature review," *World Journal of Gastroenterology*, vol. 16, no. 5, pp. 648–651, 2010.

[7] J. A. García-Velasco, M. Alvarez, A. Palumbo, A. González-González, and J. Ordás, "Rupture of an ovarian endometrioma during the first trimester of pregnancy," *European Journal of Obstetrics, Gynecology, and Reproductive Biology*, vol. 76, no. 1, pp. 41–43, 1998.

[8] M. Gregora and P. Higgs, "Endometriomas in pregnancy," *The Australian & New Zealand Journal of Obstetrics & Gynaecology*, vol. 38, no. 1, pp. 106–109, 1998.

[9] F. H. Loh, S. P. Chua, R. Khalil, and S. C. Ng, "Case report of ruptured endometriotic cyst in pregnancy treated by laparoscopic ovarian cystectomy," *Singapore Medical Journal*, vol. 39, no. 8, pp. 368-369, 1998.

[10] P. Reif, W. Schöll, P. Klaritsch, and U. Lang, "Rupture of endometriotic ovarian cyst causes acute hemoperitoneum in twin pregnancy," *Fertility and Sterility*, vol. 95, no. 6, p. 2125.e1, 2011.

[11] P. Vercellini, A. Ferrari, N. Vendola, and S. G. Carinelli, "Growth and rupture of an ovarian endometrioma in pregnancy," *International Journal of Gynaecology and Obstetrics*, vol. 37, no. 3, pp. 203–205, 1992.

[12] Y. Kurata, A. Kido, Y. Moribata et al., "Diagnostic performance of MR imaging findings and quantitative values in the differentiation of seromucinous borderline tumour from endometriosis-related malignant ovarian tumour," *European Radiology*, vol. 27, no. 4, pp. 1695–1703, 2017.

[13] M. Nishino, K. Hayakawa, K. Iwasaku, and K. Takasu, "Magnetic resonance imaging findings in gynecologic emergencies," *Journal of Computer Assisted Tomography*, vol. 27, no. 4, pp. 564–570, 2003.

[14] T. Bignardi and G. Condous, "The management of ovarian pathology in pregnancy," *Best Practice & Research. Clinical Obstetrics & Gynaecology*, vol. 23, no. 4, pp. 539–548, 2009.

2

A Case of Intertwin Membrane Hemorrhage with Spontaneous Resolution

Lily Criscione,[1] Kristen Elmezzi,[1] Saioa Torrealday,[1] Barton C. Staat,[2] and Kimberly Hickey[2]

[1]*Walter Reed National Military Medical Center, 8901 Rockville Pike, Bethesda, MD 20889, USA*
[2]*Uniformed Services University, 4301 Jones Bridge Rd., Bethesda, MD 20814, USA*

Correspondence should be addressed to Lily Criscione; lily.t.criscione.mil@mail.mil

Academic Editor: Seung-Yup Ku

Vaginal bleeding during pregnancy places women at increased risk of spontaneous abortion. Etiologies for threatened and spontaneous abortions have been well studied, but there is little information on intertwin membrane hemorrhage. We present a patient with a multiple gestation pregnancy who experienced first trimester vaginal bleeding with visualization and subsequent rapid resolution of an intertwin membrane hemorrhage. The patient had an otherwise normal pregnancy until the third trimester when she developed preeclampsia with severe features and elected for a primary cesarean section at 35 + 5 weeks. The implications of an intertwin membrane hemorrhage are not well understood, although there could be a possible correlation between the hemorrhage and the ultimate progression to preeclampsia with severe features. Despite the final diagnosis, the patient did not have any noticeable complications due to the hemorrhage both when it was discovered and in the weeks following its discovery.

1. Introduction

Vaginal bleeding during pregnancy places women at increased risk of spontaneous abortion. Etiologies for threatened and spontaneous abortions have been well studied, but there is little information on intertwin membrane hemorrhage. Intertwin membrane hemorrhage is an obstetric condition that is rarely observed; in fact, there is only one other case reported in the literature [1]. Equally to the pathophysiology of an abruption, one could postulate that an intertwin hemorrhage could increase the patient's risk of developing preterm labor or preterm prelabor rupture of membranes, as well as intrauterine growth restriction, oligohydramnios, or preeclampsia.

2. Case

A 33-year-old gravida 1 successfully conceived after ovulation induction with letrozole and intrauterine insemination. The patient's medical history was significant only for migraines. Her surgical history was notable for a laparoscopic right salpingo-oophorectomy and appendectomy for chronic right-sided pelvic pain.

The patient presented for an ultrasound at 5 + 2 weeks, which revealed 3 gestational sacs; however, only 2 contained yolk sacs. An ultrasound at 6 + 2 weeks confirmed a dichorionic twin pregnancy with 2 gestational sacs, yolk sacs, and fetal poles. At 9 + 2 weeks, she experienced vaginal bleeding followed by a second episode 4 days later. On both occasions, she was seen in the emergency room where ultrasound not only confirmed a viable twin pregnancy but also demonstrated a normal dividing membrane and no evidence of subchorionic bleeding. There was no intertwin hemorrhage noted. She continued to experience vaginal bleeding, yet subsequent evaluations were reassuring (Figure 1).

The patient presented to perinatology for her nuchal translucency ultrasound at 11 weeks. By then, her vaginal bleeding had ceased; she denied contractions, cramping, and vaginal discharge. Her ultrasound showed a 15.0 mm intertwin membrane hemorrhage (Figure 2). The recommended baby aspirin was held, and the patient was given bleeding and preterm labor precautions.

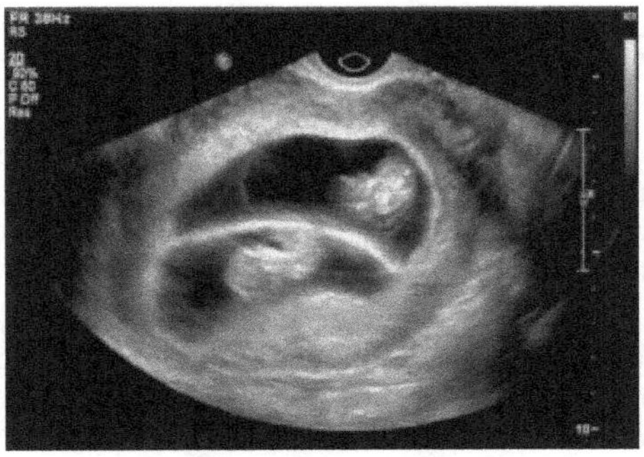

FIGURE 1: Patient at 10 + 1 weeks EGA with no evidence of abnormally thickened membrane.

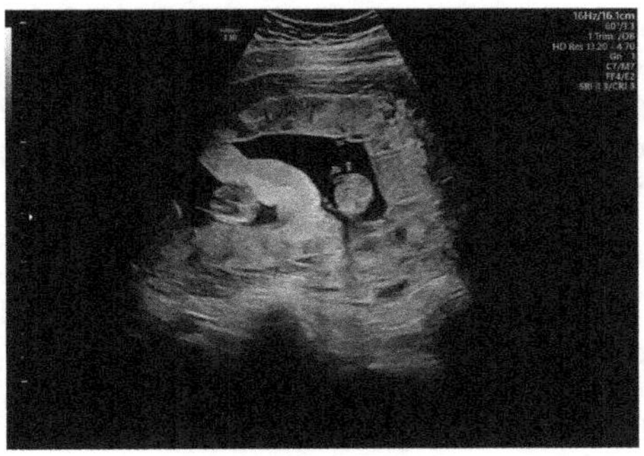

FIGURE 2: Patient at 11 + 0 weeks EGA with intertwin membrane hemorrhage, 15 mm in thickness.

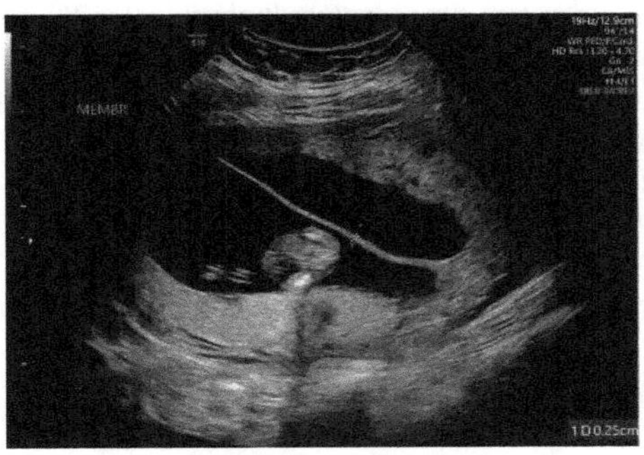

FIGURE 3: Patient at 13 + 3 weeks EGA with reabsorbed hemorrhage. Thickness now 2.5 mm.

When she returned at 13 + 3 weeks for follow-up, the hemorrhage had resolved; the spanning membranes measured 2.5 mm (Figure 3). She remained asymptomatic and denied vaginal bleeding. At her 16-week assessment, her imaging continued to be reassuring. The pregnancy progressed normally until 35 + 2 weeks, when she demonstrated mild hypertension. ALT and AST were 44 and 36, respectively; she was otherwise asymptomatic. The next day her AST and ALT were 58 and 78, and she was diagnosed with preeclampsia with severe features. Although she was offered an induction of labor, she underwent an elective primary cesarean section at 35 + 5 weeks following steroid administration for fetal lung maturity; estimated blood loss was 1 L. The cesarean was productive of two viable female infants with twin A of APGARS 8/8, weighing 2510 grams and twin B of APGARS 5/7/8, weighing 2300 grams. The twins had demonstrated appropriate growth throughout pregnancy. The patient completed a 24-hour course of magnesium following delivery; she received a transfusion of 2 units of packed red blood cells due to symptomatic anemia. She was discharged with both infants on postoperative day 5.

Upon inspection of the placentas at time of surgery, gross clot remnants between the twins' membranes were not appreciated. The pathology report showed diamniotic dichorionic nonfused placentas with an organized, dividing membrane hematoma. Placenta A's chorionic plate vessels demonstrated a possible eosinophilic or T-cell vasculitis. Neither decidual arteriopathy nor chorionic villitis was identified. Per the report, on the membrane between placenta A and B existed an area of confluent subchorionic fibrin deposition that measured 4.5 × 4.0 cm in diameter; no areas of acute hemorrhage or hematoma formation were identified.

3. Discussion

On review, there is only one other case report identifying a patient with an intertwin membrane hemorrhage visualized on ultrasound. Nevertheless, that patient's pregnancy was viable at 33 + 1 weeks when the hemorrhage was noted, and she was ultimately diagnosed with an abruption that was determined to be unstable, necessitating an emergency cesarean section. The patient did not develop subsequent sequelae from the bleed, such as preeclampsia [1]. That patient contrasts with our case, in which the patient was diagnosed with a stable hemorrhage that resolved with little discernable complications for the pregnancy. Yet with the eventual diagnosis of preeclampsia with severe features, one could postulate that the hemorrhage increased our patient's risk. Overall, both cases demonstrate ultrasound visualization of bleeding into the intertwin membrane space; however, the significance of the hemorrhages differ, in that the prior case demonstrated an abruption necessitating emergent delivery, whereas our patient, though a marginal abruption could be the underlying cause of the hemorrhage, had a bleed that was stable and ultimately resolved, enabling her to carry the pregnancy to the third trimester [1].

It is possible that when intermembrane hemorrhages occur they resolve quickly, leaving their incidence difficult to predict. Our patient was being monitored closely by multiple subspecialists and had frequent ultrasounds assessing her pregnancy's progression, increasing the opportunity of detecting transient abnormalities. With the increased use of infertility treatment modalities compounded by the increase incidence of multiple gestations within this population, perhaps more cases of intermembrane hemorrhage will be diagnosed and the sequelae will become clearer.

This irregularly thickened 15.0 mm dividing membrane was not a normal variant, as the vast majority of dichorionic twins show thickness between 1.9 and 3.6 mm [2, 3]. Differential diagnosis could include a circumvallate placenta, an amniotic band, uterine synechiae, uterine congenital abnormalities, or membranes from a vanishing twin. Due to the increased thickness, echogenicity, and relative homogeneity of the region in question as well as the transient nature, all the aforementioned possibilities are less likely than simply a hemorrhage collecting between the twins' amniotic borders.

The question that remained for our patient was the implications of the hemorrhage. She was counseled on premature preterm rupture of membranes and preterm contractions, as blood is a possible uterine irritant. Similar to the pathophysiology of an abruption, a hemorrhage in the intrauterine space can promote the release of thrombin, which acts as a uterotonic agent [4, 5]. Furthermore, thrombin ignites the inflammation cascade, which can cause further vascular degradation and possible rupture of membranes [6, 7]. Marginal abruption may not require an immediate delivery, but can result in other complications such as oligohydramnios and intrauterine growth restriction, neither of which our patient demonstrated [8]. Additionally, early vaginal bleeding in twin pregnancy has been shown to increase the overall gestation's risk of abruption, rupture of membranes, and preterm birth at less than 34 weeks [9]. Fortunately, the patient did not display preterm labor during her subsequent clinic visits, and the spontaneous resolution and reabsorption of the blood possibly returned her overall risk of preterm delivery to its baseline in a twin pregnancy [10]. Likewise, the twin pregnancy increased the patient's baseline risk for preeclampsia. The progression to preeclampsia with severe features could be correlated to the intertwin membrane hemorrhage as well, as a utero-placental malformation that allowed for the original bleed could predispose the patient to a subsequent placental disorder such as preeclampsia. Studies have shown that a history of abruption in a prior pregnancy can increase one's risk of developing preeclampsia in a following pregnancy [11].

In conclusion, intermembrane hemorrhage may be more commonplace than documented. There is a knowledge gap in regard to the prevalence of intermembrane hemorrhage and potential associated complications. Based on this case, we would recommend that intermembrane hemorrhages be managed conservatively with frequent follow-up ultrasounds and assessments for preterm labor, preterm prelabor rupture of membranes, oligohydramnios, intrauterine growth restriction, and preeclampsia. Regardless of the ambiguity that surrounds the findings and outcomes, this case is noteworthy, as it can offer guidance and counseling for future patients with intertwin membrane hemorrhages.

Acknowledgments

We would like to thank the perinatology and pathology departments at Walter Reed National Military Medical Center for their assistance in caring for this patient and in preparing this report. Furthermore, we of course would like to acknowledge the patient for her willingness to share her story; she has given written consent for publication of her case.

References

[1] M. Kacerovsky and J. Tosner, "Prenatal diagnosis of an intertwin membrane hematoma," *Journal of Clinical Ultrasound*, vol. 38, no. 7, pp. 397–399, 2010.

[2] L. A. Bracero, C. Huff, M. J. Blitz, M. J. Plata, D. J. Seybold, and M. Broce, "Ultrasound and histological measurements of dividing membrane thickness in twin gestations," *Ultrasound in Obstetrics & Gynecology*, vol. 50, no. 4, pp. 470–475, 2017.

[3] B. S. Hertzberg, A. B. Kurtz, H. Y. Choi et al., "Significance of membrane thickness in the sonographic evaluation of twin gestations," *American Journal of Roentgenology*, vol. 148, no. 1, pp. 151–153, 1987.

[4] M. A. Elovitz, J. Ascher-Landsberg, T. Saunders, and M. Phillippe, "The mechanisms underlying the stimulatory effects of thrombin on myometrial smooth muscle," *American Journal of Obstetrics and Gynecology*, vol. 183, no. 3, pp. 674–681, 2000.

[5] S.-T. Huang, F. Schatz, C. Salafia, C. Stocco, C. Lockwood, and G. Krikun, "Thrombin activation of endometrial endothelial cells: a possible role in intrauterine growth restriction," *Thrombosis and Haemostasis*, vol. 97, no. 2, pp. 245–253, 2007.

[6] A. Incebiyik, H. Uyanikoglu, N. G. Hilali, S. Sak, A. B. Turp, and M. E. Sak, "Does apoptotic activity have a role in the development of the placental abruption?," *The Journal of Maternal-Fetal & Neonatal Medicine*, vol. 30, no. 23, pp. 2871–2875, 2017.

[7] A. P. Mackenzie, F. Schatz, G. Krikun, E. F. Funai, S. Kadner, and C. J. Lockwood, "Mechanisms of abruption-induced premature rupture of the fetal membranes: Thrombin enhanced decidual matrix metalloproteinase-3 (stromelysin-1) expression," *American Journal of Obstetrics and Gynecology*, vol. 191, no. 6, pp. 1996–2001, 2004.

[8] C. V. Ananth, Y. Oyelese, V. Prasad, D. Getahun, and J. C. Smulian, "Evidence of placental abruption as a chronic process: Associations with vaginal bleeding early in pregnancy and placental lesions," *European Journal of Obstetrics & Gynecology and Reproductive Biology*, vol. 128, no. 1-2, pp. 15–21, 2006.

[9] J. A. Mcpherson, A. O. Odibo, A. I. Shanks, K. A. Roehl, G. A. Macones, and A. G. Cahill, "Adverse outcomes in twin pregnancies complicated by early vaginal bleeding," *American Journal of Obstetrics and Gynecology*, vol. 208, no. 1, pp. 56.e1–56.e5, 2013.

[10] J. A. Martin, B. E. Hamilton, S. J. Ventura et al., "Births: final data for 2009," *National Vital Statistics Reports*, vol. 60, no. 1, pp. 1–72, 2011.

[11] S. E. Parker, M. M. Werler, M. Gissler, M. Tikkanen, and C. V. Ananth, "Placental abruption and subsequent risk of preeclampsia: a population-based case-control study," *Paediatric and Perinatal Epidemiology*, vol. 29, no. 3, pp. 211–219, 2015.

3

Laparotomy for Advanced Abdominal Ectopic Pregnancy

Dereje Tegene, Sultan Nesha, Befikadu Gizaw, and Tadele Befikadu

Department of Obstetrics and Gynecology, Adama Hospital Medical College, Adama, Ethiopia

Correspondence should be addressed to Dereje Tegene; fekadutd79@gmail.com

Academic Editor: Kyousuke Takeuchi

Background. Abdominal pregnancy is the rarest and the most serious type of extrauterine pregnancy. The mainstay of treatment for advanced abdominal pregnancy is surgery. The fetus can be delivered easily, and there are two options for the management of the placenta: removal of the placenta and leave the placenta in situ. *Case Presentation.* This is a 26-year-old primigravida lady who does not recall her first day of last normal menstrual period (LNMP) but claimed to be amenorrhic for the past 9 months. She had antenatal care (ANC) follow-up at a private hospital and had obstetric ultrasound two times and told that the pregnancy was normal. Currently, she presented with absent fetal movement of one week and vaginal bleeding of 3 days duration. She had history of abdominal pain with fetal movement before one week. Upon examination, the abdomen was 34 weeks sized, with easily palpable fetal parts; fetal heartbeat was negative, with mild abdominal tenderness. The cervix was closed and uneffaced. She was investigated with ultrasound which reveals 3rd trimester abdominal ectopic pregnancy with negative fetal heartbeat. Laparotomy was done to deliver a 2000 gm female stillborn with GIII maceration from the peritoneal cavity. Placenta was removed after releasing adhesion from the bowel and omentum. She had smooth postoperative course and discharged on her 5th postoperative day. *Conclusion.* Abdominal ectopic pregnancy could be missed despite having repeated ultrasound scanning and may continue to third trimester. High index of suspicion and correlation of patient's sign and symptom is very important to make early diagnosis.

1. Introduction

Abdominal pregnancy refers to a pregnancy that has implanted in the peritoneal cavity, external to the uterine cavity and fallopian tubes [1]. An abdominal pregnancy is the rarest and the most serious type of extrauterine pregnancy [2]. It accounts 1 to 1.4 percent of all ectopic pregnancies [1, 3]. Early diagnosis of an abdominal pregnancy is difficult since it is associated with a wide range of signs and symptoms [2]. Risk factors for abdominal pregnancy include tubal damage, pelvic inflammatory disease, endometriosis, assisted reproductive techniques, and multiparity [4, 5]. The patient with advanced abdominal pregnancy may present with history of recurrent abdominal discomfort, painful fetal movement beneath the abdominal wall, the presence of fetal movements high in the upper abdomen, cessation of fetal movement, a closed and uneffaced cervix, or the failure of oxytocin to stimulate the gestational mass. Ultrasound is the most effective method for diagnosing an abdominal ectopic pregnancy [2]. The fetus can be delivered easily; the key issue is how to manage the placenta. There are two options for the management of the placenta; the first being removal of the placenta after ligating the placental blood supply, if the placental separation is not difficult [4, 6]. We have to be cautious upon removal of the placenta since it may lead to life-threatening maternal hemorrhage. The second option is leaving the placenta in situ after ligating the umbilical cord [6].

We present a case of abdominal ectopic pregnancy which progressed to third trimester and end up with fetal death. Despite having repeated ultrasound scanning, the diagnosis was missed. It emphasizes the need of high index of suspicion and correlation of patient's sign and symptom with ultrasound finding to make the early diagnosis of abdominal ectopic pregnancy. Removal of the placenta is a preferred option for the placental management, if the placental separation is not difficult. Relevant literatures were also reviewed.

2. Case Presentation

This is a 26-year-old primigravida lady who does not recall her first day of last normal menstrual period (LNMP) but claims to be amenorrhic for the past 9 months. She had no early milestones at hand. She had antenatal care (ANC) follow-up at a private hospital in Mojo town. During her ANC follow-up, she had obstetric ultrasound scanning two times, and she was told that the pregnancy was normal. Currently, she was presented with the complaint of absent fetal movement of one week and vaginal bleeding of 3 days duration; the bleeding was bright red and nonclotting. She had history of abdominal pain with fetal movement before one week. Otherwise, she had no history of nausea or vomiting. She was referred to our hospital from Bishoftu General Hospital with the diagnosis of rule out third trimester abdominal ectopic pregnancy after having an obstetric ultrasound, and the reason for referral was for better investigation and management. She was married 10 years back but unable to get pregnant despite having unprotected regular sexual intercourse for the past 10 years. She had no history of pelvic inflammatory disease (PID). She had no history of exposure to ovulation induction drugs or use of assisted reproductive technology. She had no history of chronic medical or surgical illnesses. The pregnancy was planned, wanted, and supported.

Upon physical examination, she was well looking and comfortable, and her vital signs were as follows: blood pressure = 110/70 mmHg, pulse rate = 88 bpm, respiratory rate = 20 breaths per minute, and temperature = afebrile to touch. She had pink conjunctive and nonicteric sclera. Pertinent findings were on the abdomen: the abdomen was 34 weeks sized with irregular outline and easily palpable fetal parts, fetal heartbeat (FHB) was negative, with mild abdominal tenderness, and there was no signs of fluid collection. On genitourinary system (GUS), she had normal external female genitalia, she had no active vaginal bleeding, the cervix wa[1, 7]s closed and uneffaced, there are no cervical motion tenderness and palpable adnexal mass, and upon bimanual examination, the cervix does not move with the fetal parts. She was investigated with obstetric ultrasound and reported as follows: she had singleton extrauterine pregnancy, with an empty uterus measuring 9 cm∗10 cm, FHB was negative, the placenta was attached to the posterior abdominal wall near to the blood vessels, and gestational age (GA) by femur length (FL) was 31 weeks + 3 days. The index was 3rd trimester abdominal ectopic pregnancy with fetal death (Figures 1(a) and 1(b)). Her laboratory investigation reveals the following: white blood cell = 6,290/mm^3; hemoglobin = 11.5 g/dl; platelet count = 404 × 10^3/ml, and blood group and Rh = O$^+$. Coagulation profile shows the following: PT = 15 seconds, aPTT = 28.7 seconds, and INR = 1 ratio.

With the diagnosis of primigravida + 3rd trimester abdominal ectopic pregnancy + fetal death, the plan was to admit her to the ward and to have abdominopelvic MRI to confirm the diagnosis and to assess the placental attachment with the major vessels. Since MRI was not available in our hospital and the patient could not afford the cost at a private facility, MRI was not done. The surgical team was consulted, and she was evaluated by the team. After the discussion with the surgical team, decision for laparotomy was made. After informed written consent was obtained from the patient and 4 unit of cross-matched blood was prepared, the patient was taken to the operation theater. Under general anesthesia, the abdomen was entered through the midline incision. Intraoperative findings were as follows: There was a large gestational sac containing well-formed fetus and placenta within the peritoneal cavity. The sac was adherent to the cecum and mesentery of gastrointestinal tract. There was no adhesion of the placenta with the major organs and major vessels. There was an intact 8-week-sized nongravid uterus with healthy looking left ovaries and tube. The right ovary and tube were not identified due to dense adhesion (Figures 2(a) and 2(b)).

What was done was after opening the sac, a 2000 gm female stillborn with GIII maceration was delivered (Figure 3). Meconium-stained amniotic fluid was sucked from the sac. Adhesion with the bowel and omentum was released by sharp dissection, and the placenta was taken out from the peritoneal cavity. After securing hemostasis, exploration of the bowel was made for possible bowel injury. The peritoneal cavity was lavaged with 4 liter of normal saline, and the abdomen was closed in layer. Estimated blood loss was 700 ml. The patient transferred to the ward with stable vital sign and postoperative orders. Postoperatively, the patient was on maintenance fluid, parenteral antibiotics, and standing dose of analgesia. She had smooth postoperative course, and her post-op hemoglobin was 9.4 g/dl. She was discharged on her 5th postoperative day with therapeutic dose of ferrous sulfate and appointed after 1 week. She was seen at an outpatient clinic three times and she had no new compliant.

3. Discussion

An ectopic pregnancy is a pregnancy where the blastocyst implants anywhere other than the endometrial cavity and estimated to occur in 1 to 2% of all pregnancies . Nearly 95% of ectopic pregnancies implant in the fallopian tube, while the remaining implant in other locations such as the abdomen, cesarean scar, cervix, and ovary [1]. Abdominal pregnancy refers to a pregnancy that has implanted in the peritoneal cavity, external to the uterine cavity and fallopian tubes [1]. An abdominal pregnancy is the rarest and the most serious type of extrauterine pregnancy. The reported incidence of abdominal pregnancy varies, ranging from 1 in 3,371 deliveries to 1 in 10,000 deliveries [2]. It accounts 1 to 1.4 percent of all ectopic pregnancies [1, 3].

Abdominal pregnancies are classified as primary or secondary [2]. Primary abdominal pregnancy is a result of intra-abdominal fertilization of sperm and ovum, with primary implantation in the abdomen [3, 6]. A secondary abdominal pregnancy is the most common type and is the result of early tubal abortion or rupture with secondary implantation of the pregnancy into the peritoneal cavity [2]. Rare types of secondary abdominal pregnancies have occurred after spontaneous separation of an old cesarean section scar, after uterine perforation during a therapeutic

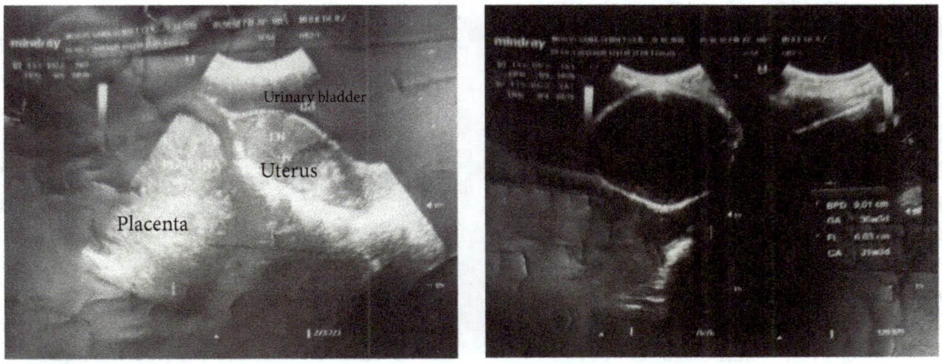

(a) (b)

FIGURE 1: (a and b) Ultrasound findings of abdominal ectopic pregnancy.

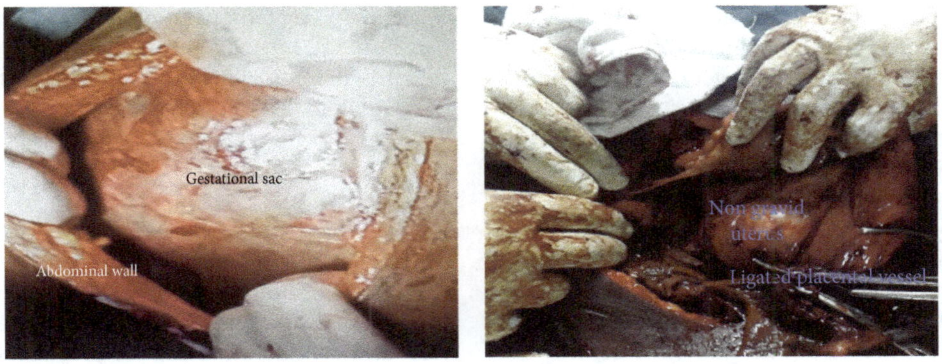

(a) (b)

FIGURE 2: (a and b) Intraoperative findings showing gestational sac with the peritoneal cavity, nongravid sized uterus, and meconium-stained bowel.

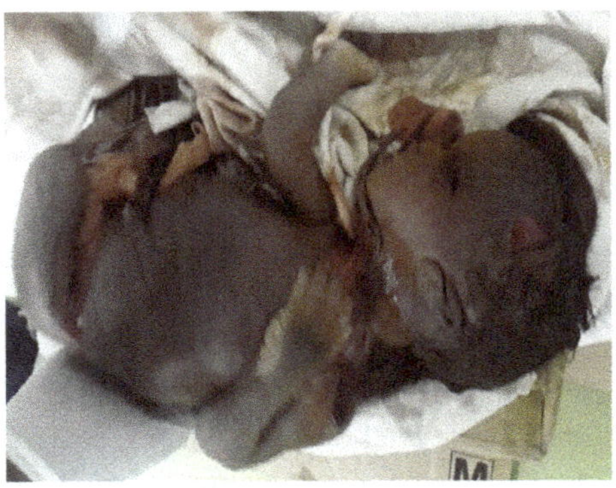

FIGURE 3: A 2000 gm female stillborn with grade-III maceration delivered from the peritoneal cavity.

or elective abortion, and after subtotal or total hysterectomy [2]. Potential sites of abdominal ectopic pregnancy include the omentum, pelvic sidewall, broad ligament, posterior cul-de-sac, abdominal organs (e.g., spleen, bowel, and liver), large pelvic vessels, diaphragm, and uterine serosa [6, 8]. The pouch of Douglas (POD) is the most common location of abdominal pregnancy followed by the mesosalpinx and omentum [8].

Early diagnosis of an abdominal pregnancy is difficult since it is associated with a wide range of signs and symptoms [2]. In a case series of 10 abdominal pregnancies, only 6/10 were diagnosed preoperatively [9]. A high index of suspicion is important for making a diagnosis of abdominal pregnancy. Risk factors for abdominal pregnancy include tubal damage, pelvic inflammatory disease, endometriosis, assisted reproductive techniques, and multiparity [4, 5].

In contrast to tubal ectopic pregnancies, abdominal pregnancies may go undetectable until an advanced gestational age. In such cases, the patient may present with history of recurrent abdominal discomfort, painful fetal movement beneath the abdominal wall, the presence of fetal movements high in the upper abdomen, cessation of fetal movement, a closed and uneffaced cervix, or the failure of oxytocin to stimulate the gestational mass, and the fetus may assume an unusual lie [2]. Nausea and vomiting may be prominent symptoms, when the pregnancy implants on bowel. Compared with tubal ectopic pregnancies, vaginal bleeding is less frequent in abdominal ectopic pregnancy; however, vaginal bleeding may occur since the endometrium still responds to hormonal changes of pregnancy [10].

Ultrasound is the most effective method for diagnosing an abdominal ectopic pregnancy and can usually identify an abdominal gestation as separate from the nonpregnant uterus [2]. Ultrasound, especially transvaginal, remains the first-line tool for diagnosing abdominal pregnancy [11].

The classic ultrasound finding is the absence of myometrial tissue between the maternal bladder and the pregnancy [6]. An empty uterus may be visualized. Other findings include poor definition of the placenta, oligohydramnios, and unusual fetal lie. An advanced abdominal gestation may be misinterpreted as being intrauterine if the ultrasonographer does not evaluate the myometrium during the examination [12]. CT scan and MRI can be useful for confirming the diagnosis, distinguishing anatomic relationships and potential vascular connections, and assessing placental adherence [13].

Abdominal pregnancies, even when advanced, are interrupted at diagnosis, as the potential for delivery of a healthy infant is poor and the risk of maternal complications is high. If the diagnosis is made late in pregnancy, a viable infant may be delivered via laparotomy. Expectant management to gain fetal maturity has been attempted and has been successful in a few cases [14]. The mainstay of treatment of advanced abdominal pregnancy is surgery, but the optimal approach has not been determined. The fetus can be delivered easily; the key issue is how to manage the placenta. There are two options for the management of the placenta: the first being removal of the placenta after ligating the placental blood supply, if the placental separation is not difficult [4, 10]. We have to be cautious upon removal of the placenta since it may lead to life-threatening maternal hemorrhage. The second option is leaving the placenta in situ after ligating the umbilical cord. The patient can then be followed without further intervention, or active intervention using arterial embolization or methotrexate can be instituted to hasten involution [6]. This is a preferred option when the placenta cannot be easily separated. Nonetheless, this approach has its own complications including abscess formation, sepsis, and delayed hemorrhage [15]. Preoperative imaging with MRI has been used successfully to determine the location and attachment of the placenta to aid in this decision [16].

The risk of maternal death from abdominal pregnancy is 7.7 times greater than the risk of maternal death from tubal ectopic pregnancy and 90 times greater than that with intrauterine pregnancy. Reported maternal mortality rates in the literature have varied in the past from 4% to 29% [2]. Maternal death is usually the result of uncontrollable hemorrhage [17]. Maternal morbidity can also be substantial, with high incidences of pelvic abscess, peritonitis, and sepsis caused by retained placental remnants. Rare instances of massive rectal bleeding or rectal passage of fetal bones secondary to the formation of celo-intestinal fistula have also been reported. Fetal mortality is notoriously high, ranging from 75% to 95% of all cases [2]. Fetal deformations and perinatal death occur more often than maternal death [17]. Common fetal abnormalities include facial and/or cranial asymmetry, joint abnormalities, hypoplastic limbs, and central nervous system malformations. Pregnancies with some vascular attachment to the uterus seem to be associated with a higher chance of fetal survival [6].

In this case, she had no identified risk factors for abdominal ectopic pregnancy. She is a primigravida with no history of PID and no exposure to assisted reproductive technology. Clinically, she had symptom suggestive of advanced abdominal ectopic pregnancy; this includes abdominal pain with fetal movement, cessation of fetal movement of 1 week duration, and vaginal bleeding of 3 days duration. Even though it is not common as tubal ectopic pregnancy, vaginal bleeding may occur in abdominal ectopic pregnancy; this is due to the endometrial response to hormonal changes of pregnancy [10]. Easily palpable fetal parts and closed and uneffaced cervix are also suggestive physical findings of abdominal ectopic pregnancy. The fetus was dead. The fetal mortality rate is very high in advanced abdominal ectopic pregnancy, reported as 75% to 95% [2]. Although ultrasound is the most effective method for the diagnosis of abdominal ectopic pregnancy, it was missed twice in our case. This can be due to the lack of experience of the radiographer and inability to evaluate the myometrium at the time of scanning. Since the placental separation was not difficult, the placenta was removed after ligating the placental vessels. There was no intra-abdominal hemorrhage. She was followed at an outpatient clinic for 3 months, and she had no complication.

4. Conclusion

This is an abdominal ectopic pregnancy in a 26-year-old woman who attempted to be pregnant for 10 years, and the pregnancy progressed to third trimester and end up with fetal death. Abdominal ectopic pregnancy could be missed despite having repeated ultrasound scanning and may continue to third trimester. High index of suspicion and correlation of patient's sign and symptom with ultrasound findings is very important to make the early diagnosis of abdominal ectopic pregnancy. Removal of the placenta is a preferred option for the placental management, if the placental separation was not difficult.

Abbreviations

AHMC: Adama Hospital Medical College
ANC: Antenatal care
FHB: Fetal heartbeat
GA: Gestational age
IUFD: Intrauterine fetal death
MRI: Magnetic resonance imaging.

Consent

Written informed consent to participate in this case report was obtained from the patient, for the publication of this case report and accompanying images.

Authors' Contributions

The concept of this case report was developed by the corresponding author. DT, SN, and BG were involved in the management and follow-up of the patient. On the preparation of the document, all authors were involved in the literature review and in critically reviewing the article. All authors read and gave final approval of the submitted manuscript.

References

[1] L. Barbara, J. S. Hoffman, L. M. Halvorson, C. A. Hamid, M. M. Corton, and J. I. Schaffer, "Ectopic Pregnancy," *William's Gynecology*, pp. 161–174, McGraw-Hill Education, New York, 2020.

[2] M. A. Damario, "Abdominal Ectopic Pregnancy," *Te Linda's Operative Gynecology*, pp. 792-793, Wolters Kluwer, Norfolk, Virginia, 2015.

[3] R. W. Dover and M. C. Powell, "Management of a primary abdominal pregnancy," *American Journal of Obstetrics & Gynecology*, vol. 172, no. 5, pp. 1603-1604, 1995.

[4] M. Ludwig, M. Kaisi, O. Bauer, and K. Diedrich, "Case report: the forgotten child—a case of heterotopic, intra-abdominal and intrauterine pregnancy carried to term," *Human Reproduction*, vol. 14, no. 5, pp. 1372–1374, 1999.

[5] D. Maas and C. Slabber, "Diagnosis and treatment of advanced extra-uterine pregnancy," *South African Medical Journal*, vol. 49, no. 48, pp. 2007–2010, 1975.

[6] R. Varma, L. Mascarenhas, and D. James, "Successful outcome of advanced abdominal pregnancy with exclusive omental insertion," *Ultrasound in Obstetrics and Gynecology: The Official Journal of the International Society of Ultrasound in Obstetrics and Gynecology*, vol. 21, no. 2, pp. 192–194, 2003.

[7] C. J. Berg, "Pregnancy-related mortality in the United States, 1991–1997," in *Obstetrics & Gynecology*, vol. 101, no. 2, pp. 289–296, 2003.

[8] V. Nama, B. Gyampoh, M. Karoshi, R. McRae, and I. Opemuyi, "Secondary abdominal appendicular ectopic pregnancy," *Journal of Minimally Invasive Gynecology*, vol. 14, no. 4, pp. 516-517, 2007.

[9] K. C. Worley, M. D. Hnat, and F. G. Cunningham, "Advanced extrauterine pregnancy: diagnostic and therapeutic challenges," *American journal of obstetrics and gynecology*, vol. 198, no. 3, pp. 297.e1–297.e7, 2008.

[10] M. S. Rahman, S. A. al-Suleiman, J. Rahman, and M. H. al-Sibai, "Advanced abdominal pregnancy-observations in 10 cases," *Obstetrics and Gynecology*, vol. 59, no. 3, pp. 366–372, 1982.

[11] J. M. Cohen, J. C. Weinreb, T. W. Lowe, and C. Brown, "MR imaging of a viable full-term abdominal pregnancy," *American Journal of Roentgenology*, vol. 145, no. 2, pp. 407-408, 1985.

[12] Y. Yagil, N. Beck-Razi, A. Amit, H. Kerner, and D. Gaitini, "Splenic pregnancy: the role of abdominal imaging," *Journal of Ultrasound in Medicine*, vol. 26, no. 11, pp. 1629–1632, 2007.

[13] M. Kitade, H. Takeuchi, I. Kikuchi, H. Shimanuki, J. Kumakiri, and K. Kinoshita, "A case of simultaneous tubal-splenic pregnancy after assisted reproductive technology," *Fertility and sterility*, vol. 83, no. 4, pp. 1042.e19–1042.e21, 2005.

[14] R. Beddock, P. Naepels, C. Gondry et al., "Diagnosis and current concepts of management of advanced abdominal pregnancy," *Gynecologie, obstetrique & fertilite*, vol. 32, no. 1, pp. 55–61, 2004.

[15] J. A. Hymel, D. S. Hughes, A. Gehlot, A. M. Ramseyer, and E. F. Magann, "Late abdominal pregnancies (≥ 20 weeks gestation): a review from 1965 to 2012," *Gynecologic and Obstetric Investigation*, vol. 80, no. 4, pp. 253–258, 2015.

[16] F. Lockhat, P. Corr, S. Ramphal, and J. Moodley, "The value of magnetic resonance imagingin the diagnosis and management of extra-uterine abdominal pregnancy," *Clinical Radiology*, vol. 61, no. 3, pp. 264–269, 2006.

[17] O. Ayinde, C. O. Aimakhu, O. A. Adeyanju, and A. O. Omigbodun, "Abdominal pregnancy at the University College Hospital, Ibadan: a ten-year review," *African Journal of Reproductive Health*, vol. 9, no. 1, pp. 123–127, 2005.

4

Duodenal Obstruction during Pregnancy

Mansooreh Haghiri,[1] Sedigheh Borna,[1] Kamran Hessami,[2,3] Ali Sharifi,[4] Seyed Mohsen Ahmadi Tafti,[5] Mahrooz Malek,[6] Nasim Pourdamghan,[7] Sedigheh Hantoushzadeh,[1] Abolfazl Shirdel Abdolmaleki,[8] and Maasoumeh Saleh[1]

[1]*Maternal, Fetal and Neonatal Research Center, Vali-e-Asr Hospital, Tehran University of Medical Sciences, Tehran, Iran*
[2]*Department of Obstetrics and Gynecology, Baylor College of Medicine, Houston, TX, USA*
[3]*Maternal-Fetal Medicine Research Center, Shiraz University of Medical Sciences, Shiraz, Iran*
[4]*Department of Surgery, Beesat Hospital, Hamadan University of Medical Sciences, Tehran, Iran*
[5]*Department of Surgery, Tehran University of Medical Sciences, Tehran, Iran*
[6]*Department of Radiology, Vali-e-Asr Hospital, Tehran University of Medical Sciences, Tehran, Iran*
[7]*Department of Obstetrics and Gynecology, Kerman University of Medical Sciences, Tehran, Iran, Kerman, Iran*
[8]*School of Medicine, Shiraz University of Medical Sciences, Shiraz, Iran*

Correspondence should be addressed to Sedigheh Hantoushzadeh; hantoushzadeh@tums.ac.ir

Academic Editor: Cem Ficicioglu

Intractable vomiting and elevated liver enzymes during pregnancy seem to be associated to the obstetric etiologies; however, other causes such as acute surgical emergencies should be considered. The patient was a 26-year-old woman at 18 weeks of gestation with intractable vomiting, intolerability of oral intake, weight loss, and absence of abdominal pain. Her physical examinations and laboratory tests had no remarkable findings except elevated liver function test (LFT) and hypokalemia. Considering the lab data and normal abdominopelvic ultrasound, magnetic resonance imaging was performed which revealed dilation of the D1-3 and collapse the D4 sections of duodenum. She underwent exploratory laparotomy which confirmed duodenal obstruction caused by Ladd's band. After the Ladd's operation, the patient started oral intake of nutritious, and her LFT decreased to normal ranges. After the last follow-up, she has had gained 18 kg and gave birth at 36 weeks of gestation due to the premature rapture of membranes and delivered a 2 kg small for gestational age otherwise healthy infant. The experience gained from this case was to consider all possibilities (such as small bowel obstruction) and evaluate them in a pregnant patient to consider other causes of nausea, vomiting, and abnormal LFTs in a pregnant patient.

1. Background

Acute intestinal obstruction during pregnancy has been described with different incidences such as 1/66,431 and 1/1500 [1]. This condition is very important and emergent during pregnancy which requires proper treatment as soon as possible as same as other abdominal emergencies [1–3]. The most common causes of mechanical obstruction in pregnancy have been reported as adhesions, volvulus, and intussusception with the prevalence of 58%, 24%, and 5%, respectively [1]. So far, some reports have highlighted malrotation as an uncommon cause of small bowel obstruction (SBO) during pregnancy [4–7]. Congenital malrotations are mostly asymptomatic in adults and have been known as a rare cause of SBO in this age group. Despite the different etiologies of SBO during pregnancy, the most common symptoms are abdominal pain (98%), vomiting (82%), and tenderness (71%) in the abdomen. Thus, abdominal pain seems to have a notable sensitivity for SBO in these cases [1].

Herein, we report a very rare case of SBO during pregnancy with persistent progressive nausea and vomiting due to duodenal obstruction caused by a previously asymptomatic congenital condition (incomplete rotation of duodenum). The clinical presentation and laboratory tests of this

TABLE 1: The results of blood laboratory test investigations at admission and postoperative.

Laboratory parameter	Before the surgery	Day 2 (postoperative)	Day *X* (postoperative)
Platelet count	256000/μL	2450000/μL	250000/μL
Aspartate aminotransferase (AST)	329 IU/L	142 IU/L	53 IU/L
Alanine aminotransferase (ALT)	745 IU/L	375 IU/L	12 IU/L
Alkaline phosphatase (ALP)	309 IU/L	240 IU/L	369 IU/L
Albumin	3 gr/dL	—	—
Total bilirubin	1.2 mg/dL	2 mg/dL	1 mg/dL
Conjugated bilirubin	0.4 mg/dL	1 mg/dL	0.2 mg/dL
Prothrombin time (PT)	12.2 seconds	14 seconds	—
INR	1.1	1.1	—
Thyroid stimulating hormone (TSH)	1.2 mIU/L	—	—
Potassium (K)	3 mEq/L	3.6 mEq/L	—
24-hour urine protein	280 mg	—	—

case were very similar to the other prevalent obstetrics-associated complications. Considering her two previous pregnancies terminated in a similar situation, the current report would bold role of proper imaging modalities and other investigations in the diagnosis and treatment of such cases.

2. Case Presentation

A 26-year-old woman (Gravida 3, Para 2, Death 2) was referred to our tertiary care center (*Vali-e-Asr Hospital*) at her 25th week of gestation (WOG) with blood pressure of 100/80 mm Hg (pulse rate 98). She complained of intractable large volume bilious vomiting, generalized weakness, progressive weight loss (13 kg so far), had an episode of bowel movement every 2 to 3 days, and inability to consume food started from 18th WOG (the patients received IV fluid therapy several times as outpatient between 18 and 25 weeks of gestation). Except for two failed pregnancies, she had no remarkable family and psychosocial history. In both of the previous pregnancies, similar presentations to her current condition were found. Those pregnancies were terminated at 26th and 22nd WOG with the diagnoses of acute fatty liver of pregnancy and HELLP syndrome, respectively.

Her first pregnancy (22 years old) had advanced with no complications until the 18th WOG when nausea and vomiting started to be more prevalent and severe as the time passed. Due to the progressive intractable vomiting, dehydration, and hypokalemia, as well as intolerance to oral intake, the patient was completely dependent on intravenous fluid and electrolytes which finally had led to weight loss and severe weakness (in another medical center). During the 25th WOG, liver function test (LFT) values started to rise along with negative laboratory results for viral hepatitis. Also, there were no criteria for autoimmune hepatitis. Since we had no more data regarding this hospitalization, the refeeding syndrome could be a suspect for the impaired LFTs [8]. Finally, the pregnancy was terminated at 26th WOG while suspecting acute fatty liver of pregnancy. Following the termination, she soon tolerated oral intake, and the LTFs returned to the normal levels after a week.

In her second pregnancy (at the age of 25), similar symptoms to the previous reemerged after the 17th WOG. Intravenous (IV) hydration plus mineral supplement replacement were not able to meet the patient's maintenance needs. Meanwhile, the symptoms became more severe, and LFTs increased with a very quickly and during hospitalization period. The second pregnancy was terminated around 22nd WOG with suspicion of HELLP syndrome. Considering the complications during both pregnancies, the patient was referred to a gastroenterologist for evaluation of Wilson's disease, autoimmune hepatitis, and Crohn's disease. The multidisciplinary workup did not show any remarkable finding of such sort. Before her third pregnancy, she was evaluated by a well-experienced rheumatologist as well, which they did not find any abnormal issue (according to the patient's statement). In the third pregnancy and before referring to our center (around the 22nd WOG), the patient was switched to intravenous nutrition replacement since oral intake was intolerable (by general practitioners because of their suspicion to hyperemesis gravidarum). At the same time and when the patient was under treatment with dexamethasone and full dose of ondansetron with steady clinical status, laboratory results showed a progressive increase in liver enzymes. At the time of admission to our center, the patient's physical examinations, fetal heart rate, and primary laboratory investigations (such as complete blood count, blood sugar, 24-hour urine protein, amylase, lipase, and viral tests) revealed no remarkable finding except for LFTs and potassium levels (Table 1). Also, abdominopelvic ultrasound and Doppler flow of inferior vena cava (IVC), portal, and hepatic veins were normal. As the next step, upper gastrointestinal endoscopy was performed which showed no significant findings such as peptic ulcer or pyloric obstruction. Considering the following results, magnetic resonance imaging (MRI) without contrast revealed marked dilation of the stomach and duodenum up to the third part of duodenum, D3 level as well as collapse in D4 part (Figures 1(a) and 1(b)). Thus, the obstruction site suggested to be between D3 and D4.

After deteriorated clinical status and solid evidence of duodenal obstruction, laparotomy was indicated. The

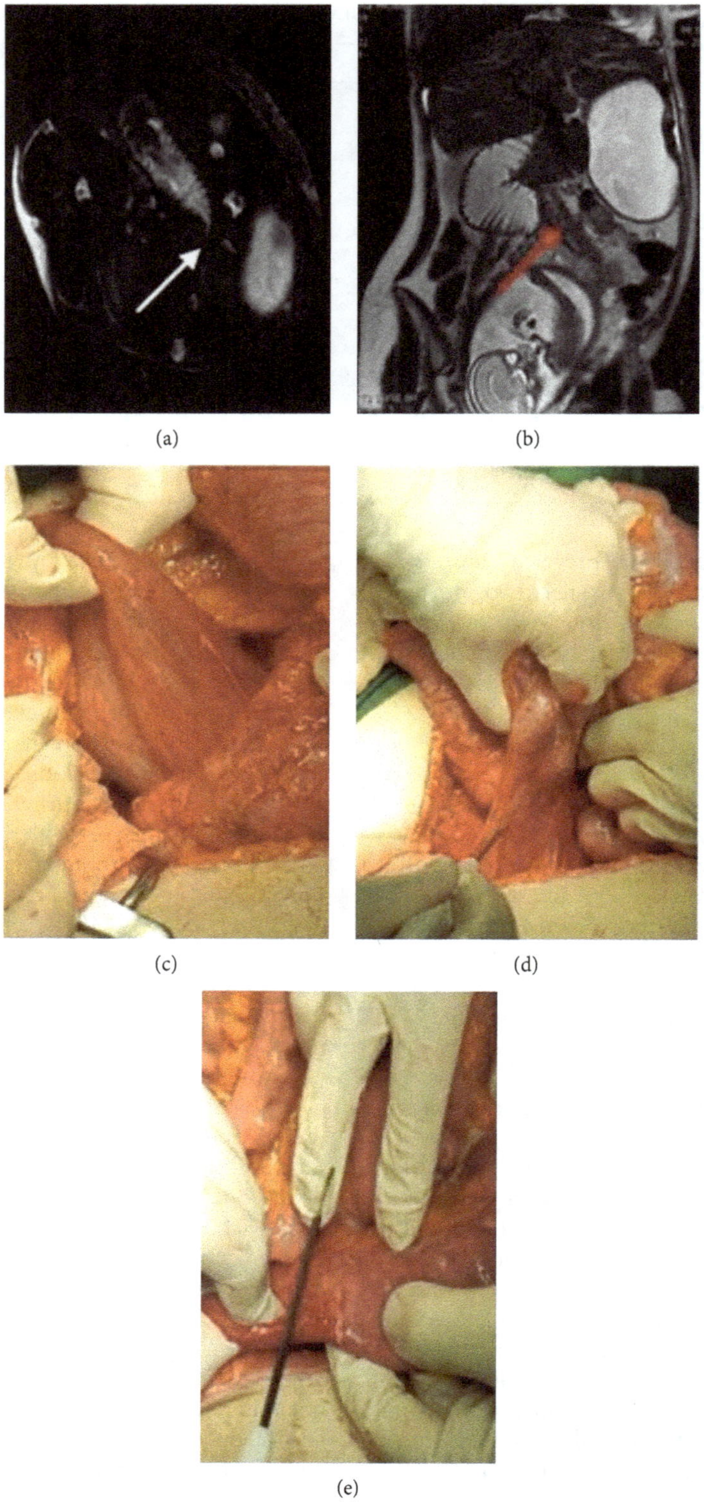

Figure 1: (a) Transverse oblique (patient is lying on a side) view marked dilation of the stomach and duodenum up to D3 level (the arrow is the point of stenosis). (b) The site of Ladd's bands (red arrow), uterus, and duodenum. (c) Dilated duodenum under cecum. (d) Peritoneal Ladd's bands. (e) Released peritoneal band in the site of stenosis.

transition zone of duodenal obstruction was observed at the junction of peritoneal bands passing across the third part of the duodenum. At the proximal portion of Ladd's band, D3 was significantly dilated while the distal part, D4, was completely collapsed lying on the right side (Figures 1(c)–1(e)). The peritoneum to the right of the ascending colon was incised, and the anteriorly situated bands were stripped to release the duodenum (Figure 1(e)). After the surgery (Ladd's procedure), the patient remained stable and was admitted to intensive care unit (ICU). After two days, the elevated LFTs were decreased by about 50% compared to the presurgery levels (Table 1). She was discharged from ICU after two days with favorable postoperative recovery and normal oral intake. After being discharged, she was followed up to three weeks after labor. During the follow-ups, she gained 18 kg until the time of delivery (cesarean delivery). She gave birth at the 36th week of gestation as a result of the premature rupture of the membrane. The Apgar score and weight of her neonate were 9/10 and 2 kg (small for gestational age), respectively, and both mother and neonate were discharged after labor with no problem or complaint.

3. Discussion and Conclusions

Herein, we reported a rare case of duodenal obstruction during pregnancy caused by Ladd's band. One of the most challenging issues, in this case, was the absence of abdominal pain observed in up 98% of pregnant women with the same condition [1]. Thus, considering the absence of abdominal pain in this patient and presence of more common pathologies with nausea and vomiting (accompanied with elevated LFTs) during the second trimester of pregnancy (such as acute fatty liver of pregnancy and HELLP syndrome), obstruction became a neglected diagnosis in her past pregnancies terminated with other diagnoses. This time, considering all of the already mentioned tests performed for rolling out other possible conditions, MRI was carried out which increased the suspicion of the duodenal obstruction. After the surgery (Ladd's procedure), symptoms and abnormal laboratory tests were also resolved, and results returned to the normal ranges.

According to our knowledge, so far, only two cases of duodenal obstruction caused by malrotation following the Ladd's band pain have been reported. However, there have been different major differences [9, 10]. As Yin et al. have explained, the symptoms of their primigravid case were started at 9th WOG with nausea, vomiting, and intolerance to oral intake. Her clinical symptoms worsen, and serum transaminase levels increased (AST: 100-243 U/L and ALT: 297-536 U/L) which led to hospitalization in the 24th WOG. Similar to the current report, their case declared no abdominal pain accompanied by any of the other symptoms. Following the MRI, they performed laparotomy which confirmed congenital bowel malrotation and Ladd's band. Unlike our case, however, they found no signs of obstruction, bowel ischemia, and volvulus; hence, the Ladd's procedure was not performed for their case. She was just treated with parenteral nutrition and was discharged 6 days after the surgery. Also, their six-month follow-up did not reveal any gastrointestinal (obstetrics not mentioned) issues [9]. Furthermore, Pelikan et al. reported extreme nausea and vomiting in a pregnant woman at 38th WOG with nausea, vomiting, and abdominal pain (unlike our case). Ultrasound and gastroscopy were normal, and in despite the obtained results, all the laboratory tests, including LTFs, were normal. After the labor, an abdominopelvic computed tomography (CT) scan (with IV and oral contrast) was performed for the patient which showed intestinal malrotation due to volvulus. During the laparotomy, they incised the Ladd's bands, and in the ascending colon, the mesenteric veins were found thrombosed. Thus, they performed right colectomy accompanied by ileocolic anastomosis due to the suspicion of the tissue viability [10].

Malrotation of the midgut is an abnormal intestinal rotation and fixation in the embryological development of the gastrointestinal tract. While the majority of such abnormalities remain asymptomatic during adulthood, the symptomatic cases are usually encountered in the clinical setting of duodenal obstruction or midgut volvulus [11]. All and all, this was a case of confirmed duodenal obstruction that commonly goes without abdominal pain but only retching and vomiting which seems to be common findings for this level of obstruction. The most remarkable "takeaway lesson" [12] of this case is not to neglect (any) possible diagnoses in a patient, especially pregnant women with no abdominal pain but progressive vomiting accompanied by impaired LTFs. In such cases, MRI should be used more to reach a correct diagnosis as it has helped before in the rare conditions during pregnancy [13]. Also, it should be noted that during pregnancy (especially second and third trimesters), anatomical and physiological changes could alter asymptomatic conditions to symptomatic issues found to be threatening for both mother and fetus.

Abbreviations

SBO: Small bowel obstruction
WOG: Weeks of gestation
LFT: Liver function test
ICU: Intensive care unit.

Consent

The patient kindly signed a written consent form freely for publishing/using of her medical data.

Acknowledgments

We thank the multidisciplinary team, especially Dr. Basirat (Department of Gastroenterology Imam Khomeini Hospital Complex, Tehran University of Medical Sciences, Tehran, Iran) for his kind cooperation in management of the case. Also, we are very grateful for the kind permission of the patient to share her data.

References

[1] P. W. Perdue, H. W. Johnson Jr., and P. W. Stafford, "Intestinal obstruction complicating pregnancy," *American Journal of Surgery*, vol. 164, no. 4, pp. 384–388, 1992.

[2] P. K. Hsu, P. Y. Yang, W. W. Su, and Y. Y. Chen, "Small bowel obstruction caused by infant compression during pregnancy," *Digestive and Liver Disease*, vol. 52, no. 11, pp. 1370-1371, 2020.

[3] A. Daimon, Y. Terai, Y. Nagayasu et al., "A case of intestinal obstruction in pregnancy diagnosed by MRI and treated by

intravenous hyperalimentation," *Case reports in obstetrics and gynecology*, vol. 2016, Article ID 8704035, 4 pages, 2016.

[4] S. Siwatch, M. T. Noor, U. Dutta, R. Kochhar, A. Behera, and K. Singh, "Endoscopic management of a pregnant lady with duodenal obstruction due to malrotation with midgut volvulus," *Tropical gastroenterology.*, vol. 32, no. 4, pp. 339–341, 2012.

[5] I. Vassiliou, A. Tympa, M. Derpapas, G. Kottis, and N. Vlahos, "Small bowel ischemia due to jejunum volvulus in pregnancy: a case report," *Case reports in obstetrics and gynecology*, vol. 2012, Article ID 485863, 2 pages, 2012.

[6] Z.-H. Zheng, J.-L. Huang, H.-B. Wei, J.-P. Liu, and Y. Huang, "Adult congenital intestinal malrotation accompanied by midgut volvulus: report of eight cases," *International journal of clinical and experimental medicine*, vol. 7, no. 6, pp. 1614–1618, 2014.

[7] A. S. G. Antunes, B. Peixe, and H. Guerreiro, "Midgut volvulus as a complication of intestinal malrotation in pregnancy," *ACG case reports journal*, vol. 4, no. 1, p. e9, 2017.

[8] R. H. Harris, G. Sasson, and P. S. Mehler, "Elevation of liver function tests in severe anorexianervosa," *The International Journal of Eating Disorders*, vol. 46, no. 4, pp. 369–374, 2013.

[9] Y. Yin, C. Li, C. Xu et al., "Intestinal obstruction due to congenital malrotation complicating a multiple pregnancy: a rare case report," *The Journal of the Pakistan Medical Association*, vol. 67, no. 2, pp. 308–310, 2017.

[10] H. Pelikan, J. Stoot, S. Meens-Koreman, and J. Teijink, "Congenital intestinal malrotation masquerading as hyperemesis gravidarum," *International Journal of Gynaecology and Obstetrics*, vol. 102, no. 1, pp. 74-75, 2008.

[11] M. Haqqani, M. Seetharaman, R. Teo et al., "Midgut malrotation complicated by small bowel obstruction in an 80-year-old woman: a case report," *International Journal of Surgery Case Reports*, vol. 63, pp. 89–93, 2019.

[12] J. J. Gagnier, G. Kienle, D. G. Altman et al., "The CARE guidelines: consensus-based clinical case reporting guideline development," *BML Case Reports*, vol. 2013, article bcr2013201554, 2013.

[13] G. Augustin, I. Separovic, and D. Bajramovic, "Chilaiditi sign and Chilaiditi syndrome in pregnancy," *The Journal of Emergency Medicine*, vol. 59, no. 2, pp. e73–e76, 2020.

5

Paratubal Cystectomy in a Pregnant Woman using the Single-Incision Laparoscopic Surgery (SILS) Technique

Luke William Nelson and Elliot MacKenzie

Dunedin Public Hospital, 201 Great King Street, Dunedin 9010, New Zealand

Correspondence should be addressed to Luke William Nelson; luke.nelson@southerndhb.govt.nz

Academic Editor: Maria Grazia Porpora

Introduction. The proliferation of prenatal ultrasound has enhanced the detection of adnexal masses during pregnancy. The presentation necessitates a clear approach to investigation and treatment that balances both maternal and fetal risk. Laparoscopy is a safe approach to surgical management in the pregnant patient, and SILS may contribute to minimising perioperative complications. *Case Presentation.* We present the case of a 21-year-old female in her second trimester of pregnancy presenting with a large 20 cm right adnexal cyst. We proceeded with laparoscopic cystectomy via the SILS technique. There were no intraoperative complications, and she recovered well postoperatively. *Conclusion.* Laparoscopic resection of adnexal lesions is safe during pregnancy and should be favoured over the open approach. SILS minimises incision sites and has potential for reduction in perioperative morbidity.

1. Introduction

The proliferation of prenatal ultrasound has enhanced the detection of adnexal masses during pregnancy. With an incidence of 2%, the presentation necessitates a clear approach to investigation and treatment that balances both maternal and fetal risk [1]. In determining the appropriate management strategy, namely, intervention vs. conservative, there are considerations idiosyncratic to the pregnant patient that should be accounted for. The absence of malignant features on imaging and stable size may obviate the need for intervention and allow for conservative management [2].

Historical concerns regarding safety of laparoscopy in pregnancy have now largely been assuaged. There still exist considerations unique to the pregnant patient. For example, the gravid uterus may be susceptible to puncture during blind insufflation [3].

Single-incision laparoscopic surgery (SILS) is an emerging approach to laparoscopy. It confers improved cosmesis and, by limiting the surgery to a single-entry point, reduces the potential for infection and bleeding [4]. Its chief disadvantages include a greater technical challenge and longer operative duration [5].

We present a case report of a 21-year-old pregnant woman who underwent a right paratubal cystectomy at 18 weeks gestation using a SILS approach.

2. Case Presentation

Our patient was a 21-year-old female who presented with a wanted pregnancy at 14 + 3 weeks gestation complicated by abdominal pain and vomiting. She had a medical history of 2 previous first trimester miscarriages and a raised body mass index of 33. She was taking appropriate folic acid supplementation. On examination, she had a palpable mass in the right lower abdominal quadrant, with associated tenderness and guarding. A vaginal examination was unremarkable, and the cervical os was closed. She had normal blood pressure and pulse. Her serum hCG was 15900.

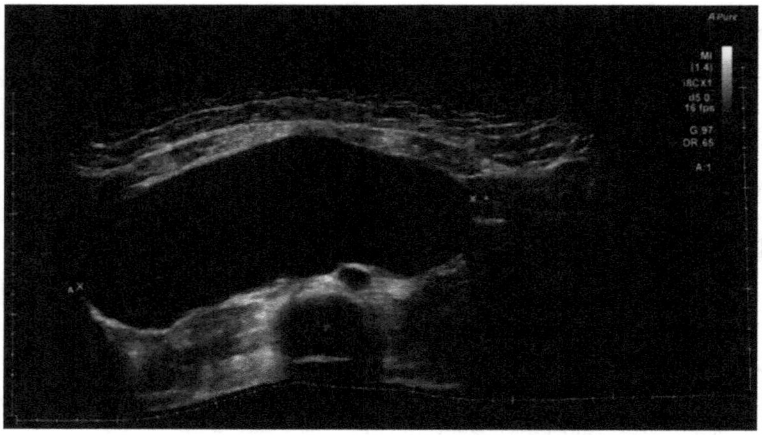

Figure 1: Transverse ultrasound view of the right adnexa, demonstrating the cyst. Note its homogenous echotexture.

She proceeded to have a pelvic ultrasound which demonstrated a single live intrauterine pregnancy consistent with a gestational age of 14 + 3 weeks and a large right adnexal mass measuring 201 × 148 × 73 mm (1129 cc), likely arising from the right ovary. There were no septations, solid components, or abnormal vascularity noted (Figure 1).

She was admitted overnight for analgesia and antiemesis and discharged the next day following improvement in her symptoms. A planned MRI was conducted as an outpatient when she was 17 + 2 weeks gestation (Figure 2). This demonstrated interval growth of the cyst from the previous ultrasound scan and concurred with the presumptive diagnosis of a large right simple cyst measuring 190 × 170 × 100 mm (1680 cc).

The patient was referred to our gynaecological-oncology multidisciplinary team. It was determined that the cyst was benign in appearance, but surgical resection was necessitated. Cystectomy was favoured over drainage, for concerns regarding reaccumulation.

We proceeded to take her to theatre for laparoscopic right adnexal cystectomy at 18 + 2 weeks gestation. The operation was conducted under general anaesthesia by endotracheal intubation in Trendelenburg position with a urinary catheter in situ. Due to her gravid state, no transvaginal uterine manipulation was performed. Following skin preparation and application of sterile drapes, we made a 15 mm incision at the umbilicus. A SILS port (Applied Medical Gelseal) was placed at the umbilicus, through which we insufflated the peritoneal cavity with carbon dioxide. Via the SILS port, a 30-degree laparoscope and 2 working instruments were inserted. A large right adnexal mass extending to reach the liver was visualised and determined to be paratubal in origin (Figure 3).

Both ovaries and left fallopian tube were normal. Peritoneal washings were taken. A sharp incision was made on the cyst capsule followed by water-jet hydrodissection using a standard laparoscopic suction irrigation system under pressure. Following near complete dissection within its capsule, leaving base attached to maintain orientation, the cyst was punctured sharply with laparoscopic scissors under suction tip and suction immediately placed into cyst cavity. 1300 millilitres of clear serous fluid were drained without spill. Patient size, gravid uterus, and instrument length then limited reach deep into pelvis from the umbilicus position to allow cyst excision and control of haemostasis at its base via the SILS port alone; hence, an accessory 5 mm port was placed in the left flank. We then proceeded to complete the excision of the cyst capsule using Ligasure bipolar device, delivering it extracorporeally via the SILS port. The right-sided fallopian tube was elongated and partially twisted. We untwisted the right fallopian tube following the cystectomy. Otherwise, both the right and left fallopian tubes and ovaries were normal and left intact bilaterally (Figure 4).

Pneumoperitoneum was released, and the SILS port was removed from the abdomen. The rectus sheath at the umbilicus was sutured with 0 Vicryl, and overlying skin was sutured with 3/0 Monocryl. The left-sided accessory port site was repaired with 3/0 Monocryl.

The estimated blood loss was approximately 75 millilitres, and no intraoperative complications arose. She had an uneventful postoperative course and was discharged the next day.

Histology confirmed the diagnosis of a benign serous cystadenoma. The patient was followed up at 22 + 2 weeks gestation, and her pregnancy was progressing well.

3. Discussion

The finding of an ovarian cyst during pregnancy presents a dilemma to the obstetrician. Should it be necessitated, surgery must be used judiciously and timed so that fetal risk is minimised. Amongst such patients, there is a preponderance of functional cysts. This is reflected by a 70% spontaneous resolution rate by the 2nd trimester [6]. Nevertheless, 1-6% of adnexal masses in pregnancy are malignant and necessitate timely resection and staging [7].

3.1. Diagnosis and Selection for Surgery. Ultrasound is the mainstay of investigation of ovarian masses in pregnancy, allowing the obstetrician to stratify patients according to features suggestive of malignancy [8]. Tumour markers such as the glycoprotein CA-125 are of reduced applicability in the pregnant patient and may rise as a consequence of pregnancy itself [9, 10]. MRI can provide a useful adjunct to

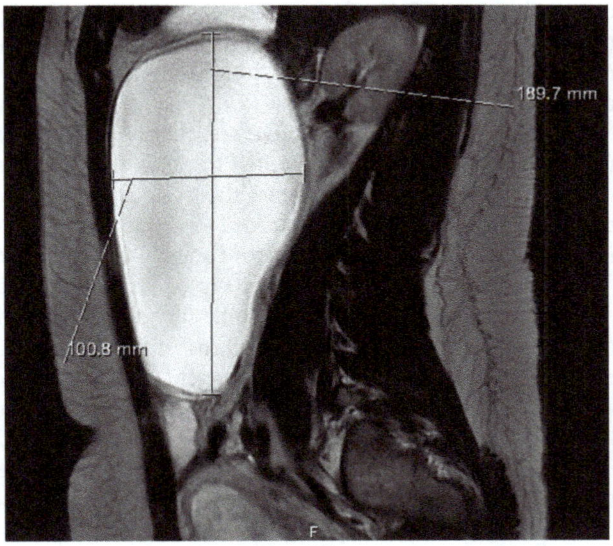

FIGURE 2: Sagittal view (MRI) of the right adnexal cyst. Note its simple appearance.

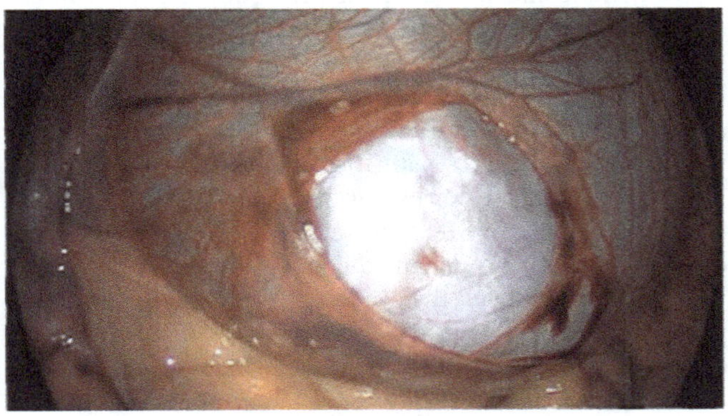

FIGURE 3: The partially dissected right adnexal cyst.

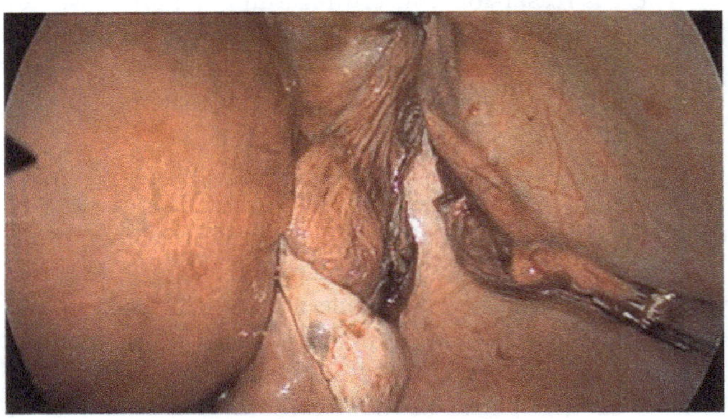

FIGURE 4: The right adnexa following complete excision of the cyst. Note the normal right ovary and gravid uterus.

diagnosis, through further characterisation of mass morphology [11]. Both methods are safe and do not expose the fetus to the effects of ionising radiation [12].

Our patient had radiographic features highly suggestive of a benign simple cyst. However, imaging alone cannot fully replace pathological staging [13]. As such, pregnant patients with features of ovarian malignancy are a group who require surgical intervention. Alongside increasing the suspicion of malignancy, ovarian masses that are large (>10 cm) or increasing in size pose a risk of torsion or obstructed labour and are an indication for surgery [14]. Another important consideration is the risk of emergency surgery in the event of ovarian torsion and its apparent predisposition towards preterm birth [15].

Such risks must be balanced with the risks inherent to the surgery itself, both to fetus and mother. Delaying surgery until the second trimester affords time for resolution of functional cysts and avoids spontaneous first trimester miscarriage being falsely linked to the operation. Furthermore, organogenesis has largely concluded as well as the pregnancy's reliance upon the corpus luteum for progesterone [1, 16, 17].

In keeping with current practice, we performed the operation in the patient's second trimester for the aforementioned reasons. Additionally, operating before the third trimester reduces the technical burden that a large gravid uterus may place upon the surgeon. Our management included review by our gynaecologic-oncology multidisciplinary team. This is concordant with Vernooij et al. [18] who determined that mean survival time for ovarian malignancy is improved through consultation with a gynaecological oncology service [18].

3.2. Laparoscopy and Pregnancy. Multiple studies have corroborated the safety of laparoscopic management of adnexal masses in pregnant patients [19–21]. Compared to an open approach, laparoscopy may mitigate the risks of thromboembolism and maternal hypoventilation by offering earlier mobilisation and less reliance upon postoperative opioid analgesia, respectively [22]. Concerns regarding the risk of preterm birth when operating in the third trimester may be unfounded given that the preterm birth rate ranges between 7.3 and 11.7% in the general population [23, 24].

3.3. Pneumoperitoneum. An animal study performed by Barnard et al. [25] demonstrated reduced placental perfusion in the presence of maternal pneumoperitoneum [25]. Encouragingly, fetal perfusion and blood gas values were not adversely affected. These findings are yet to be confirmed or refuted by human studies. In light of its uncertain significance, multiple sources advocate for limiting the operating pneumoperitoneum to below 15 or even 12 mmHg [26–28]. Intra-abdominal pressures should be titrated to account for the already deleterious effect that the gravid uterus has upon visualisation [29].

3.4. Electrosurgical Instrumentation. Several case series have incorporated electrosurgical instruments into their laparoscopic surgeries on pregnant women without operative complications [15, 30, 31]. We used the bipolar tissue sealing device Ligasure to excise the cyst, without intraoperative or postoperative complication. The envelopment of the fetus in amniotic fluid is believed to be protective from energy-related injury. As with any application of electrosurgery, care should be taken to avoid inadvertent trauma. This is especially salient in the pregnant patient in whom there is a paucity of evidence regarding its usage [16].

3.5. Uterine Manipulation and Tocolysis. Cervical manipulation of the pregnant uterus has the propensity to induce premature contractions, and as such, is contraindicated. Intra-abdominal surgery, particularly in the third trimester, may lead to uterine contractions [32]. However, Walsh et al. [33] demonstrated no reduction in preterm birth with prophylactic tocolysis [33]. As such, we did not manipulate the uterus during the course of our surgery, and tocolysis was not employed.

3.6. SILS. SILS is a novel approach to minimal access surgery. A single-entry point is placed, typically at the umbilicus, through which the laparoscope and all instruments are inserted [34]. Its efficacy and safety have been demonstrated across the spectrum of surgical disciplines [35].

Prospective studies comparing SILS to standard laparoscopic management of adnexal lesions are lacking. Several studies have demonstrated the feasibility and safety of SILS for adnexal lesions [36, 37]. A recent retrospective study demonstrated longer operative times when SILS was applied to adnexal lesions [38], whilst shorter operating times have been described by other applications of the technique [39]. Nevertheless, the potential for improved cosmesis and perioperative outcome should not be discounted based on scarcity of evidence.

Delay in widespread adoption of SILS may be in part due to its technical challenges. Convergence of all instruments through one port can reduce the working space available [40]. Furthermore, movement of the camera can be restricted by its proximity to the working instruments [4].

The applicability of SILS to the treatment of a variety of adnexal diseases has been established. Marcelli et al. [41] exhibited good success rates for SILS salpingectomy for ectopic pregnancy. Despite prolonging operative time, patients treated with SILS had shorter hospital stays than those who underwent conventional multiport laparoscopy [41]. Similarly, Loh et al. (2017) found outcomes from SILS management of ectopic pregnancy to be at least equivalent with conventional laparoscopy [42]. Dursun et al. [43] successfully treated 14 women with benign adnexal masses using SILS in combination with standard laparoscopic instruments. Optimisation of instrument and surgeon position compensated for difficulties encountered with instrument collision [43]. In the future, this issue may be avoided entirely with the advent of instruments designed specifically for SILS. Common to existing research surrounding SILS, these studies were marred by small sample sizes. Xiao et al. (2020) have since demonstrated the feasibility of SILS in laparoscopic management of adnexal disease, myomectomy, and cervical cerclage, specifically in the pregnant woman [44].

The importance of cosmesis cannot be understated given that the population who undergo laparoscopy for benign gynaecological disease largely consist of young women. By virtue of a single incision site, SILS has the potential to maximise patient satisfaction postoperatively [45]. Additionally, utilising the umbilicus as the sole incision site limits the potential for immediate and long-term postoperative pain [46].

In our case, due to locomotive restrictions and instrument length size, we were compelled to place an additional port into the left flank to remove the cyst capsule at the end. This was further compounded by the inability to manipulate the uterus due to its gravid state. Our experience is echoed in other reports on the usage of SILS in adnexal cysts. Rezai et al. [47] noted the difficulty faced through not being able to alter the gravid uterus' impact upon the operating field [47]. Also, 24% of patients in a study by Huang et al. [38] required the addition of an accessory port [38]. We were still able to excise the lesion using the SILS port in tandem with the accessory port, avoiding the placement of an additional trocar into the abdomen. It could also be argued that additional port placement after a large cyst decompression in the presence of a gravid uterus gives a safety margin on trauma to the uterus derived from an increased space created as in our case. Bariatric surgery size instruments could be utilised if the concern is instrument size alone. We did not have these available to us.

Ross et al. [48] proposed several potential drawbacks to the use of SILS. The presence of preexisting pelvic adhesions and excessive extra- and intraperitoneal fat may exacerbate the intrinsic difficulties with instrument triangulation [48]. This may render previous surgery and a raised BMI relative contraindications to SILS. However, in our experience, the elevated BMI of the patient did not substantially alter the use of SILS. Moreover, the availability of longer instruments may have averted the need to place an accessory port. This is a technical consideration which could be ameliorated with the development and dispersion of instruments specific to the SILS technique. On the discovery of extensive adhesions or an abdomen that is not amenable to SILS, there is always the recourse to convert to standard laparoscopy.

There is reasonable concern regarding the propensity of SILS to cause umbilical hernia due to the larger incision size for entry. The overall risk of port site hernia is a difficult entity to quantify, a systematic review estimated its prevalence as 0.5% for all laparoscopic surgery [49]. Gunderson et al. (2013) looked specifically at SILS, and adjusting for confounding variables, derived an umbilical hernia rate of 0.5% [50]. Nevertheless, there is not significant literature to reliably refute the hypothetical increased risk of herniation with SILS. In our case, we made a 15 mm incision at the umbilicus. We feel that given that this is only marginally larger than the Hasson entry technique incision the potential benefits of SILS outweigh the theoretical increased risk of umbilical hernia [51]. Overall, the application of SILS reduces the total number of incision sites and potential locations for herniation. Furthermore, fewer trocar insertions expose the patient to less risk of intra-abdominal trauma, bleeding, and pain.

Potential issues with instrument triangulation and obtaining adequate fulcrum in order to manipulate tissue adequately were countered by the flexibility of the Gelseal SILS port. This flexibility affords the surgeon adequate instrument articulation; hence, we do not foresee significant challenges in intracorporeal suturing. Furthermore, the presence of a large volume cyst did not restrict our use of SILS as we decompressed the cyst prior to its removal. We expect that with the increasing prevalence of SILS, adaptations to its unique challenges will proliferate.

4. Conclusion

Laparoscopic resection of adnexal lesions is safe during pregnancy and should be favoured over the open approach. SILS minimises incision sites and has potential for reduction in perioperative morbidity. The scope to add additional ports if needed makes SILS a feasible primary approach to laparoscopic cystectomy in the pregnant patient.

Consent

Informed consent has been obtained from the patient.

Disclosure

This study was performed as part of employment at our institution: Dunedin Public Hospital.

References

[1] J. Haan, M. Verheecke, and F. Amant, "Management of ovarian cysts and cancer in pregnancy," *Facts, Views and Vision in Obstetrics and Gynaecology*, vol. 7, no. 1, pp. 25–31, 2015.

[2] K. M. Schmeler, W. W. Mayo-Smith, J. F. Peipert, S. Weitzen, M. D. Manuel, and M. E. Gordinier, "Adnexal masses in pregnancy: surgery compared with observation," *Obstetrics and Gynaecology*, vol. 105, 5, Part 1, pp. 1098–1103, 2005.

[3] M. B. Reedy, H. L. Galan, W. E. Richards, C. K. Preece, P. A. Wetter, and T. J. Kuehl, "Laparoscopy during pregnancy. A survey of laparoendoscopic surgeons," *Journal of Reproductive Medicine*, vol. 42, no. 1, pp. 33–38, 1997.

[4] N. Greaves and J. Nicholson, "Single incision laparoscopic surgery in general surgery: a review," *Annals of the Royal College of Surgeons of England*, vol. 93, no. 6, pp. 437–440, 2011.

[5] S. A. Antoniou, O. O. Koch, G. A. Antoniou et al., "Meta-analysis of randomized trials on single-incision laparoscopic versus conventional laparoscopic appendectomy," *American Journal of Surgery*, vol. 207, no. 4, pp. 613–622, 2014.

[6] R. L. Giuntoli, R. S. Vang, and R. E. Bristow, "Evaluation and management of adnexal masses during pregnancy," *Clinical Obstetrics and Gynaecology*, vol. 49, no. 3, pp. 492–505, 2006.

[7] K. E. Webb, K. Sakhel, S. P. Chauhan, and A. Z. Abuhamad, "Adnexal mass during pregnancy: a review," *American Journal of Perinatology*, vol. 32, no. 11, pp. 1010–1016, 2015.

[8] P. Aggarwal and S. Kehoe, "Ovarian tumours in pregnancy: a literature review," *European Journal of Obstetrics, Gynaecology and Reproductive Biology*, vol. 155, no. 2, pp. 119–124, 2011.

[9] L. Rucker, Z. Walker, and B. Casey, "Case report: management of an early third trimester large adnexal mass in a singleton pregnancy," *Obstetrics and Gynaecology Cases–Reviews*, vol. 8, no. 1, p. 190, 2021.

[10] G. S. Leiserowitz, "Managing ovarian masses during pregnancy," *Obstetrical and Gynaecological Survey*, vol. 61, no. 7, pp. 463–470, 2006.

[11] I. A. Yakasai and L. A. Bappa, "Diagnosis and management of adnexal masses in pregnancy," *Journal of Surgical Technique and Case Report*, vol. 4, no. 2, pp. 79–85, 2012.

[12] J. G. Ray, M. J. Vermeulen, A. Bharatha, W. J. Montanera, and A. L. Park, "Association between MRI exposure during pregnancy and fetal and childhood outcomes," *Journal of the American Medical Association*, vol. 316, no. 9, pp. 952–961, 2016.

[13] A. Shaaban and M. Rezvani, "Ovarian cancer: detection and radiologic staging," *Clinical Obstetrics and Gynaecology*, vol. 52, no. 1, pp. 73–93, 2009.

[14] M. K. Montes de Oca, S. K. Dotters-Katz, J. A. Kuller, and R. A. Previs, "Adnexal masses in pregnancy," *Obstetrical and Gynaecological Survey*, vol. 76, no. 7, pp. 437–450, 2021.

[15] G. S. R. Lee, S. Y. Hur, J. C. Shin, S. P. Kim, and S. J. Kim, "Elective vs. conservative management of ovarian tumors in pregnancy," *International Journal of Gynaecology and Obstetrics*, vol. 85, no. 3, pp. 250–254, 2004.

[16] E. Ball, N. Waters, N. Cooper et al., "Evidence-based guideline on laparoscopy in pregnancy," *Facts, Views and Visions in Obstetrics and Gynaecology*, vol. 11, no. 1, pp. 5–25, 2019.

[17] T. W. Sadler, *Langman's Medical Embryology*, Lippincott Williams and Wilkins, Philadelphia, 11th edition, 2010.

[18] F. Vernooij, P. Heintz, E. Witteveen, and Y. van der Graaf, "The outcomes of ovarian cancer treatment are better when provided by gynecologic oncologists and in specialized hospitals: a systematic review," *Gynaecologic Oncology*, vol. 105, no. 3, pp. 801–812, 2007.

[19] P. Mathevet, K. Nessah, D. Dargent, and G. Mellier, "Laparoscopic management of adnexal masses in pregnancy: a case series," *European Journal of Obstetrics, Gynaecology and Reproductive Biology*, vol. 108, no. 2, pp. 217–222, 2003.

[20] A. G. Rizzo, "Laparoscopic surgery in pregnancy: long-term follow-up," *Journal of Laparoendoscopic and Advanced Surgical Techniques*, vol. 13, no. 1, pp. 11–15, 2003.

[21] Y. Lenglet, H. Roman, B. Rabishong et al., "Laparoscopic management of adnexal masses during pregnancy," *Gynaecology, Obstetrics and Fertility*, vol. 34, no. 2, pp. 101–106, 2006.

[22] S. Morton, N. Cooper, J. Walravens-Evans, M. S. Nair, A. Karthikeyan, and W. Yoong, "Operative laparoscopy in advanced pregnancy beyond 20 weeks," *The Obstetrician and Gynaecologist*, vol. 22, no. 3, pp. 237–241, 2020.

[23] National Institute for Health and Care Excellence, "Preterm labour and birth," 2015, October 2021 https://www.nice.org.uk/guidance/ng25.

[24] K. B. Markham and M. Klebanoff, "Prevention of preterm birth in modern obstetrics," *Clinics in Perinatology*, vol. 41, no. 4, pp. 773–785, 2014.

[25] J. M. Barnard, D. C. Chaffin, S. Droste, A. Tierney, and T. Phernetton, "Fetal response to carbon dioxide pneumoperitoneum in the pregnant ewe," *Obstetrics and Gynaecology*, vol. 85, no. 5, pp. 669–674, 1995.

[26] Society of American Gastrointestinal and Endoscopic Surgeons, *Guidelines for the Use of Laparoscopy during Pregnancy*, 2017, October 2021 https://www.sages.org/publications/guidelines/guidelines-for-diagnosis-treatment-and-use-of-laparoscopy-for-surgical-problems-during-pregnancy/.

[27] M. Candiani, S. Maddalena, M. Barbieri, S. Izzo, D. Alberico, and S. Ronzoni, "Adnexal masses in pregnancy: fetomaternal blood flow indices during laparoscopic surgery," *Journal of Minimally Invasive Gynaecology*, vol. 19, no. 4, pp. 443–447, 2019.

[28] M. Ko, T. Lai, and S. Chen, "Laparoscopic management of complicated adnexal masses in the first trimester of pregnancy," *Fertility and Sterility*, vol. 92, no. 1, pp. 283–287, 2009.

[29] D. Nasioudis, D. Tsilimigras, and K. P. Economopoulos, "Laparoscopic cholecystectomy during pregnancy: a systematic review of 590 patients," *International Journal of Surgery*, vol. 27, pp. 165–175, 2016.

[30] S. H. Park, M. I. Park, J. S. Choi, J. H. Lee, H. O. Kim, and H. Kim, "Laparoscopic appendectomy performed during pregnancy by gynecological laparoscopists," *European Journal of Obstetrics, Gynaecology and Reproductive Biology*, vol. 148, no. 1, pp. 44–48, 2010.

[31] J. C. Chung, G. S. Cho, E. J. Shin, H. C. Kim, and O. P. Song, "Clinical outcomes compared between laparoscopic and open appendectomy in pregnant women," *Canadian Journal of Surgery*, vol. 56, no. 5, pp. 341–346, 2013.

[32] F. R. Nezhat, S. Tazuke, C. H. Nezhat, D. S. Seidman, D. R. Phillips, and C. R. Nezhat, "Laparoscopy during pregnancy: a literature review," *Journal of The Society of Laparoscopic and Robotic Surgeons*, vol. 1, no. 1, pp. 17–27, 1997.

[33] C. A. Walsh, T. Tang, and S. R. Walsh, "Laparoscopic versus open appendicectomy in pregnancy: a systematic review," *International Journal of Surgery*, vol. 6, no. 4, pp. 339–344, 2008.

[34] S. Saeed and S. Miraj, "Single-incision laparoscopy surgery: a systematic review," *Electronic Physician*, vol. 8, no. 10, pp. 3088–3095, 2016.

[35] E. Chouillard, S. Alsabah, R. Daher et al., "Single-incision laparoscopy could be better than standard laparoscopy in right colectomy for cancer," *Journal of Laparoendoscopic and Advanced Surgical Techniques*, vol. 26, no. 5, pp. 371–378, 2016.

[36] P. F. Escobar, M. A. Bedaiwy, A. N. Fader, and T. Falcone, "Laparoendoscopic single-site (LESS) surgery in patients with benign adnexal disease," *Fertility and Sterility*, vol. 93, no. 6, pp. 2074.e7–2074.e10, 2010.

[37] M. A. Bedaiwy, D. Sheyn, L. Eghdami et al., "Laparoendoscopic single-site surgery for benign ovarian cystectomies," *Gynaecologic and Obstetric Investigation*, vol. 79, no. 3, pp. 179–183, 2015.

[38] K. J. Huang, K. T. Lin, C. J. Wu, Y. X. Li, W. C. Chang, and B. C. Sheu, "Single incision laparoscopic surgery using conventional laparoscopic instruments versus two-port laparoscopic surgery for adnexal lesions," *Scientific Reports*, vol. 11, no. 1, p. 4118, 2021.

[39] T. Shiraishi, T. Tominaga, T. Nonaka et al., "A learning curve in using organ retractor for single-incision laparoscopic right colectomy," *Scientific Reports*, vol. 11, no. 1, p. 6546, 2021.

[40] P. Garg, S. Misra, J. D. Thakur, and J. Song, "Single incision laparoscopic surgery ovarian cystectomy in large benign ovarian cysts using conventional instruments," *Journal of Minimal Access Surgery*, vol. 7, no. 4, pp. 232–235, 2011.

[41] M. Marcelli, C. Lamourdedieu, A. Lazard, L. Cravello, M. Gamerre, and A. Agostini, "Salpingectomy for ectopic pregnancy by transumbilical single-site laparoscopy with the SILS system," *European Journal of Obstetrics, Gynaecology and Reproductive Biology*, vol. 167, no. 1, pp. 67–70, 2012.

[42] A. Loh, M. P. Torrizo, and Y. W. Ng, "Single incision laparoscopic surgery for surgical treatment of tubal ectopic pregnancy: a feasible alternative to conventional laparoscopy," *Journal of Gynaecologic Surgery*, vol. 33, no. 2, pp. 61–67, 2017.

[43] P. Dursun, T. Tezcaner, H. B. Zeyneloglu, I. Alyazici, A. Haberal, and A. Ayhan, "Adnexal masses treated using a combination of the SILS port and noncurved straight laparoscopic instruments: Turkish experience and review of the literature," *Minimally Invasive Surgery*, vol. 2013, Article ID 836380, 8 pages, 2013.

[44] J. Xiao, K. Fu, K. Duan, J. Wang, S. Sunkara, and X. Guan, "Pregnancy-preserving Laparoendoscopic Single-site Surgery for Gynecologic Disease: A Case Series," *Journal of Minimally Invasive Gynaecology*, vol. 27, no. 7, pp. 1588–1597, 2020.

[45] F. R. Borle, B. Mehra, and A. Singh, "Comparison of cosmetic outcome between single-incision laparoscopic cholecystectomy and conventional laparoscopic cholecystectomy in rural Indian population: a randomized clinical trial," *Indian Journal of Surgery*, vol. 77, no. S3, pp. 877–880, 2015.

[46] B. S. M. Chern, S. Lakhotia, C. K. Khoo, and A. Y. M. Siow, "Single incision laparoscopic surgery in gynecology: Evolution, current trends, and future perspectives," *Gynaecology and Minimally Invasive Therapy*, vol. 1, no. 1, pp. 9–18, 2012.

[47] S. Rezai, A. C. Hughes, E. Wang et al., "Laparoendoscopic single-site cystectomy in pregnancy for a benign Mullerian serous cystadenofibroma: a case report with review of literature," *Obstetrics and Gynaecology International Journal*, vol. 9, no. 4, pp. 234–236, 2018.

[48] S. B. Ross, W. C. Clark, C. A. Morton, and A. S. Rosemurgy, "Access for Laparoendoscopic Single Site Surgery," *Diagnostic and Therapeutic Endoscopy*, vol. 2010, Article ID 943091, 7 pages, 2010.

[49] H. A. Swank, I. M. Mulder, C. F. Chapelle, J. B. Reitsma, J. F. Lange, and W. A. Bemelman, "Systematic review of trocar-site hernia," *British Journal of Surgery*, vol. 99, no. 3, pp. 315–323, 2012.

[50] C. C. Gunderson, J. Knight, J. Ybanez-Morano et al., "The Risk of Umbilical Hernia and Other Complications with Laparoendoscopic Single-Site Surgery," *Journal of Minimally Invasive Gynaecology*, vol. 19, no. 1, pp. 40–45, 2012.

[51] A. K. Sangrasi, A. I. Memon, M. M. Memon, M. R. Abbasi, A. A. Laghari, and J. N. Qureshi, "A safe quick technique for placement of the first access port for creation of pneumoperitoneum," *Journal of the Society of Laparoscopic and Robotic Surgeons*, vol. 15, no. 4, pp. 504–508, 2011.

6

A Case of a Patient with Adhesive Small Bowel Obstruction in Pregnancy after Extensive Myomectomy for Diffuse Uterine Leiomyomatosis

Yuri Suminaga, Mana Taki, Haruko Okamoto, Yosuke Kawamura, Yusuke Sagae, Masumi Sunada, Yoshitsugu Chigusa, Akihito Horie, Masaki Mandai, and Haruta Mogami

Department of Gynecology and Obstetrics, Kyoto University, Kyoto, Japan

Correspondence should be addressed to Mana Taki; takimana@kuhp.kyoto-u.ac.jp

Academic Editor: Daniel Martin

Background. Diffuse uterine leiomyomatosis is a rare disease in which countless, poorly defined, and small nodules are present in most parts of the uterine myometrium. It frequently occurs in fertile women and causes infertility. A deep, median, longitudinal incision of the uterine corpus with the opening of the endometrial cavity, "extensive myomectomy," is required to restore fertility. However, myomectomy may also be a risk factor for perinatal complications. We present a rare case of adhesive small bowel obstruction after extensive myomectomy for diffuse uterine leiomyomatosis. *Case.* A 37-year-old primigravida presented with sharp epigastric pain and vomiting at 21-week gestation. The patient had a history of extensive myomectomy for diffuse uterine leiomyomatosis. Abdominal radiography revealed moderate air fluid levels in the small intestine, and the patient was diagnosed with adhesive small bowel obstruction. The patient was also diagnosed with placenta previa. Bowel rest with intestinal tube was continued until delivery. Cesarean section was performed at 32-week gestation due to (i) prolonged fasting and total parenteral nutrition for conservative treatment and (ii) fear of sudden massive bleeding from placenta previa. Because the ileum was strongly adherent to the uterine scar from the previous myomectomy, adhesiolysis and enterectomy were performed. The placenta was uncomplicatedly delivered and the hemorrhage was well-controlled. *Conclusions.* Pregnancy with a history with extensive myomectomy for diffuse uterine leiomyomatosis should be carefully monitored because of the occasional occurrence of adhesive small intestine obstruction during pregnancy.

1. Introduction

Diffuse uterine leiomyomatosis is a rare and benign disease that results in enlargement of the uterus with almost complete replacement of the uterine myometrium by innumerable, poorly defined, and small nodules ranging from microscopic to 3 cm in size [1–3]. It frequently occurs in fertile women and causes infertility [4, 5]. Typical myomectomy is insufficient for diffuse uterine leiomyomatosis; a deep, median, and longitudinal incision of the uterine corpus with the opening of the endometrial cavity is required, and "extensive myomectomy" is performed to restore fertility [4, 6]. However, myomectomy could also increase the risk of other perinatal complications including postoperative adhesions.

Small bowel obstruction in pregnancy is a rare perinatal complication with an incidence of 0.001–0.003% and is a life-threatening situation for mothers and fetuses [7–10]. Small bowel obstruction is primarily caused by adhesions, hernias, inflammatory diseases, and malignancies. Adhesion is the leading cause of small bowel obstruction, even during pregnancy. A history of abdominal surgery is the most common cause of adhesions, leading to adhesive small bowel obstruction during pregnancy. Small bowel obstruction is defined as a partial or complete blockade of the small intestine [11]. The symptoms are mainly abdominal pain, vomiting, constipation, and distension, and worsen during pregnancy. Most patients are conservatively treated with nasogastric or intestinal tubes and total parenteral nutrition (TPN), whereas surgical intervention during pregnancy is sometimes required if the small intestine is strangulated. Increased maternal mortality and fetal loss have been reported in the literature [8].

In this report, we present a rare case of adhesive small bowel obstruction a year after extensive laparotomic myomectomy for diffuse uterine leiomyomatosis.

2. Case Report

A 37-year-old primiparous woman presented at 21-week gestation with sharp epigastric pain and vomiting. She underwent extensive laparotomic myomectomy with a longitudinal incision of the anterior and posterior wall of the uterus for diffuse uterine leiomyomatosis and removal of 49 nodules 9 months before pregnancy that resulted from artificial insemination (Figure 1). She was afebrile and had normal blood pressure and pulse rate. She had epigastric tenderness, and her uterus was soft with no abnormal signs. Abdominal radiography revealed mild air and fluid levels in the small intestine. Sonography showed total placenta previa. She was admitted to our hospital with adhesive small intestinal obstruction and total placenta previa, which could be a postoperative complication of her previous myomectomy. One week of intravenous fluids and bowel rest improved her symptoms, and she was discharged.

She was re-admitted again at 26-week gestation for abnormal genital bleeding due to placenta previa. The patient had no abdominal pain and normal appetite. Three days later, the patient experienced sharp epigastric pain, vomiting, distention, and constipation. Abdominal radiography showed moderate air fluid levels in the small intestine, and she was diagnosed with worsening adhesive small bowel obstruction. Bowel rest and intravenous fluids were started at the same time that tocolysis was needed because of the increasing uterine contraction caused by vomiting. Over the next 72 h, she developed fever with worsening symptoms, in which small intestine obstruction promoted bacterial translocation. Computed tomography (CT) revealed consecutive dilatation of the proximal small intestine and collapsed distal ileum adjacent to the fundus of the uterus without free air (Figure 2). The patient was managed using an intestinal tube and antibiotics. However, her abdominal pain did not resolve, and accordingly, her uterine contraction, genital bleeding, and fever increased. We discussed this with gastroenterologists and thought that it would be better to continue the conservative therapy, without surgical treatment. We inserted the intestinal tube deeper into the adhesion site (total 245 cm in length) at 28-week gestation, and her symptoms, including fever and uterine contraction, gradually resolved. Unexplained oligohydramnios occurred 4 days after fever, but gradually resolved within 10 days as her symptoms improved.

Ultrasonography revealed a clear retroplacental hypoechoic zone, which did not suggest the presence of placenta accreta spectrum (PAS), whereas magnetic resonance imaging showed placental recess (a wedge-shaped contraction of the placental surface and uterine outer rim accompanying a T2 dark band), which is a predictive sign of PAS (Figure 3) [12]. Also, the placenta was present on the scar of the previous extensive myomectomy. If PAS is present, hysterectomy must be performed urgently in some cases [13]. However, hysterectomy is difficult to perform when the small intestine is attached to the uterus. Therefore, we scheduled her cesarean section for 32^{+4}-week gestation because (i) fasting and TPN were too long and strong patient psychological stress and (ii) fear of massive bleeding due to placenta previa, which frequently occurs around 34 to 36-week gestation. An intra-aortic balloon occlusion catheter was inserted before a cesarean section to avoid massive hemorrhage in case of PAS. A cesarean section under general anesthesia was performed, and she gave birth to a healthy male weighing 1807 g (46.88 percentile) with an Apgar score of 4 at 1 min and 6 at 5 min. The placenta was spontaneously delivered without manual removal, and uterine hemorrhage was well controlled by prophylactic intrauterine balloon tamponade without inflating the intra-aortic balloon occlusion catheter. The total blood loss was 3100 g, and the patient received a blood transfusion. During laparotomy, there were ileal loops strongly adhered to the uterine scar of the myomectomy, but there was no volvulus of the small intestine. The patient underwent adhesiolysis and enterectomy. The patient recovered uneventfully, without recurrent bowel obstruction.

3. Discussion

Diffuse uterine leiomyomatosis is a rare condition in which innumerable, poorly defined, and small leiomyomas replace most parts of the myometrium, leading to uterine enlargement of uterus [1, 14]. This rare condition affects women of reproductive age, and is associated with menstrual pain, menorrhagia, and infertility [5]. Hysterectomy is the only definitive treatment because it is not easy to perform myomectomy on numerous nodules with indistinct margins [2]. In order to restore fertility in patients with diffuse uterine leiomyomatosis, many treatments have been tried as alternatives to hysterectomy. The uterine artery embolization (UAE) may be an effective alternative to hysterectomy and one of seven patients treated by UAE became pregnant 5 months after UAE treatment [15], although pregnancy after UAE treatment is controversial. High intensity focused ultrasound (HIFU) treatment has also been used as an alternative to hysterectomy [16]. Purohit et al. reported that HIFU treatment reduced 67.6% of uterine volume and improved normal menstruation, although they did not have pregnancy outcomes after HIFU treatment. Gonadotropin-releasing hormone analog (GnRHa) is widely used for diffuse uterine leiomyomatosis, and successful pregnancies after GnRHa administration has been reported, but it is primarily administered before myomectomy to control bleeding during myomectomy [5]. Hysteroscopic myomectomy has also been reported to recover fertility in patients with diffuse uterine leiomyomatosis [17, 18].

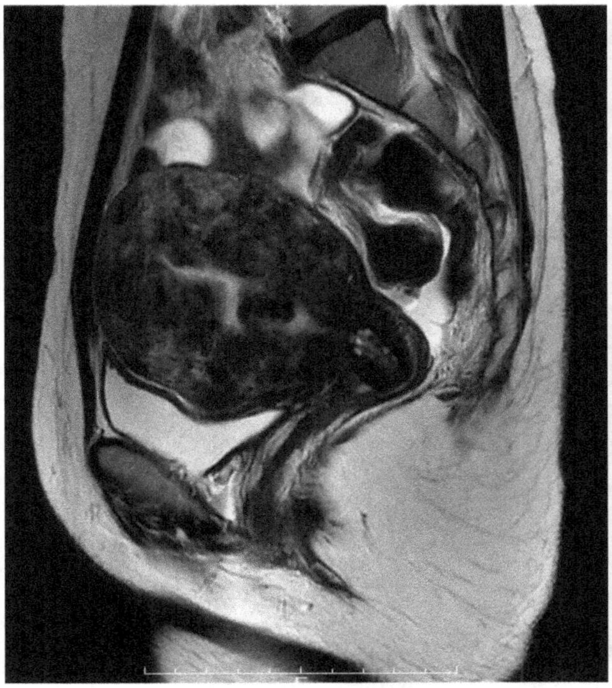

(a)

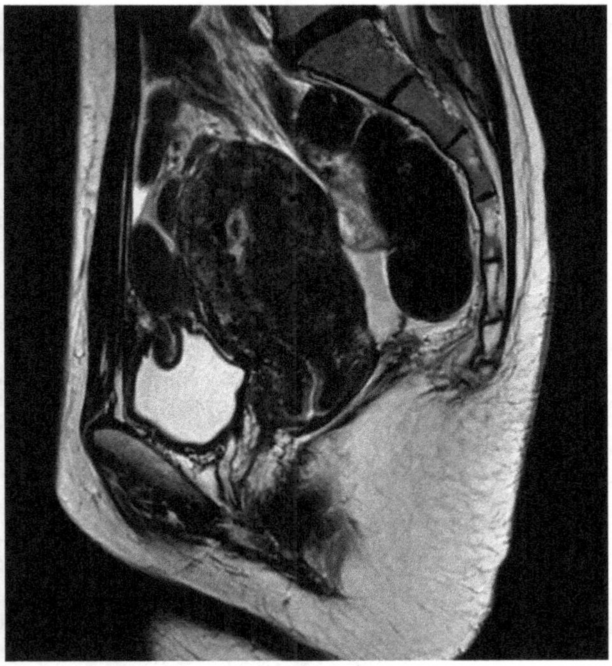

(b)

FIGURE 1: MRI T2-weighted findings of diffuse uterine leiomyomatosis (a) before and (b) after extensive myomectomy.

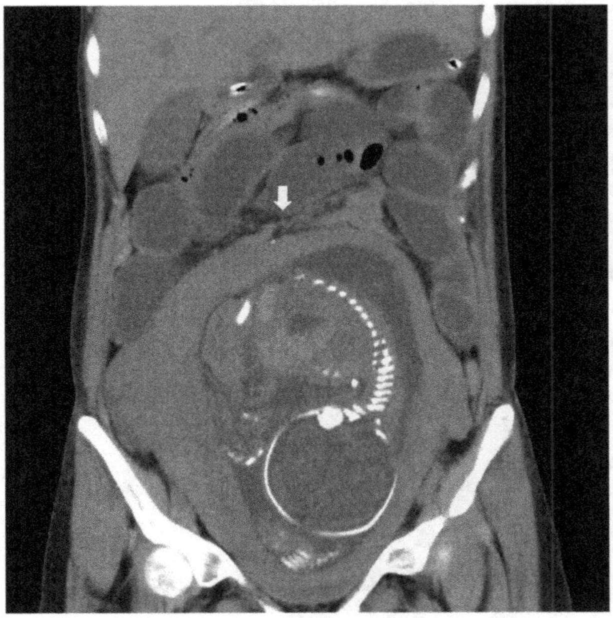

FIGURE 2: CT findings of adhesive small intestine at 26-week gestation. An arrow indicates adhesion site.

We have currently performed a new surgical treatment, extensive myomectomy to restore fertility in women with diffuse uterine leiomyomatosis. In this procedure, the uterus is deeply dissected longitudinally with complete opening of the uterine cavity after tourniquet for hemostasis [4, 6]. Since this surgical procedure has only recently begun to be reported, it is unclear to what extent it improves fertility. It has been reported that the pregnancy rate after myomectomy is lower the greater the number of myomas enucleated [19, 20]. In the future, it is necessary to compare the degree of fertility improvement between conventional myomectomy and this new procedure in patients with diffuse uterine leiomyomatosis. This method results in a more extensive uterine scar that may cause perinatal complications, including uterine rupture. Furthermore, myomectomy causes peritoneal adhesions that make cesarean section more difficult.

Small bowel obstruction during pregnancy is a very rare disease, with an incidence of 0.0014%–0.0034% [21]. A review of small bowel obstruction in pregnancy showed that 50% of all cases were caused by adhesions [8]. Surgical treatment was performed in 91% of adhesive small bowel obstructions because conservative treatment failed in 81% of cases. The problem lies in the high fetal mortality rate. The risk of fetal loss was 17% in patients with adhesive small bowel obstruction, whereas the rate of maternal mortality was 2% [8]. In the previous report, fetal deaths occurred when the maternal condition was severe and required emergency laparotomy in 2nd and 3rd trimester [22]. It suggests that the high fetal mortality rate is related to fetal-maternal infection rather than due to preterm delivery. In our case, the baby was born prematurely at 32-week gestation and grew without problems. However, unexplained oligohydramnios occurred for 10 days between 28- to 30-week gestations when the mother developed fever. A nonstress test and ultrasonography showed no abnormal fetal signs, except for oligohydramnios. Amniotic fluid gradually increased as the mother's condition improved with conservative treatment. Maternal dehydration may be the cause of oligohydramnios.

Myomectomy is considered a risk factor for PAS, which is a rare life-threatening condition of pregnancy [13]. PAS is

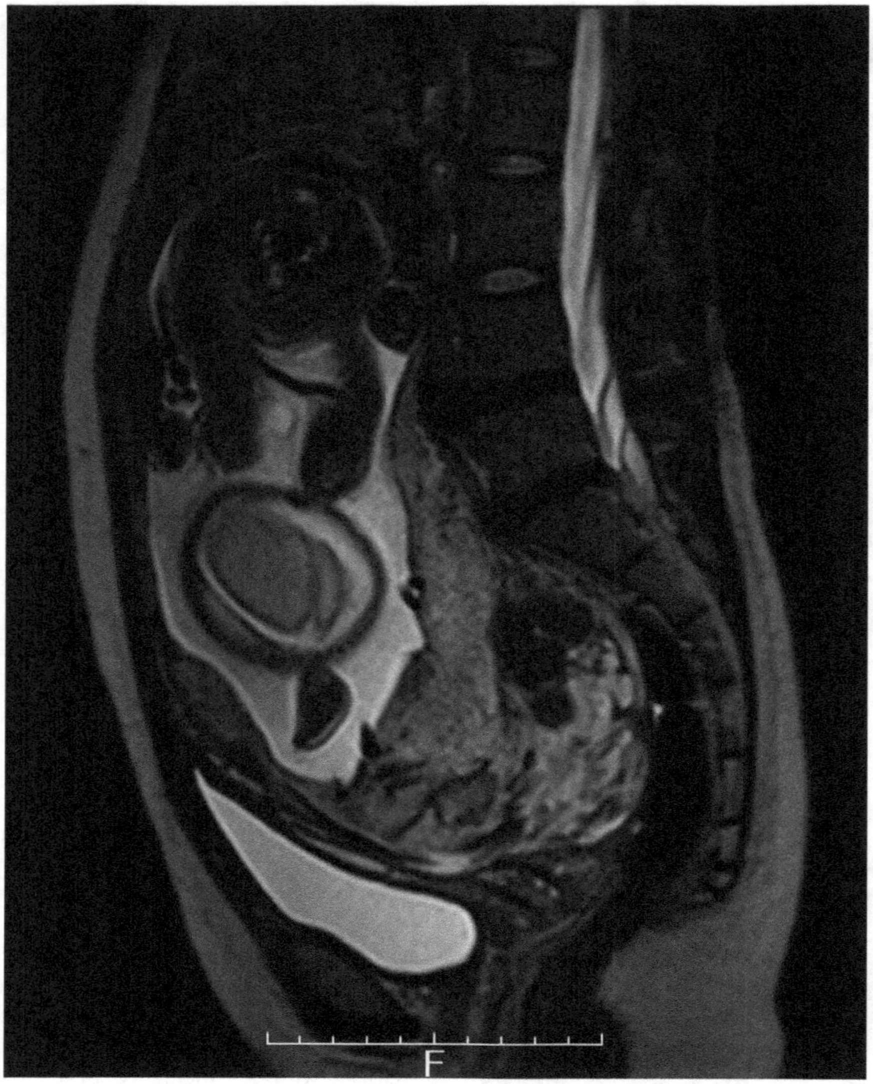

(a)

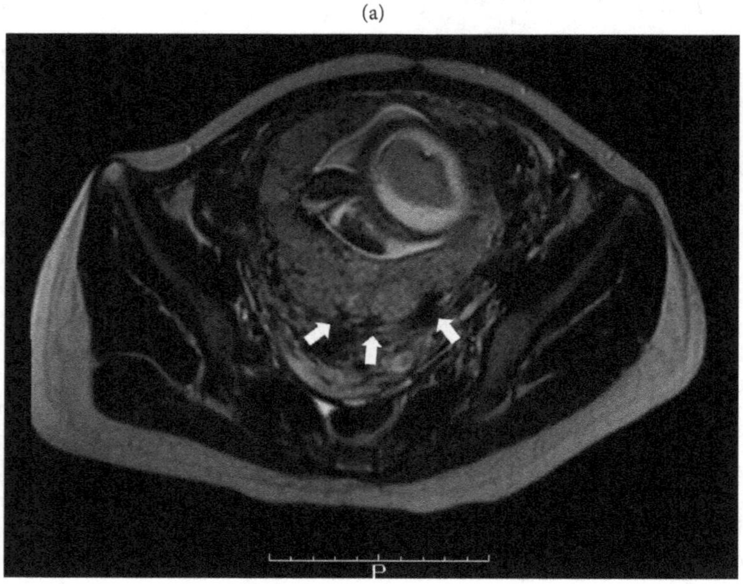

(b)

Figure 3: MRI findings of placenta previa. (a) Sagittal and (b) axial image. Arrows represent placental recess (a wedge-shaped contraction of the placental surface and uterine outer rim accompanying a T2 dark band).

the abnormal attachment of placental villi to the myometrium, which includes placenta accreta (attachment to the myometrium without decidua), placenta increta (invasion into the uterine myometrium), and placenta percreta (deeper invasion into surrounding organs, such as the bladder). Compared to conventional myomectomy, extensive myomectomy results in much longer uterine scar into endometrium, which may increase the risk of PAS. In our case, IVF pregnancy is also a risk factor of placenta anomalies [23]. The main clinical problem is massive bleeding, which occurs when the placenta does not detach after delivery. Hysterectomy is sometimes required when massive bleeding is not controlled by other hemostatic procedures. Placenta Accreta Spectrum Ultrasound Scoring System (PASUSS) can estimate the severity of PAS and can be a useful tool to predict massive bleeding during PAS [24].

Our case was a rare combination of placenta previa and adhesive small bowel obstruction, for which we were unable to perform immediate hysterectomy. We planned to perform a cesarean section with an intra-aortic balloon catheter to avoid emergent hysterectomy due to massive bleeding. Fortunately, the placenta detached normally, and intra-aortic balloon occlusion was not used. The total blood volume during the cesarean section and enterectomy was lower than expected. A lesson from our case was to perform immediate full preparation for the cesarean section. As previously described, small bowel obstruction during pregnancy is associated with a high risk of fetal loss [8]. When the maternal and fetal condition worsens, immediate laparotomy and fetal delivery are necessary to end the pregnancy.

This is the first case report of adhesive small bowel obstruction during pregnancy after extensive myomectomy for diffuse uterine leiomyomatosis, which is our strength of the case. However, the fertility-improving effects of extensive myomectomy are still unknown. Also, perinatal complications after extensive myomectomy will be reported. It is necessary to compare the degree of fertility improvement and perinatal complications between conventional myomectomy and this new procedure in patients with diffuse uterine leiomyomatosis.

We report a case of two rare complications, adhesive small bowel obstruction and placenta previa, presumably due to aggressive myomectomy for diffuse uterine leiomyomatosis. The placenta was not adherent to the scar of the previous extensive myomectomy in our case. However, the scar of extensive myomectomy is larger and deeper than that of conventional myomectomy, which may increase the risk of adhesive small bowel obstruction and PAS. Adhesive small bowel obstruction can lead to severe maternal conditions, sometimes resulting in fetal death. Pregnant women after extensive myomectomy should be managed with the possibility of adhesive small bowel obstruction in mind and the degree of placental adhesion to the scar should be evaluated.

Consent

Informed patient consent has been obtained.

References

[1] B. Lapan and L. Solomon, "Diffuse leiomyomatosis of the uterus precluding myomectomy," *Obstetrics and Gynecology*, vol. 53, Supplement 3, pp. 82S–84S, 1979.

[2] C. A. Silva, F. Rosa, M. Rito, and T. M. Cunha, "Diffuse leiomyomatosis: a rare cause of a diffusely enlarged uterus," *Radiology Case Reports*, vol. 17, no. 5, pp. 1536–1539, 2022.

[3] A. Coskun, O. Ozdemir, M. A. Vardar, G. Kiran, D. Arikan, and C. Ersoz, "A case with diffuse uterine leiomyomatosis and review of the literature," *Clinical and Experimental Obstetrics & Gynecology*, vol. 35, no. 3, pp. 227–230, 2008.

[4] Y. Otsubo, M. Nishida, Y. Arai, R. Ichikawa, and M. Sakanaka, "Diffuse uterine leiomyomatosis in patient with successful pregnancy following new surgical management," *Archives of Gynecology and Obstetrics*, vol. 290, no. 4, pp. 815–818, 2014.

[5] R. Purohit, J. G. Sharma, and S. Singh, "A case of diffuse uterine leiomyomatosis who had two successful pregnancies after medical management," *Fertility and Sterility*, vol. 95, no. 7, pp. 2434.e5–2434.e6, 2011.

[6] I. Konishi, "Diffuse Leiomyomatosis: Complete Myomectomy for Innumerable Small Nodules to Achieve Fertility Sparing and Childbearing," *The Surgery Journal*, vol. 6, pp. S50–S57, 2020.

[7] W. W. Beck, "Intestinal obstruction in pregnancy," *Obstetrics and Gynecology*, vol. 43, no. 3, pp. 374–378, 1974.

[8] P. J. Webster, M. A. Bailey, J. Wilson, and D. A. Burke, "Small bowel obstruction in pregnancy is a complex surgical problem with a high risk of fetal loss," *Annals of the Royal College of Surgeons of England*, vol. 97, no. 5, pp. 339–344, 2015.

[9] S. Meyerson, T. Holtz, M. Ehrinpreis, and R. Dhar, "Small bowel obstruction in pregnancy," *The American Journal of Gastroenterology*, vol. 90, no. 2, pp. 299–302, 1995.

[10] S. Rauff, S. K. Chang, and E. K. Tan, "Intestinal obstruction in pregnancy: a case report," *Case Reports in Obstetrics and Gynecology*, vol. 2013, Article ID 564838, 2 pages, 2013.

[11] F. Catena, S. di Saverio, F. Coccolini et al., "Adhesive small bowel adhesions obstruction: evolutions in diagnosis, management and prevention," *World Journal of Gastrointestinal Surgery*, vol. 8, no. 3, pp. 222–231, 2016.

[12] A. Delli Pizzi, A. Tavoletta, R. Narciso et al., "Prenatal planning of placenta previa: diagnostic accuracy of a novel MRI-based prediction model for placenta accreta spectrum (PAS) and clinical outcome," *Abdominal Radiology*, vol. 44, no. 5, pp. 1873–1882, 2019.

[13] R. M. Silver and D. W. Branch, "Placenta accreta spectrum," *The New England Journal of Medicine*, vol. 378, no. 16, pp. 1529–1536, 2018.

[14] L. Fedele, S. Bianchi, G. Zanconato, S. Carinelli, and N. Berlanda, "Conservative treatment of diffuse uterine leiomyomatosis," *Fertility and Sterility*, vol. 82, no. 2, pp. 450–453, 2004.

[15] J. Koh, M. D. Kim, D. C. Jung et al., "Uterine artery embolization (UAE) for diffuse leiomyomatosis of the uterus: clinical and imaging results," *European Journal of Radiology*, vol. 81, no. 10, pp. 2726–2729, 2012.

[16] X. Zhang, T. Tian, J. Zhu et al., "High intensity focused ultrasound treatment for diffuse uterine leiomyomatosis: a feasibility study," *International Journal of Hyperthermia*, vol. 37, no. 1, pp. 1060–1065, 2020.

[17] I. Mazzon, A. Favilli, M. Grasso, D. Morricone, G. C. di Renzo, and S. Gerli, "Is 'cold loop' hysteroscopic myomectomy a better option for reproduction in women with diffuse uterine leiomyomatosis? A case report of successful repeated pregnancies," *Journal of Obstetrics and Gynaecology Research*, vol. 41, no. 3, pp. 474–477, 2015.

[18] H. Zhao, B. Yang, H. Li, Y. Xu, and L. Feng, "Successful pregnancies in women with diffuse uterine leiomyomatosis after hysteroscopic management using the hysteroscopy endo operative system," *Journal of Minimally Invasive Gynecology*, vol. 26, no. 5, pp. 960–967, 2019.

[19] R. Sudik, K. Hüsch, J. Steller, and E. Daume, "Fertility and pregnancy outcome after myomectomy in sterility patients," *European Journal of Obstetrics, Gynecology, and Reproductive Biology*, vol. 65, no. 2, pp. 209–214, 1996.

[20] S. Kameda, M. Toyoshima, K. Tanaka et al., "Utility of laparoscopic uterine myomectomy as a treatment for infertility with no obvious cause except for uterine fibroids," *Gynecology and Minimally Invasive Therapy*, vol. 7, no. 4, pp. 152–155, 2018.

[21] V. Sivanesaratnam, "The acute abdomen and the obstetrician," *Baillière's Best Practice & Research. Clinical Obstetrics & Gynaecology*, vol. 14, no. 1, pp. 89–102, 2000.

[22] P. W. Perdue, H. W. Johnson, and P. W. Stafford, "Intestinal obstruction complicating pregnancy," *American Journal of Surgery*, vol. 164, no. 4, pp. 384–388, 1992.

[23] S. Capriglione, C. Ettore, C. Terranova et al., "Analysis of ultrasonographic and hystopathologic features of placental invasiveness," *The Journal of Maternal-Fetal & Neonatal Medicine*, pp. 1–8, 2021.

[24] Y. Wang, Y. Zhou, L. Zeng, L. Chen, and Y. Zhao, "Analysis of risk factors for massive intraoperative bleeding in patients with placenta accreta spectrum," *BMC Pregnancy and Childbirth*, vol. 22, no. 1, p. 116, 2022.

7

Prenatal Diagnosis of Umbilical Cord Ulcer: A Report of Two Cases

Daisuke Katsura, [1] Suzuko Moritani, [2] Shunichiro Tsuji, [1] Kaori Hayashi, [1] Kazutaka Yamada, [1] Shinsuke Tokoro, [1] Kounosuke Suzuki, [1] Fuminori Kimura, [1] and Takashi Murakami [1]

[1] *Department of Obstetrics and Gynecology, Shiga University of Medical Science Hospital, Setatsukinowa-cho, Otsu, Shiga 520-2192, Japan*
[2] *Department of Diagnostic Pathology, Shiga University of Medical Science Hospital, Setatsukinowa-cho, Otsu, Shiga 520-2192, Japan*

Correspondence should be addressed to Daisuke Katsura; katsuo14@belle.shiga-med.ac.jp

Academic Editor: Giovanni Monni

Umbilical cord ulcer is related to fetal intestinal atresia or meconium; perforation of the ulcer causes fetal deterioration leading to fetal and neonatal death owing to fetal hemorrhage. However, to the best of our knowledge, a method to diagnose umbilical cord ulcer prenatally is not available. No reports exist about the prenatal findings before perforation of umbilical cord ulcer using ultrasonography. We encountered two cases of umbilical cord ulcer showing ultrasonographic finding of a linear echo around the umbilical cord. Umbilical cord ulcers with an exposed umbilical cord artery in the first case and with perforation of the artery in the second case were diagnosed postnatally. When we encounter such ultrasonographic finding, especially with polyhydramnios and high amniotic bile acid concentration in cases of fetal intestinal atresia, risk of perforation of the umbilical cord ulcer should be included in the differential diagnosis.

1. Introduction

Umbilical cord ulcer (UCU) was first reported by Blanc and Allan [1]. It is related to fetal intestinal atresia and occurs in 5.6% of fetuses with intestinal atresia [2]. Congenital intestinal atresia, with an estimated incidence of approximately 1 in 5000 live births, shows ultrasonographic findings of gastrointestinal dilatation such as a double, triple, or multiple bubble sign [3]. The perinatal mortality rate in fetuses with intestinal atresia was approximately 10% [4]. In addition, UCU has been reported to be caused by meconium [5]. The mortality rate in fetuses with UCU was approximately 46% [6]. As UCU perforation causes acute fetal blood loss leading to fetal death, an emergency delivery is often required [1, 2]. However, as the fetal condition deteriorates rapidly after perforation, delivery before perforation is desirable. The degree of UCU is graded based on its width: from the desquamation of the epithelium (grade 1) and detachment of the basal lamina (grade 2) to the thinning of Wharton's jelly with widespread grade 2 changes (grade 3) and exposed umbilical artery or vein (grade 4), in addition to perforation [7]. Therefore, it may be valuable to diagnose UCU and determine the risk of perforation prenatally. Ultrasonographic and amniotic findings for such diagnoses have been discussed; however, they have not been established yet. Herein, we present our experience of two interesting cases with the same ultrasonographic findings: one case of UCU grade 4 and one case of UCU perforation.

2. Case Presentation

2.1. Case 1. A 31-year-old woman with polyhydramnios at 31 weeks of gestation was admitted to our hospital owing to threatened premature labor. Fetal ultrasound examination revealed that the maximum vertical pocket (MVP) was 8.0 cm, amniotic fluid index (AFI) was 30 cm, and estimated fetal weight (EFW) was 1556 g (26.4 gestational age percentile). The double bubble sign was observed in

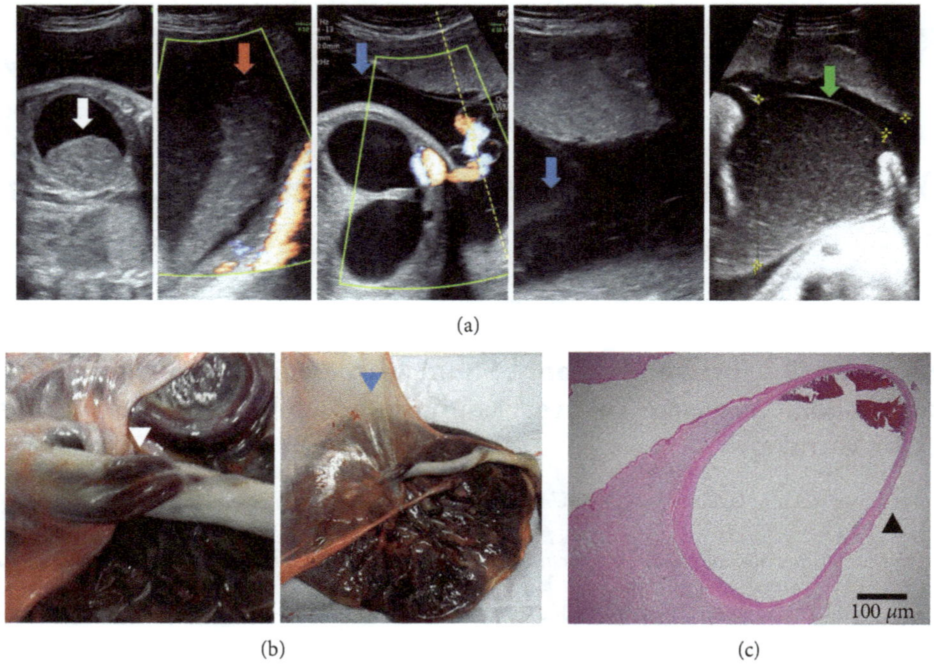

FIGURE 1: Case 1. (a) Ultrasonographic findings at 36 weeks of gestation. Heterogeneous high echoic mass-like debris within the fetal stomach (white arrow) and uterus (red arrow). Linear echo findings around the umbilical cord (blue arrow) and chorioamniotic membrane separation (green arrow). (b) Macroscopic findings. Umbilical ulcer with exposed umbilical cord artery (white arrowhead). The amniotic and chorionic membranes were separated on the surface of the placenta (blue arrowhead). (c) Original magnification. Loss of the amniotic membrane, degeneration of the umbilical cord stroma, and exposure of the umbilical cord artery (black arrowhead, hematoxylin and eosin; H&E, ×40).

the fetal abdomen, and fetal duodenal atresia was diagnosed. Because the patient had frequent uterine contractions and cervical dilatation, amnioreduction was performed at 31 weeks and at 32 weeks of gestation. During the first amniocentesis, we performed amniotic diagnosis for karyotyping and made a diagnosis of trisomy 21. The patient was provided information about the genetics and clinical course of trisomy 21. The amniotic bile acid concentration was 16.6 μmol/L and 16.5 μmol/L during the first and second amniocenteses, respectively. Thereafter, the patient's condition was stable.

At 36 weeks of gestation, fetal ultrasound findings showed heterogeneous high echoic mass-like debris within the uterus and fetal stomach, linear echo around the umbilical cord, and chorioamniotic membrane separation (Figure 1(a)). Because these findings were not confirmed 5 days earlier, fetal heart rate was fully monitored on the cardiotocogram. The umbilical artery pulsatility index (UmA PI), middle cerebral artery (MCA) PI, and MCA peak systolic velocity (PSV) were 1.33, 2.14, and 79.75 cm/s (1.49 MoM), respectively, in the fetal Doppler. Although the fetal heart rate pattern remained reassuring on cardiotocogram, we could not deny the risk of UCU perforation considering these findings and performed a cesarean section around 12 hours later. The amniotic fluid was not blood tinged.

A female infant weighing 2282 g with Apgar scores of 7 and 9 at 1 and 5 min, respectively, umbilical artery pH of 7.352, and hemoglobin concentration (Hb) of 13.0 g/dL was delivered. After birth, a large amount of bile-like yellowish brown fluid was aspirated from the infant's stomach, and her respiratory and circulatory states were stable. She had mild anemia but did not require any treatment. Although fetal hemoglobin and alpha-fetoprotein levels were not measured, fetomaternal transfusion was suggested as the cause of anemia because there was no bleeding, no blood group incompatibility, and no other apparent cause. The infant underwent an operation for duodenal atresia at 2 days after birth. Duodenal atresia type IIIa, distal from the ampulla of Vater, was diagnosed. The postoperative course was uneventful and the infant was discharged at age 39 days.

Macroscopically, two UCUs with exposed umbilical artery were observed at the umbilical cord surface attached to the placenta (Figure 1(b)). The amniotic and chorionic membranes were separated from the surface of the placenta (Figure 1(b)). Histopathological examination revealed amniotic membrane loss, umbilical cord stroma degeneration, and umbilical artery exposure (Figure 1(c)).

2.2. Case 2. A 38-year-old woman with polyhydramnios at 30 weeks of gestation was admitted to our hospital owing to threatened premature labor. On fetal ultrasound examination, the MVP, AFI, and EFW were 12.2 cm, 31.5 cm, and 1388 g (26.3, gestational age percentile), respectively. The double bubble sign was observed in the fetal abdomen, and fetal duodenal atresia was diagnosed. Because the patient had abdominal distension and frequent uterine contractions, amnioreduction was performed. At this point, the amniotic bile acid concentration was 25.3 μmol/L. Thereafter, her condition was stable.

At 34 weeks of gestation, it was difficult to confirm the fetal heart rate on cardiotocogram. On fetal ultrasound examination, heterogeneous high echoic mass-like debris

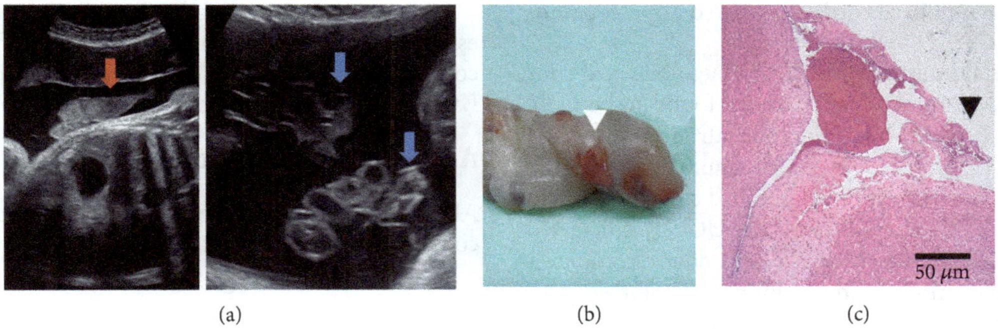

Figure 2: Case 2. (a) Ultrasonographic findings at 36 weeks of gestation. Heterogeneous high echoic mass-like debris within the uterus (red arrow) and linear echo finding around the umbilical cord (blue arrow). (b) Macroscopic findings. Umbilical ulcer with perforation of umbilical cord artery (white arrowhead). (c) Original magnification. Focal perforation of the umbilical cord artery with thinning of Wharton's jelly (black arrowhead, H&E, ×100).

within the uterus and linear echo findings around the umbilical cord were detected (Figure 2(a)). These findings were not confirmed 2 days earlier. Fetal myocardium movement seemed weak, UmA PI of 0.97, MCA reversed end-diastolic velocity, and MCA PSV of 25 cm/s were seen, and the fetal heart rate was 80-110 bpm as observed by fetal Doppler. We speculated fetal circulatory insufficiency due to fetal hemorrhage caused by UCU perforation; we performed an emergency cesarean section. The amniotic fluid was blood tinged. After surgery, from the images, the calculated left and right ventricle myocardial performance index was 0.67 and 0.70, respectively, and the left and right ventricle fractional shortening was 10% and 9%, respectively.

A female infant weighing 2086 g was delivered; the infant required resuscitation with intubation, heart massage, and epinephrine. Her Apgar scores were 1, 3, 3, and 5 at 1, 5, 10, and 15 min, respectively. Her umbilical artery pH was 7.157, base excess was -9.6, and Hb was 7.9 g/dL. Results of the neonatal laboratory tests were as follows: Hb, 6.9 g/dL; platelets at birth and one day later, 12.8×10^4 μL and 3.1×10^4 μL, respectively; fibrinogen, 30 mg/dL; prothrombin time—international normalized ratio, 6.29; and D-dimer, 21.8 μg/mL. Neonatal anemia and disseminated intravascular coagulation were observed. The infant received repeated blood transfusions and was placed on conventional mechanical ventilation. The Thompson score was 12, and the case was classified as severe encephalopathy. Brain diffusion-weighted magnetic resonance imaging showed diffuse hyperintensity throughout the cerebral cortex, which suggested diffuse hypoxic-ischemic necrosis and hypoxic ischemic encephalopathy. Chromosomal abnormality was not confirmed.

Macroscopically, one UCU with umbilical artery perforations and one UCU with exposed umbilical artery were observed at the umbilical cord surface attached to the placenta and fetus (Figure 2(b)). Histopathological examination revealed focal perforation of the umbilical cord artery with thinning of Wharton's jelly (Figure 2(c)).

3. Discussion

Prenatal diagnosis of UCU and assessment of the risk of perforation of UCU using ultrasonography are yet to be established. To our knowledge, these are the first report of UCU cases with ultrasonographic findings that were suggestive of a risk of UCU perforation. The finding of linear echo around the umbilical cord might be helpful as a marker to predict UCU perforation.

Although the causes of UCU are unclear, congenital abnormalities of the umbilical cord epithelium, ischemia caused by abnormal spasm of the umbilical vessels, and degeneration caused by digestive enzymes in fetal vomiting [8] may be potential causes. These factors alone or in combination might cause UCUs [8]. Congenital abnormalities of the umbilical cord epithelium might be related to chromosomal anomalies, structural anomalies, fetal growth restriction, abnormal insertion of the umbilical cord, and umbilical cord abnormalities, such as noncoiled umbilical cord, umbilical cord cysts, umbilical vein varices, and single umbilical artery [9]. In a previous report, bile toxicity was suggested as the cause of UCU based on pathological findings that revealed activated macrophages containing pigment granules within the ulcer bed, necrotic areas of Wharton's jelly, and fetal membranes [10]. Not only digestive enzymes but also meconium reportedly cause ischemia and degeneration of umbilical vessels, leading to the development of UCU [5].

Regarding the heterogeneous high echoic mass seen on ultrasound, amniotic fluid sludge indicating the presence of bacteria and intra-amniotic inflammation could be responsible for it [11]. However, intra-amniotic inflammation was not found in both our cases. Therefore, we speculated that the heterogeneous high echoic mass-like debris within the fetal stomach and uterus indicated a high-density mass, including digestive enzymes, such as bile acid, caused by intestinal atresia as in case 1, in which nonbloody amniotic fluid and bile-like fluid were aspirated from the stomach; there was linear echo finding around the umbilical cord, and chorioamniotic membrane separation indicated exposure to highly concentrated bile acid. However, the debris within the uterus in case 2 might indicate blood clot because of bloody amniotic fluid. Considering the ultrasonographic findings of UCU, spontaneous bleeding from the umbilical cord [12] and a hazy substance flowing near the fetal navel in the amniotic cavity [13] have been reported. In these cases, the UCU had ruptured already. Although our cases showed similar ultrasonographic findings, case 1 was of UCU with exposed umbilical cord artery and case 2 was of UCU with perforation of the umbilical cord artery based on histopathological findings.

In cases of fetal intestinal atresia, although bile acid concentration in the amniotic fluid has been found to be high, the relationship between bile acid concentration and UCU remains unclear [14, 15]. However, Nakamura et al. reported that UCU was associated with high bile acid concentration in the amniotic fluid [4]. They showed that UCU was detected in more than 90% of cases with bile acid concentrations ≥ 10 μmol/L in the amniotic fluid [4]. In intestinal atresia with polyhydramnios, we measure bile acid concentration when amnioreduction. If the bile acid concentration is ≥10 μmol/L, hospitalization continues, cardiotocogram is performed twice daily for 40 minutes, and ultrasonography is performed twice a week. In our cases, the amniotic bile acid concentration was ≥10 μmol/L. In addition, UCU perforation was reported after 26 weeks of gestation [2, 4, 10], which covers the time (30.0 ± 3.5 (25-7) weeks of gestation) of polyhydramnios development in fetal intestinal atresia [16]. Polyhydramnios might suggest that the umbilical cord is exposed to a high concentration of digestive enzymes, which may be considered as a risk factor for UCU.

Regarding common sites of UCU, there are various reports of UCU occurring on the fetal side [17], on the placental side [5], or as a line or spot along umbilical artery [6]. UCUs were confirmed in the placental side in case 1 and in the fetal and placental side in case 2. The location of UCU might be related to the degree of exposure to digestive enzymes and may depend on the location of the placenta, umbilical cord, and fetus.

We have carefully incorporated ultrasound findings after managing the present two cases; subsequently, we experienced four cases of fetal duodenal atresia. All cases had amnioreduction, and the bile acid concentration was ≥10 μmol/L except in one case. One case with high bile acid concentration had UCU grade 2, and the other cases had no UCU. None of these cases had chromosomal anomalies and any unusual findings including the ultrasonographic findings. Therefore, our ultrasonographic finding might reflect perforation and UCU grade 4. Although UCU grade 4 was associated with intrauterine fetal death [4], we could save the fetus, and it appeared that there was a time delay between confirming these findings and UCU perforation. However, the degree to which these findings represent the risk of UCU perforation could be the subject of a future study. In addition, although we detected these ultrasonographic finding of linear echo around the umbilical cord and chorioamniotic membrane separation, these are insufficient for an accurate diagnosis of UCU. Amnioreduction might cause these ultrasonographic findings because chorioamniotic membrane separation is induced by medical intervention, such as amniocentesis and fetal surgery [18]. Chorioamniotic membrane separation has been reportedly related to chromosome abnormalities [19]. Therefore, further data are needed to clarify the efficacy of these ultrasonographic findings, and it is necessary to comprehensively evaluate these ultrasonographic findings. Careful judgment considering gestational age is required for delivery because premature delivery increases neonatal morbidity.

In summary, in case of such ultrasonographic findings, especially with polyhydramnios and high amniotic bile acid concentration in cases of fetal intestinal atresia, the risk of UCU perforation should be considered.

Authors' Contributions

All authors have significantly contributed and agree with the content of the manuscript.

References

[1] W. A. Blanc and G. W. Allan, "Intrafunicular ulceration of persistent omphalomesenteric duct with intra- amniotic hemorrhage and fetal death," *American Journal of Obstetrics and Gynecology*, vol. 82, no. 6, pp. 1392–1396, 1961.

[2] T. Kimura, N. Usui, S. Kamata et al., "Umbilical cord ulcer associated with fetal jejunal atresia: report of 2 cases," *Fetal Diagnosis and Therapy*, vol. 18, no. 3, pp. 144–147, 2003.

[3] M. Yamanaka, M. Ohyama, M. Koresawa, M. Kawataki, I. Ohsaki, and Y. Tanaka, "Umbilical cord ulceration and intestinal atresia," *European Journal of Obstetrics & Gynecology and Reproductive Biology*, vol. 70, no. 2, pp. 209–212, 1996.

[4] N. Nakamura, K. Ozawa, S. Wada et al., "Umbilical cord ulcer and intrauterine death in fetal intestinal atresia," *Fetal Diagnosis and Therapy*, vol. 46, no. 5, pp. 313–318, 2019.

[5] G. Altshuler, M. Arizawa, and G. Molnar-Nadasdy, "Meconium-induced umbilical cord vascular necrosis and ulceration: a potential link between the placenta and poor pregnancy outcome," *Obstetrics and Gynecology*, vol. 79, 5, Part 1, pp. 760–766, 1992.

[6] M. Ohyama, Y. Itani, H. Ishikawa, and Y. Tanaka, "Is umbilical cord ulcer associated with congenital upper intestinal atresia so rare? Japanese case series and review of the literature," *Fetal Diagnosis and Therapy*, vol. 28, no. 4, pp. 236-237, 2010.

[7] M. Ichinose, T. Takemura, K. Andoh, and M. Sugimoto, "Pathological analysis of umbilical cord ulceration associated with fetal duodenal and jejunal atresia," *Placenta*, vol. 31, no. 11, pp. 1015–1018, 2010.

[8] R. W. Bendon, R. W. Tyson, V. J. Baldwin, K. A. Cashner, F. Mimouni, and M. Miodovnik, "Umbilical cord ulceration and intestinal atresia: a new association?," *American Journal of Obstetrics and Gynecology*, vol. 164, no. 2, pp. 582–586, 1991.

[9] A. Weissman and A. Drugan, "Sonographic findings of the umbilical cord: implications for the risk of fetal chromosomal anomalies," *Ultrasound in Obstetrics & Gynecology*, vol. 17, no. 6, pp. 536–541, 2001.

[10] M. Ohyama, Y. Itani, M. Yamanaka et al., "Umbilical cord ulcer: a serious in utero complication of intestinal atresia," *Placenta*, vol. 21, no. 4, pp. 432–435, 2000.

[11] R. Romero, C. Schaudinn, J. P. Kusanovic et al., "Detection of a microbial biofilm in intraamniotic infection," *American Journal of Obstetrics and Gynecology*, vol. 198, no. 1, pp. 135.e1–135.e5, 2008.

[12] A. Nijagal, L. Rand, R. Goldstein, L. Poder, and D. Miniati, "Intrauterine umbilical cord hemorrhage with associated jejunal atresia captured by real-time ultrasound," *American Journal of Obstetrics and Gynecology*, vol. 200, no. 3, pp. e5–e6, 2009.

[13] K. Miyachi, A. Kikuchi, M. Kitsunezaki et al., "Sudden fetal

hemorrhage from umbilical cord ulcer associated with congenital intestinal atresia," *The Journal of Obstetrics and Gynaecology Research*, vol. 33, no. 5, pp. 726–730, 2007.

[14] G. Délèze, D. Sidiropoulos, and G. Paumgartner, "Determination of bile acid concentration in human amniotic fluid for prenatal diagnosis of intestinal obstruction," *Pediatrics*, vol. 59, pp. 647–650, 1977.

[15] Y. Ohhama, "Pitfall of perinatal care for the fetus who suffered from upper gastrointestinal obstruction," *Japanease Journal of Pediatric Surgery*, vol. 33, p. 1073-1037, 2001.

[16] T. Fukami, M. Goto, S. Matsuoka et al., "The relation between causes and onset time of polyhydramnios," *Clinical and Experimental Obstetrics & Gynecology*, vol. 44, no. 1, pp. 113–115, 2017.

[17] S. S. Chan, A. P. Lau, K. F. To, T. Y. Leung, T. K. Lau, and T. N. Leung, "Umbilical cord ulceration causing foetal haemorrhage and stillbirth," *Hong Kong Medical Journal*, vol. 14, no. 2, pp. 148–151, 2008.

[18] M. Takano, M. Nakata, S. Murata, M. Sumie, and M. Morita, "Chorioamniotic membrane separation after fetoscopic laser photocoagulation," *Fetal Diagnosis and Therapy*, vol. 43, no. 1, pp. 40–44, 2018.

[19] O. Erol, M. Erol, and M. Karaca, "Complete chorioamniotic separation and persistence of a yolk sac associated with triploidy," *Journal of Obstetrics and Gynaecology Canada*, vol. 35, no. 10, pp. 914–916, 2013.

Novel Role of Dehydrated Human Amnion/Chorion Membrane in Healing of Denuded Ureter in Robot-Assisted Excision of Endometriosis

Osamah Hasan,[1] **Grant S. Johnson**,[2] **James J. Siegert**,[2] **Francisco Garcini**,[3] **and Thai T. Nguyen**[4]

[1]*Midwestern University Chicago College of Osteopathic Medicine, 555 31st St, Downers Grove, IL 60515, USA*
[2]*Franciscan Health, 20201 South Crawford Avenue, Olympia Fields, IL 60461, USA*
[3]*Silver Cross Hospital, 1890 Silver Cross Boulevard, Suite 210, New Lenox, IL 60451, USA*
[4]*Advanced Urology Associates, 1541 Riverboat Center Drive, Joliet, IL 60431, USA*

Correspondence should be addressed to Osamah Hasan; ohasan15@midwestern.edu

Academic Editor: Seung-Yup Ku

Ureteral injury is an uncommon but potentially morbid complication following any open or endoscopic pelvic procedure. Gynecologic surgeries alone make up 50 percent of nonurologic ureteral injuries leading to prolonged hospital stays, secondary interventions, and potential loss of renal function. The use of AmnioFix ® a processed dehydrated, immunologically privileged cellular amniotic membrane allograft has been well established in urologic and gynecologic procedures. These allografts contain human extracellular matrix components, growth factors, and cytokines that mediate inflammation and facilitate would healing. We report the first application of AmnioFix on a denuded ureter during a case of robotic-assisted excision of endometriosis. We include a literature review and discussion on the management outcomes of iatrogenic injury to the ureters.

1. Case Description

A 35-year-old Caucasian female with extensive history of pelvic surgery but without prior urological history underwent robotic-assisted laparoscopic excision of endometriosis by gynecological surgery team secondary to chronic pelvic pain with suspected endometriosis. On initial laparoscopic evaluation of pelvic contents, visible vermiculation of bilateral ureters was noted as well as suspected findings of endometriosis-like lesions covering the pelvic peritoneum. The pelvic peritoneum was excised with sparing of the urinary bladder. Careful ureterolysis was performed bilaterally, during which the distal left ureter was found to be partially denuded, spanning 2 cm in length (Figure 1). An intraoperative urologic consultation was requested, and denuded ureteral injury was confirmed by urology on laparoscopic evaluation. Given no evidence of ureteral laceration or obvious extravasation of urine from left ureter, no cystoscopy or contrast studies were performed. A 2 cm x 12 cm AmnioFix membrane was wrapped three times around the left ureter using laparoscopic robotic assistance (Figures 2 and 3). The procedure was completed without anesthesia complications and the patient was discharged on postoperative day one in stable condition.

The patient was seen by her gynecologist on postoperative day six after experiencing lower urinary tract symptoms and was subsequently started on PO antibiotic therapy. However, her symptoms did not improve, and she developed new left flank pain which brought her back to the hospital for further evaluation on postoperative day seven. She underwent noncontrast CT imaging of the abdomen and pelvis demonstrating moderate left hydroureteronephrosis to the level of the distal ureter. She underwent cystoscopy with left retrograde pyelogram demonstrating 1.5 cm distal ureteral stricture with moderate hydroureteronephrosis (Figure 4). Continued contrast injection showed a small amount of extravasation from the vicinity of the narrowed ureteral segment (Figure 5). However, the site of extravasation could

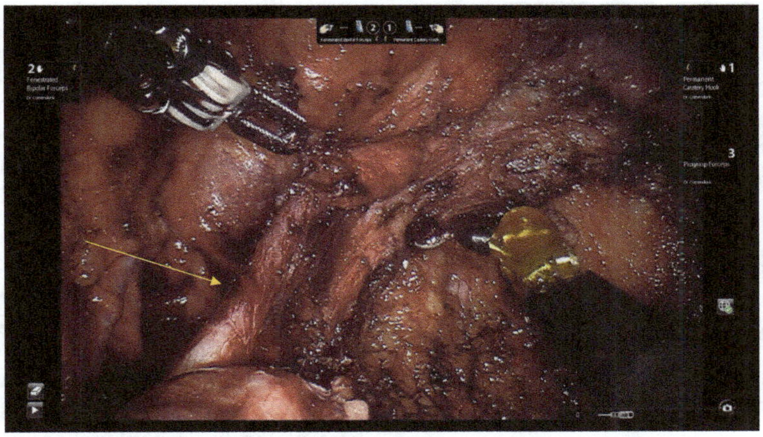

FIGURE 1: Intraoperative finding of left ureteral injury with subserosal hematoma (yellow arrow).

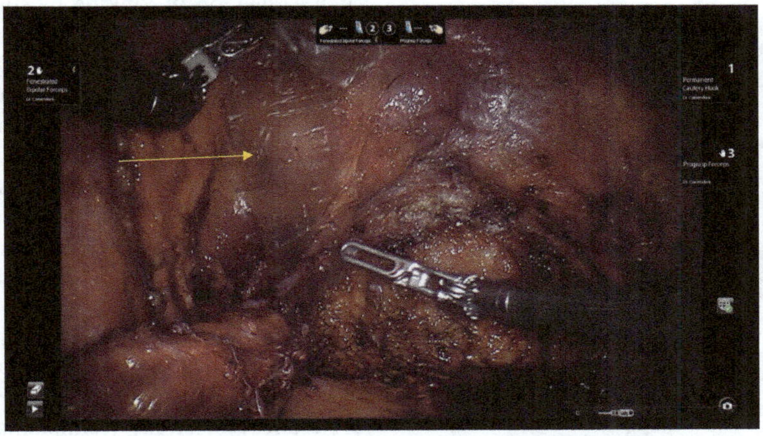

FIGURE 2: AmnioFix membrane wrapped around the site of left ureteral injury. AmnioFix membrane identified by yellow arrow.

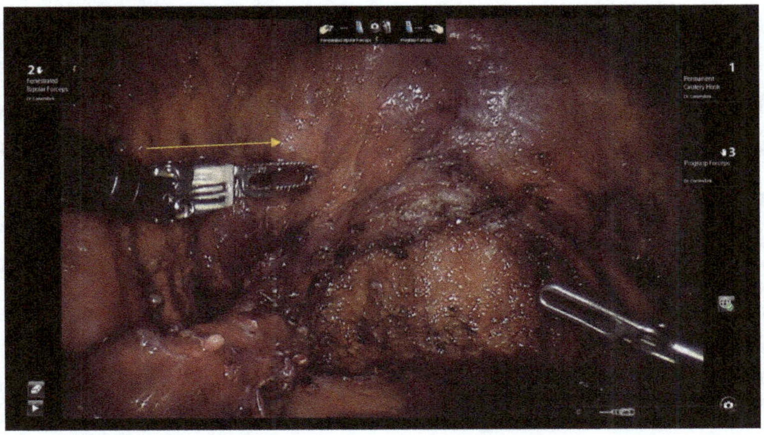

FIGURE 3: Left ureter following AmnioFix membrane placement. AmnioFix membrane identified by yellow arrow.

not be delineated. A guidewire was passed through the left ureter and into left renal pelvis without resistance and a left ureteral stent was placed. Her pain improved, and she was discharged home.

Patient was readmitted one month later secondary to nausea, vomiting, and lower urinary tract symptoms at which time she was found to have enterococcus urinary tract infection. Cross section imaging of the abdomen and pelvis was unremarkable without fluid collections. Left ureteral stent was noted to be in appropriate position. She was discharged home with antibiotic therapy with outpatient follow-up in two weeks at which time her ureteral stent was removed.

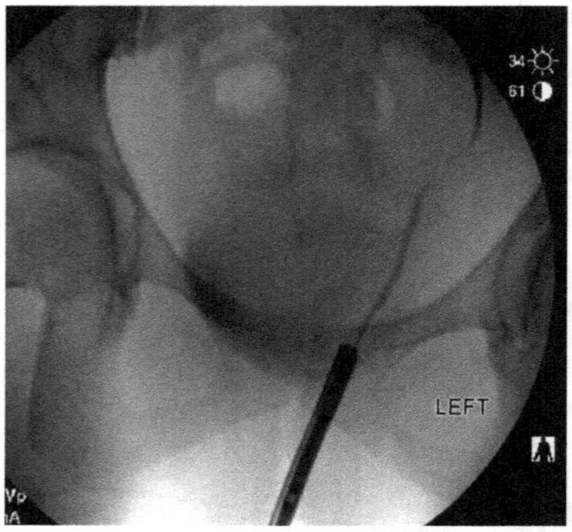

FIGURE 4: Left retrograde pyelogram shows 1.5 cm distal ureteral stricture with mild hydroureteronephrosis.

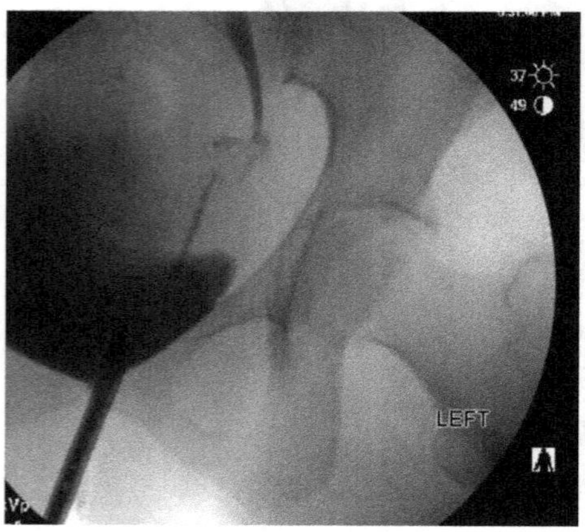

FIGURE 5: Mild extravasation noted on the left ureter with continued contrast injection.

The patient did not report renal colic or abdominal pain following ureteral stent removal. A Lasix renal scan was performed three months following ureteral injury which demonstrated normal perfusion and excretion by 20 minutes without signs of left ureteral obstruction (Figures 6 and 7). Differential renal function was 45% left kidney and 55% right kidney. Repeat CT urogram performed 4 months after injury demonstrated no obstructive uropathy or contrast extravasation. Patient was recommended repeat Lasix renal scan in 1 year. The patient reported no symptoms during the interim.

2. Discussion

2.1. Incidence, Etiology, and Management of Ureteral Injury. While iatrogenic ureteral injuries are an uncommon complication of any abdominal or pelvic surgery, the incidence ranges from 0.2% to 1% [1]. Gynecologic procedures alone make up 50% of the ureteral injuries [1]. Lower anterior resection of the colon and abdominal perineal resection are responsible for 9% of ureteral injuries [2]. Assessment of an accurate incidence rate is likely hampered by unrecognized or unreported ureteric injuries [3]. Injury often occurs secondary to the close proximity of the ureter to the peritoneum and can occur in both complex and straightforward intra-abdominal and retroperitoneal surgery. Certain factors increase the risk of ureteral injury: endometriosis/endometriolysis, adhesions/adhesiolysis, distorted pelvic anatomy, coexistent bladder injury, lymphadenectomy, and vesicourethral anastomosis [3, 4].

The ureter is susceptible to injury along its entire course. However, the distal third of the ureter, from the pelvic brim to the bladder, is most frequently injured. Studies demonstrate that the most common site of injury is lateral to the uterine vessels [5]. Other common sites include the base of the infundibulopelvic ligament, at the level of the uterosacral ligament, and at the uterovesical junction [1]. Ureteric trauma can be injured from various mechanisms such as ligation or kinking by suture, crushing by a clamp, partial or complete transection, diathermy, or ischemia from devascularization. Signs and symptoms of ureteral injury usually include flank pain, hematuria, fever, retroperitoneal urinoma, and postoperative anuria [1].

In cases of suspected ureteral injury, intravenous pyelogram or contrast CT scan can assess for ureteric integrity and drainage. Intraoperative methods include infusion of indigo carmine with IV furosemide to assess for urinary extravasation [6]. Partial ureteral lacerations (i.e., ureteric defect <2.5 cm) are commonly managed by endoscopic placement of the stent for 2-6 weeks [7]. While approximately 50% of patients with lacerations showed no signs of obstruction at follow-up after stenting, the other half ultimately required ureteroneocystostomy (reimplantation) [7]. In our patient, a cystoscopy with retrograde pyelogram was performed to identify the anatomic site of obstruction. She was noted to have urinary extravasation and subsequently underwent ureteral stent placement.

2.2. Uses of AmnioFix in Surgical Applications. AmnioFix is composed of dehydrated human amnion/chorion membrane (dHACM), which is an immunoprivileged allograft containing an array of cytokines and growth factors that regulate processes involved in inflammation and wound healing. The dHACM allograft comes in multiple configurations and sizes to allow for its heterogenous use in internal and external applications. Various applications of AmnioFix have been well-described in literature. Subach et al. applied dHACM in patients undergoing lumbar fusion with posterior instrumentation effectively preventing epidural fibrosis and facilitating dissection in revision spinal surgery [8]. Mrugala et al. reported accelerated would healing after application of dHACM in five case reports in patients with chronic, nonhealing ulcers [9]. Dulemba et al. observed no adhesion formation in 14 of 15 cases of women undergoing robotic laparoscopy [10]. Patel et al. observed accelerated return of continence and potency in patients following nerve-sparing robot-assisted radical prostatectomy after the application of dHACM on the prostatic neurovascular bundle [11]. Ortega et al. in a poster presentation from a retrospective multicenter study showed dHACM significantly reduced the number

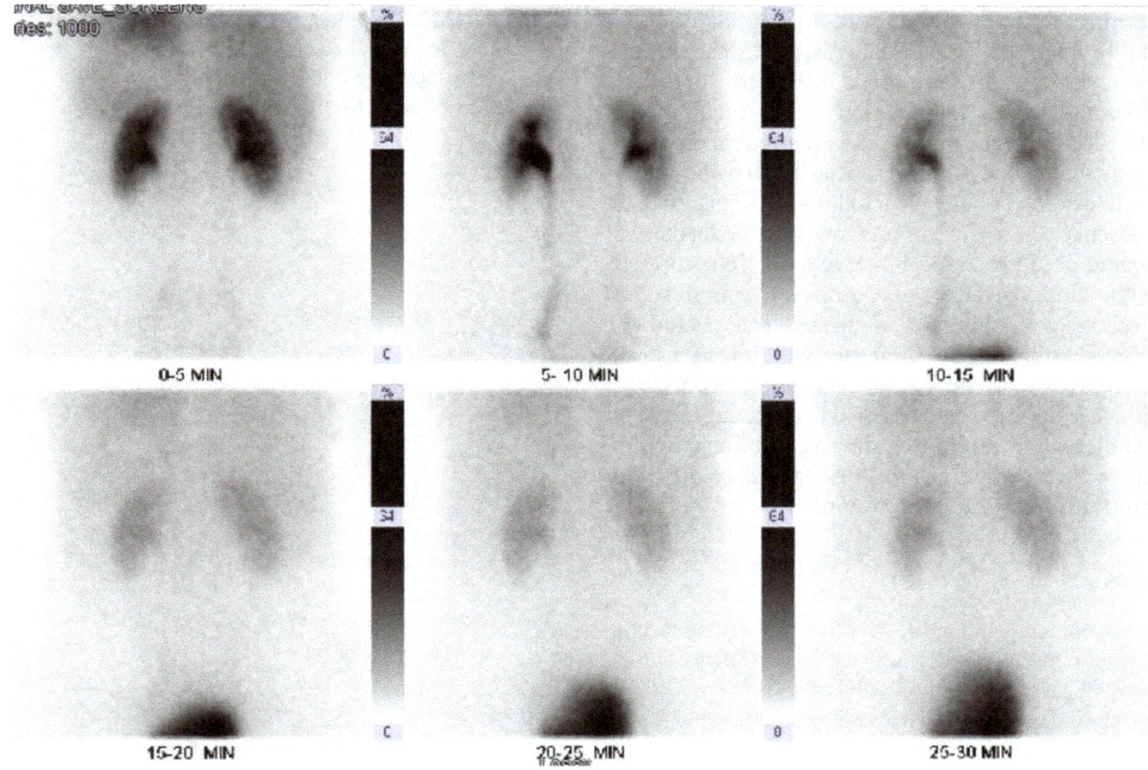

FIGURE 6: Renal scan: initial findings show mild asymmetrical activity in the left ureter compared to the right. However, washout at 20 min is symmetrical bilaterally without any signs of obstruction.

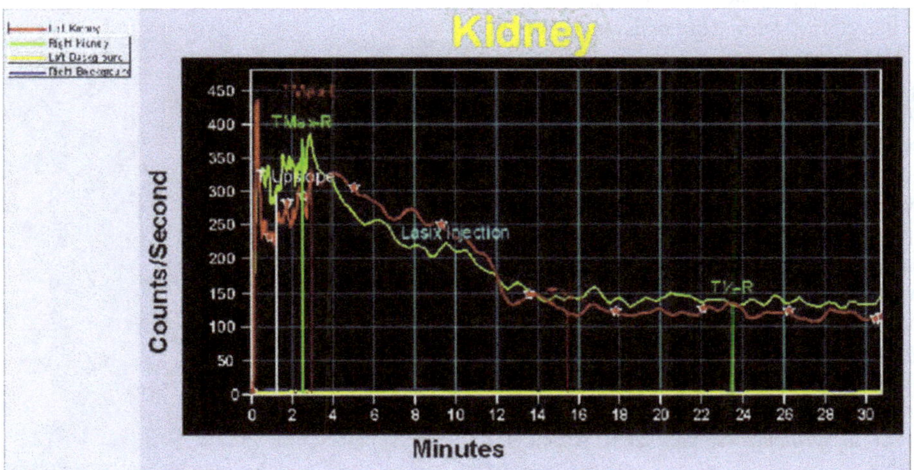

FIGURE 7: Renogram findings identical for left (red) and right (green) kidney: symmetrical downward slope consistent with no signs of obstruction bilaterally.

of anastomotic leaks following colon resection [12]. These studies applied the dHACM in a unique format. Similarly, we employed AmnioFix in a novel manner with the express purpose of accelerating ureteric healing after ureteral denudement. Initial follow-up indicates that our patient has not required repeat intervention following ureteral stent removal and had a normal renal Lasix scan. The clinical goal was to apply AmnioFix in the hopes that the inherent growth factors would assist in healing, decrease ureteral stricture formation, and therefore avoid additional future surgical intervention such as ureteral reimplantation with neocystotomy.

3. Conclusion

Surgeons should be able to identify ureteral injury as soon as possible to improve surgical outcomes. The possibility of ureteric injury should be immediately considered if patients do not make satisfactory postoperative recovery or present with concerning signs or symptoms. Radiographic inquiries are essential to form the basis of diagnosis. This case report proposes a novel role for AmnioFix in ureteric injury in addition to standardized intervention as indicated. Given our patient's delayed injury and need for ureteral stenting, there is a possibility that AmnioFix exacerbated the injury or prolonged healing. Long term follow-up is planned to assess the absence or presence of ureteral stricture formation and subsequent need for surgical intervention. To accurately determine the clinical efficacy and utility of AmnioFix for ureteric healing, a randomized controlled trial would be required. Factors that might limit the widespread use of AmnioFix are high cost and lack of randomized controlled studies. This case hopes to assist surgeons in management of iatrogenic ureteral injuries by providing an additional option that could provide expedited healing, decrease morbidity, and ideally avoid future surgical intervention.

References

[1] S. Jha, A. Coomarasamy, and K. K. Chan, "Ureteric injury in obstetric and gynaecological surgery," *The Obstetrician & Gynaecologist*, vol. 6, no. 4, pp. 203–208, 2004.

[2] M. A. ST Lezin and M. L. Stoller, "Surgical ureteral injuries," *Urology*, vol. 38, no. 6, pp. 497–506, 1991.

[3] J. W. Daly and K. A. Higgins, "Injury to the ureter during gynecologic surgical procedures," *Surgery, Gynecology, and Obstetrics*, vol. 167, pp. 19–22, 1988.

[4] J. K. Jhaveri, F. J. Penna, M. Diaz-Insua, W. Jeong, M. Menon, and J. O. Peabody, "Ureteral injuries sustained during robot-assisted radical prostatectomy," *Journal of Endourology*, vol. 28, no. 3, pp. 318–324, 2014.

[5] J. H. Ridely, "Gynecologic Surgery: Errors, Safeguards, Salvage," p. 110, Lipincott Williams & Wilkins, Philadelphia, 1981.

[6] J. K. Jhaveri, F. J. Penna, M. Diaz-Insua et al., "Ureteral injuries sustained during robot-assisted radical prostatectomy," *Journal of Endourology*, vol. 28, no. 3, pp. 318–324, 2014.

[7] V. Minas, N. Gul, T. Aust, M. Doyle, and D. Rowlands, "Urinary tract injuries in laparoscopic gynaecological surgery; prevention, recognition and management," *The Obstetrician & Gynaecologist*, vol. 16, no. 1, pp. 19–28, 2014.

[8] B. R. Subach and A. G. Copay, "The use of a dehydrated amnion/chorion membrane allograft in patients who subsequently undergo reexploration after posterior lumbar instrumentation," *Advances in Orthopedics*, vol. 2015, Article ID 501202, 6 pages, 2015.

[9] A. Mrugala, A. Sui, M. Plummer et al., "Amniotic membrane is a potential regenerative option for chronic non-healing wounds: A report of five cases receiving dehydrated human amnion/chorion membrane allograft," *International Wound Journal*, vol. 13, no. 4, pp. 485–492, 2015.

[10] J. Dulemba, P. Mirzakhani, and N. B. Istwan, "Evaluation of dehydrated human amnion/chorion membrane as an adhesion barrier in women undergoing robotic laparoscopy," *Gynecology & Obstetrics*, 2016.

[11] V. R. Patel, S. Samavedi, A. S. Bates et al., "Dehydrated human amnion/chorion membrane allograft nerve wrap around the prostatic neurovascular bundle accelerates early return to continence and potency following robot-assisted radical prostatectomy: Propensity score-matched analysis," *European Urology*, vol. 67, no. 6, pp. 33–35, 2015.

[12] F. R. Ortega, J. Cohen, D. Choat, and E. Minnard, "Dehydrated human amnion chorion membrane in colorectal anastomoses: A retrospective multi-center study," *Journal of the American College of Surgeons*, vol. 225, no. 4, p. e66, 2017.

9

An Unusual Presentation of COVID-19 Associated Multisystem Inflammatory Syndrome in Adults (MIS-A) in a Pregnant Woman

Mohamed Rishard,[1,2] Suren Perera,[2] Kushan Jayasinghe,[2] Amila Rubasinghe,[2] Sanjaya Athapaththu,[2] Malindu Edirisinghe,[2] Prabhodana Ranaweera,[1,2] Tushani Ranawaka,[1] Athula Kaluarachchi,[1,2] Priyankara Jayawardana,[2] and Zacky Haniffa[2]

[1]*Department of Obstetrics and Gynecology, Faculty of Medicine, University of Colombo 25, Kynsey Road, Colombo 08, Sri Lanka*
[2]*De Soysa Hospital for Women Kynsey Road, Colombo 08, Sri Lanka*

Correspondence should be addressed to Mohamed Rishard; rishi7875@yahoo.com

Academic Editor: Manvinder Singh

Based on available literature, pregnant women are at an increased risk of severe illness from severe acute respiratory syndrome coronavirus 2 (SARS-CoV-2) infection, compared to nonpregnant women. Consequences of coronavirus disease 2019 (COVID-19) in pregnancy have many implications in women's lives other than unfavorable obstetric outcomes. In addition to managing acute respiratory illness and symptoms, caregivers should be equipped to detect and manage the short-term, intermediate, and long-term consequences of SARS-CoV-2 infection as well. Many pregnant women can remain asymptomatic and continue their pregnancy without being diagnosed. Pregnancy outcomes and consequences of SARS-CoV-2 infected yet asymptomatic mothers have not been very well explained. Reports of a new multisystem inflammatory syndrome in children (MIS-C) and multisystem inflammatory syndrome in adults (MIS-A) following COVID-19 have been described. However, MIS-A in pregnancy is an extremely rare presentation that can cause a huge diagnostic dilemma to caregivers. We describe the successful management of a pregnant woman with MIS-A following SARS-CoV-2 infection.

1. Introduction

The world's healthcare paradigms have been changed within a short period of time, by the new disease coronavirus disease 2019 (COVID-19) as a result of the novel severe acute respiratory syndrome coronavirus 2 (SARS-CoV-2) viral infection, which has infected millions of people all over the world and caused 2.9 million deaths by April 2021 [1].

Pregnancy and manifestations of COVID-19 are still not well understood. This has led to a huge dilemma among the caregivers. Understanding the spectrum of its manifestations is mainly based on case reports, and new information is added to existing literature on this area.

At the beginning, it was thought that pregnant women were not at higher risk than nonpregnant women [2]. However, in a multinational cohort study, COVID-19 in pregnancy was associated with significant increase in severe maternal morbidity and mortality. It has been shown that pregnant women with COVID-19 are at 22 times increased risk of maternal death [3].

Although many recover from acute infection, some patients experience the consequences requiring further follow-up and specialized care. These post-COVID-19 conditions may present with many overlapping symptoms, and correct diagnosis may become a huge challenge. Moreover, they may present with or without any evidence of overt SARS-CoV-2 infection. Multisystem inflammatory syndrome in children (MIS-C) and multisystem inflammatory syndrome in adults (MIS-A) following COVID-19 have been described [4]. MIS-A is defined by extrapulmonary organ dysfunction and absence of respiratory illness [4]. Although outcomes of MIS-A in pregnant women following pregnancy are not well known, this condition leads to a critical condition requiring multidisciplinary team involvement.

We present an unusual presentation of MIS-A following SARS-CoV-2 infection in pregnancy.

2. Case Presentation

A 28-year-old pregnant mother in her second pregnancy was transferred at 30 + 6 weeks of gestational age with a history of acute onset high grade fever with chills and difficulty in breathing for a period of two days. Her antenatal period had been uneventful up until then. She had delivered by cesarean section due to pregnancy induced hypertension in the first pregnancy.

On examination, she was febrile; her pulse rate was 140 beats per minute and had a respiratory rate of 40 cycles per minute. Lung bases were clear.

Rapid antigen test for SARS-CoV-2 showed a negative result, and three consecutive samples for SARS-CoV-2 reverse transcriptase polymerase chain reaction (SARS-CoV-2 RT-PCR) resulted inconclusive. She was managed in the high dependency unit under multidisciplinary care. Since she was breathless, high flow oxygen was given along with other supportive measures. From fourth to eighth day of illness, she became increasingly tachycardic and tachypneic with high fever, left-sided cervical lymphadenopathy, and rising inflammatory markers. White blood cell count was 13×10^9/L; platelet count was 120×10^9/L. Blood picture revealed an absolute lymphocytosis. Her blood and urine cultures showed no significant growth. 2D echocardiogram showed a grade two diastolic dysfunction with an ejection fraction of 50% with a mild pericardial effusion and elevated troponin I (0.401 ng/L). Her chest X-ray showed a mild pleural effusion. She was not in a position to mobilize for computed tomography scan of the chest. She was commenced on intravenous Ceftriaxone and Oseltamivir despite sterile blood culture reports. SARS CoV-2 specific total antibody including IgG became positive indicating a previous exposure. Her initial arterial blood gas revealed a compensated respiratory alkalosis. She was able to maintain a saturation of 95% on room air. Her liver and renal functions remained normal throughout.

Despite repeated blood, urine, and sputum cultures being sterile, her procalcitonin levels were elevated 2.03 ng/mL (normal < 0.5), CRP was 321, and ESR was 120 mm in the 1st hour. Cardiologist reconfirmed cardiac dysfunction with an ejection fraction of 50%, with mild pericardial effusion, elevated troponin I (0.045 ng/mL), and elevated BNP levels (335 pg/mL). With the evidence of myocardial injury, digoxine, bisoprolol, and asprin were added. Her lower limb compression Doppler was normal, and 2D echo was negative for right heart strain; hence, computed tomography pulmonary angiogram (CTPA) was not carried out considering the risks and clinical status. She was investigated for dengue, influenza, HIV, typhoid, legionella, mycoplasma, leptospirosis, connective tissue disorders, and excluded.

However, she was commenced on therapeutic dose of low molecular weight heparin. By day 12 of illness, she improved remarkably. She was mobilized and discharged. One week later, she presented with gradual onset left-sided lower motor type facial nerve palsy which subsided with a course of steroids and physiotherapy.

During the course of her management, it became evident that this was a novel clinical presentation of MIS-A. On detail inquiry, she recalled a possible COVID-19 exposure 4 weeks ago, when she came in contact with a few people who had fever; however, their COVID-19 status was unconfirmed.

At 37 weeks of gestation, she developed severe pregnancy induced hypertension and delivered a baby boy weighing 2.46 kg by a cesarean section.

3. Discussion

It is not yet clear how and why adults develop MIS-A following SARS-CoV-2 infection. However, it is believed to be due to SARS-CoV-2-induced hyperinflammatory reaction [5]. Extrapulmonary dysfunction in COVID-19 is believed to occur as a result of damage to the endothelium and thromboinflammation and disruption to the regulatory mechanisms of immune responses and renin angiotensin-aldosterone system [6] Table 1.

The temporal relationship between SARS-CoV-2 infection and MIS-A is not clear. However, a case series states that 2-5 weeks following typical COVID-19 symptoms and symptoms of MIS-A could occur [7]. Our patient could recall a potential exposure 4 weeks prior; this was tallying with her serological markers too. A repeatedly inconclusive result on multiple SARS-CoV-2 RT-PCR samples may be obtained due to a virological cause such as when either one of the two targets but not both are above the threshold for positivity or when there is some reactivity in the assay which may not suffice to yield a positive result or nonspecific binding of PCR primer during the late phases of PCR cycles [8]. Thus, a clinical correlation of the symptoms, history of exposure, and serological evidence of antibodies of this unvaccinated lady is likely to depict a past infection of COVID-19.

Features to diagnose MIS-A include "a severe illness requiring hospitalization in a person aged ≥21 years; a positive test result for current or previous SARS-CoV-2 infection (nucleic acid, antigen, or antibody) during admission or in the previous 12 weeks, severe dysfunction of one or more extra pulmonary organ systems (e.g., hypotension or shock, cardiac dysfunction, arterial or venous thrombosis or thromboembolism, or acute liver injury); laboratory evidence of severe inflammation (e.g., elevated CRP, ferritin, D-dimer, or interleukin-6); and absence of severe respiratory illness (to exclude patients in which inflammation and organ dysfunction might be attributable simply to tissue hypoxia)" [7]. Our patient presented with acute onset shortness of breath with evidence of myocarditis and laboratory evidence of severe inflammation and had met all diagnostic criteria of MIS-A.

At the time of initial presentation, her clinical presentation was complex. Initially, her symptoms mimicked the clinical picture of acute pneumonia or pulmonary embolism. Then, with the evidence of cardiac injury and elevated inflammatory markers, nonsignificant changes in

Table 1: Summary of investigations.

	Day 0	Day 3	Day 7	Reference ranges
Hemoglobin (g/dL)	11.4	9.3	9.2	11.0–16.0
Platelets ($10^3/\mu L$)	120	187	377	150-450
White blood cells ($10^3/\mu L$)	13.6	18	19	4-10
C reactive protein (mg/dL)	321	291	43.4	<6
Erythrocyte sedimentation rate (ESR) 1st Hr in mm	98	120		
Procalcitonin (ng/mL)		2.03		<0.5
Serum ferritin (ng/mL)		171.5		12-190
High sensitive D-dimers (ng/mL)		1249		<250
High sensitive troponin I (ng/mL)	0.401	0.045		<0.015
Brain natriuretic peptide (BNP) (pg/mL)		335		<28
Elevated liver enzymes	No	No		
Serum creatinine (micromol/L)	56	62	49	49-95
ECG	Sinus tachycardia	Sinus tachycardia	Sinus rhythm	
2D echo	Grade two diastolic dysfunction with an ejection fraction of 50% with a mild pericardial effusion, possible myocarditis	EF 50%, thin rim of effusion	Good biventricular function, no trans thoracic echo evidence of pulmonary embolism Ejection fraction 55-60%	
Chest X-ray	Mild left pleural effusion	Improved		

chest X-ray, the working diagnosis was changed in the line of MIS-A. This is not an unusual situation as they present with a heterogeneous clinical picture. Similarly, many factors can lead to a delayed diagnosis in adults. These include less severe cardiac involvement, negative diagnostic testing at the time of the presentation, limited diagnostic role for antibody testing, diagnostic difficulty with preexisting cardiac disease, COVID-19-related acute myocardial injury having a higher incidence, and multiple causes.

According to data available, many had multiple negative SARS-CoV-2 RT-PCR during cardiac presentations (mean 4.6), and some had a recent history of COVID-19 and recovery afterwards [9]. In one case series, out of 11 cases of MIS-A patients, 10 patients showed positive SARS-CoV-2 RT-PCR test results; seven of them had positive antibodies during the same time [7].

Although serological testing is an option in patients with negative SARS-CoV-2 RT-PCR tests, kinetics of serological markers is not well known. However, there is evidence to show that supplementing with serological tests when there is a negative or unequivocal test could help in the management of patients as well managing contacts [10]. Tests to quantify serum specific antibodies against SARS-CoV-2 are not freely available in all settings. This could be a big challenge in settings where prevalence of COVID-19 is high. This could mean that caregivers should empirically commence treatment in such cases without depending on the antibody status if there is a strong suspicion of multisystem involvement even without evidence of acute SARS-CoV-2 infection. In our patient, high values of cardiac markers and 2D echocardiogram findings were adequately favoring the diagnosis of myocardial injury.

Another useful distinguishing feature is thrombocytopenia which occur as a result of mediators being secreted in the process of eradication of the virus (mainly to stimulate CD8+ cells to kill viral infected cells), which would inadvertently suppress bone marrow function and activate platelets [11]. However, our patient's complete blood count did not show a significant drop in the platelet count.

Many hospitalized COVID-19 patients suffer from myocardial injury. It is believed that the SARS-CoV-2 virus can directly affect the heart. Injury which indirectly occur due to an inflammatory cascade during SARS-CoV-2 infection can also cause cardiac damage. The extent depends on the viral load, the capacity of the host to mount an immune response, and presence of other comorbidities [12]. However, myocardial injury in pregnancy following COVID-19 has been not being well reported. Various physiological changes that occur in pregnancy may make the women more vulnerable to cardiac injury [13]. One report suggests that myocardial injury and left ventricular dysfunction in pregnant women pose a significant risk of maternal death up to 13.3% due to malignant arrhythmias [14]. When positive troponin concentrations are found, it indicates severe illness and poor outcomes in patients with COVID-19. These patients are five times more likely to need ventilation and suffer arrhythmias [15]. Hence, caregivers treating pregnant women with COVID-19 must screen for possible myocardial injury and follow them up in order to avoid serious complications. This would require a huge workforce in low resource settings and may require careful evaluation and selection criterion before requesting cardiac assessment for COVID-19 affected pregnant women. Troponin elevation and high BNP levels in COVID-19 are associated with adverse outcomes and mortality. Values of these two markers should play a key role when managing pregnant women with COVID-19.

Given the associated risks of venous thromboembolism in pregnancy, we commenced therapeutic dose of low molecular heparin. Chau et al. in their case series had commenced therapeutic dose of low molecular heparin in 7 cases [16]. Morris et al. reported that in their case series almost all adults had cardiac dysfunction as a feature and most commonly treated with intravenous immunoglobulin, corticosteroids, and inotropes or vasopressors [7].

Multisystem inflammatory syndrome in adults and in pregnant women has improved with immunoglobulin therapy and corticosteroids [17]. In one case series, rapid and profound improvement in cardiac function occurred soon after initiation of supportive, antimicrobial, or immunomodulatory therapy [10]. In our case, we commenced intravenous broad-spectrum antibiotic and antiviral treatment despite sterile cultures. This was empirical rather than evidence based. However, we believe that we could have commenced steroids as well. Our suspicion about ongoing septic focus prevented us from starting steroids in our patient.

There are reports of facial nerve palsy around the time of SARS-CoV-2 infection and even one month after diagnosis of SARS-CoV-2 infection. This is believed to occur due to an autoimmune pathogenesis [18].

Our patient presented with a complex clinical picture of sepsis, cardiac injury, and Bell's palsy following possible asymptomatic COVID-19, and she met all the diagnostic criteria for MIS-A. All this multifaceted pathophysiology and multiorgan involvement require multidisciplinary team involvement.

There are reports that shows, women who tend to endure COVID-19 symptoms are specially those who are living with social deprivation and those with preexisting comorbidities [19]. This indicates that pregnant women should be educated regarding symptoms of COVID-19, and adequate supportive measures should be provided when they are found to be positive for SARS-CoV-2. This should include psychological support and family support.

Although our patient's clinical condition required an intensive care unit, the team was left with the choice of managing her in the high dependency unit setting due to unavailability of an ICU bed. This situation may prevail or even worsen in the future. She developed severe pregnancy induced hypertension and had to undergo caesarean section. This can be very well attributed to already known pregnancy outcomes of COVID-19.

Clinical vigilance, prompt diagnosis using available resources, and multidisciplinary team involvement are key factors in managing COVID-19-related complications in low resource settings. Caregivers in the primary care services including general practitioners should expect more cases with similar clinical pictures in future. A uniform centralized reporting system is needed to collect data regarding various COVID-19-related conditions to enlighten the caregivers with correct information.

4. Conclusion

Clinicians should have a high level of clinical suspicion of MIS-A in any patient presenting with unusual multisystem involvement. Features of myocarditis, fever, and elevated inflammatory markers should prompt the caregivers to correlate with COVID-19 specific serology in the absence of positive SARS-CoV-2 RT-PCR results or obvious history of infection.

High inflammatory markers and fever should not delay the commencement of steroids or immunotherapy. Although antigen, RT-PCR, or serology is mandatory for diagnosis of MIS-A, in the context of a resource limited setup, it may be prudent to start empirical treatment for cases with strong clinical suspicion, preventing undue delays in diagnosis and prompt treatment with steroids and immunoglobulins.

BNP and troponin levels will yield valuable information in pregnant women with cardiac involvement.

Clinicians also should be aware to take in to consideration the physiological changes in pregnancy when interpreting COVID-19-related investigations and clinical parameters that are better described for the nonpregnant population.

Distinguishing the overlapping symptoms of this new disease entity from other medical conditions affecting gravid women can be very challenging and may lead to a diagnostic dilemma. Hence, a good knowledge of various presentations of COVID-19, careful evaluation of the clinical picture, understanding the physiological changes of pregnancy, and their influences on various investigations are vital in managing COVID-19-related complications.

Consent

Informed written consent has been obtained from the patient to publish case details.

References

[1] E. Dong, H. Du, and L. Gardner, "An interactive web-based dashboard to track COVID-19 in real time," *The Lancet Infectious Diseases*, vol. 20, no. 5, pp. 533-534, 2020.

[2] E. H. Adhikari, W. Moreno, A. C. Zofkie et al., "Pregnancy outcomes among women with and without severe acute respiratory syndrome coronavirus 2 infection," *JAMA Network Open*, vol. 3, no. 11, article e2029256-e, 2020.

[3] J. Villar, S. Ariff, R. B. Gunier et al., "Maternal and neonatal morbidity and mortality among pregnant women with and without COVID-19 Infection," *JAMA Pediatrics*, vol. 175, no. 8, pp. 817–826, 2021.

[4] "Multisystem inflammatory syndrome in adults (MIS-A) case definition information for healthcare providers," 2021, https://www.cdc.gov/mis/mis-a/hcp.html.

[5] J. H. Rubens, N. P. Akindele, M. M. Tschudy, and A. C. Sick-Samuels, "Acute COVID-19 and multisystem inflammatory syndrome in children," *BMJ*, vol. 372, article n385, 2021.

[6] A. Gupta, M. V. Madhavan, K. Sehgal et al., "Extrapulmonary

manifestations of COVID-19," *Nature Medicine*, vol. 26, no. 7, pp. 1017–1032, 2020.

[7] S. B. Morris, N. G. Schwartz, P. Patel et al., "Case series of multisystem inflammatory syndrome in adults associated with SARS-CoV-2 infection - United Kingdom and United States, March-August 2020," *MMWR. Morbidity and Mortality Weekly Report*, vol. 69, no. 40, pp. 1450–1456, 2020.

[8] S. Bhattacharya, A. Vidyadharan, and V. Joy, "Inconclusive SARS-COV-2 reverse transcription-polymerase chain reaction test reports: interpretation, clinical and infection control implications," *Journal of The Academy of Clinical Microbiologists*, vol. 22, no. 1, pp. 59–61, 2020.

[9] R. Bajaj, H. C. Sinclair, K. Patel et al., "Delayed-onset myocarditis following COVID-19," *The Lancet Respiratory Medicine*, vol. 9, no. 4, pp. e32–e34, 2021.

[10] Q.-X. Long, B.-Z. Liu, H.-J. Deng et al., "Antibody responses to SARS-CoV-2 in patients with COVID-19," *Nature Medicine*, vol. 26, no. 6, pp. 845–848, 2020.

[11] W. S. Yeo and Q. X. Ng, "Distinguishing between typical Kawasaki disease and multisystem inflammatory syndrome in children (MIS-C) associated with SARS-CoV-2," *Medical Hypotheses*, vol. 144, article 110263, 2020.

[12] G. Giustino, S. P. Pinney, A. Lala et al., "Coronavirus and Cardiovascular Disease, Myocardial Injury, and Arrhythmia:," *Journal of the American College of Cardiology*, vol. 76, no. 17, pp. 2011–2023, 2020.

[13] S. Ellington, P. Strid, V. T. Tong et al., "Characteristics of women of reproductive age with laboratory-confirmed SARS-CoV-2 infection by pregnancy status - United States, January 22-June 7, 2020," *MMWR. Morbidity and Mortality Weekly Report*, vol. 69, no. 25, pp. 769–775, 2020.

[14] B. R. Mercedes, A. Serwat, L. Naffaa et al., "New-onset myocardial injury in pregnant patients with coronavirus disease 2019: a case series of 15 patients," *American Journal of Obstetrics and Gynecology*, vol. 224, no. 4, p. 387.e1-.e9, 2021.

[15] M. Bansal, "Cardiovascular disease and COVID-19," *Diabetes & Metabolic Syndrome: Clinical Research & Reviews*, vol. 14, no. 3, pp. 247–250, 2020.

[16] V. Q. Chau, G. Giustino, K. Mahmood et al., "Cardiogenic shock and hyperinflammatory syndrome in young males with COVID-19," *Circulation: Heart Failure*, vol. 13, no. 10, article e007485, 2020.

[17] M. Gulersen, C. Staszewski, E. Grayver et al., "Coronavirus disease 2019 (COVID-19)-related multisystem inflammatory syndrome in a pregnant woman," *Obstetrics and Gynecology*, vol. 137, no. 3, pp. 418–422, 2021.

[18] E. H. Dahl, K. A. Mosevoll, D. Cramariuc, C. A. Vedeler, and B. Blomberg, "COVID-19 myocarditis and postinfection Bell's palsy," *BMJ Case Reports*, vol. 14, no. 1, article e240095, 2021.

[19] S. E. Daugherty, Y. Guo, K. Heath et al., "Risk of clinical sequelae after the acute phase of SARS-CoV-2 infection: retrospective cohort study," *BMJ*, vol. 373, article n1098, 2021.

10

Case Report of a Rare Nonpuerperal Uterine Inversion Managed with Uterosacral Ligament Hysteropexy

Ali Azadi,[1,2] **Alexandra Wolfe**,[3] **and Greg J. Marchand**[4]

[1]*University of Arizona, College of Medicine, 475 N 5th St, Phoenix, AZ 85004, USA*
[2]*Star Urogynecology, 14155 N 83rd Ave, Suite 138, Peoria, AZ 85381, USA*
[3]*OMS-IV Midwestern University, 19555 N 59th Ave, Glendale, AZ 85308, USA*
[4]*The Marchand Institute for Minimally Invasive Surgery, 10238 E Hampton Ave, Suite 212, Mesa, AZ 85209, USA*

Correspondence should be addressed to Alexandra Wolfe; awolfe11@midwestern.edu

Academic Editor: John P. Geisler

Nonpuerperal uterine inversions are rare. Typically occurring in older women, they are most commonly due to transcervical mass expulsion. Diagnosis is often difficult because of vague symptomatology, presentation, and unknown course of the pathology. Surgical correction is often necessary in the presence of active bleeding or prolapse severity causing urinary retention. This case of nonpuerperal inversion presented to the emergency department with vaginal bleeding and mass protrusion. The examination was consistent with POPQ stage IV prolapse and uterine inversion secondary to cervical expulsion of multiple uterine fibroids. Because of full cervical dilation and concerns of ureteral injury with an extirpative procedure, vaginal myomectomy was performed with concomitant robotic uterosacral ligament hysteropexy. The operative procedure and postoperative course were uncomplicated, and discharge occurred on post-op day 1. She remained asymptomatic at the 6-month follow-up encounter. Though uterine preservation has been performed in cases of uterine inversion to maintain fertility, there are no reported cases of concomitant hysteropexy being completed for correction of POPQ stage IV prolapse simultaneously encountered. Additionally, the novel robotic approach has not been documented. This case illustrates the short-term success of robotic uterosacral hysteropexy as an additional option of care with potentially less morbidity when compared to hysterectomy for advanced stage uterine prolapse with nonpuerperal uterine inversion.

1. Introduction

While puerperal uterine inversions are an uncommon gynecologic event, nonpuerperal uterine inversions are extremely rare, reported 229 times between 1947 and 2017 [1]. Nonpuerperal inversions are caused by benign corpus uterine tumors 57.2% of the time, typically leiomyomas as demonstrated in this case. Their etiology is often multifactorial, due to rapid growth of the tumor, fundal location, thinning of the fundal wall, cervical dilation, and subsequent uterine expulsion [1]. Manual traction and increased intra-abdominal pressure can also contribute [2]. Women most often present with vaginal discharge, irregular uterine bleeding, pelvic discomfort, and anemia [3]. Depending on the acuity of the inversion, manual repositioning alone is possible. However, in chronic inversions, and those involving tumor growth, surgical intervention is often necessary [4]. Considering the average age of women who experience nonpuerperal inversion is above 45 years old, typically women have completed child bearing [5]. In 86.5% of patients, hysterectomy is performed for uterine inversion and is the most common corrective operative technique. This case presentation illustrates the success of surgical correction with a potentially less morbid procedure when POPQ stage IV prolapse is simultaneously encountered with nonpuerperal inversion [2].

2. Case Presentation

A 66-year-old without significant past medical or surgical history except pelvic organ prolapse presented to the emergency department complaining of vaginal bleeding and a

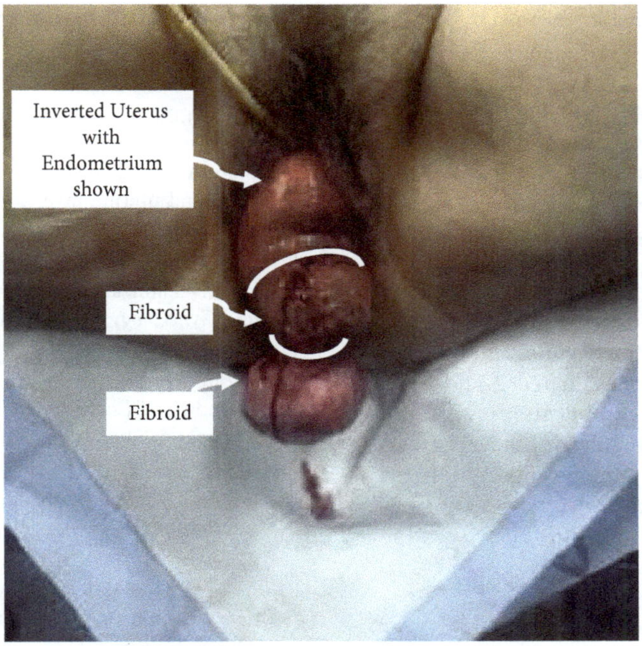

FIGURE 1: Preoperative uterine masses with complete uterovaginal prolapse and uterine inversion.

mass protruding outside of the vaginal introitus. She had managed her chronic prolapse condition for the prior 5 years with self-reduction of the prolapse. The prolapse was not affecting her quality of life and she had not sought medical treatment prior to this emergency department encounter. An acute increase in vaginal bulge and associated vaginal bleeding precipitated the emergency encounter.

Upon presentation, an actively bleeding 15 cm mass was noted to be protruding from the vaginal introitus. Vital signs were stable, and the admission Hgb was 8 mg/dl. She was noted to be in urinary retention. With further evaluation and indwelling catheter placement, a decision was made to transfuse 2 units of packed red blood cells.

Closer examination of the vaginal mass revealed complete uterovaginal prolapse with uterine inversion (Figure 1). Two distinct masses consistent with uterine myomas were noted and found to have broad-based attachment to the inverted endometrial cavity. Active bleeding was encountered, and the patient was counseled and consented for surgical management. Because of the complete cervical dilation and advanced stage of prolapse, it was felt that total hysterectomy would be associated with greater risk of morbidity due to ureteral injury; therefore, a decision was made for uterine preservation. The patient expressed desire for native tissue correction of the prolapse.

Typical preoperative work was completed, and after adequate general endotracheal anesthesia was obtained, an examination under anesthesia confirmed the preoperative diagnosis. Starting vaginally, endometrial sampling was performed, and Ligassure® was utilized to obtain hemostasis and divide the broad-based masses from their insertion site. The prolapse was then manually reduced. A uterine manipulator was inserted and utilized to elevate the uterus to normal anatomic position.

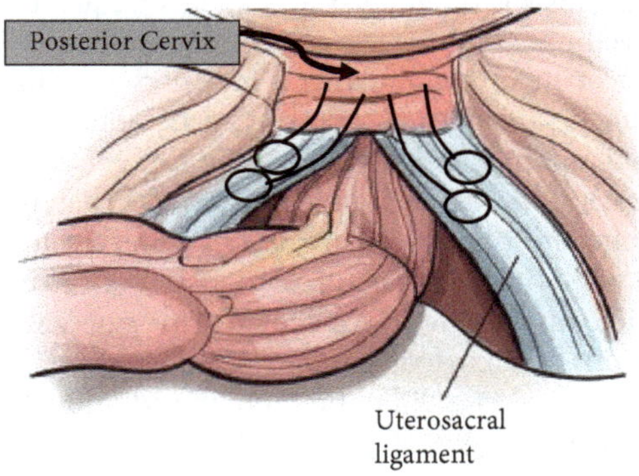

FIGURE 2: Uterosacral ligament hysteropexy [6].

Abdominal trocars were placed in a typical fashion, and the uterosacral ligaments were identified under tension. The peritoneum over both ligaments was opened and bilateral ureters were identified laterally. A monofilament polypropylene suture was passed from lateral to medial at the level of the ischial spines bilaterally. Each suture was then passed from lateral to medial of the posterior surface of the cervix with inclusion of the uterosacral ligament insertion site. Both sutures were then secured with care to avoid air knots.

A second suture of polydioxanone (delayed absorbable) was placed in a similar fashion 1 cm distal to the original suture placement bilaterally (Figure 2). These sutures were secured with close observation for ureteral compromise. Good apical support was obtained with point C -6. Cystourethroscopy was performed, and bilateral ureteral efflux was confirmed.

Overnight observation was performed with discharge the following morning after meeting post-op criteria. Minimal bleeding was noted. The Foley catheter was kept in place

Table 1: Stages of genital inversion [1].

Stage	Description
1	Incomplete inversion, fundus is within the uterine cavity
2	Complete inversion, fundus is protruding through the cervix
3	Total inversion, fundus is protruding through the vulva
4	Total inversion, fundus is protruding through the vulva with vagina involved

overnight and was discontinued the next day after a successful voiding trial. The patient was evaluated 2 and 6 weeks postoperatively. No immediate complications were noted, and she was asymptomatic. Pathology confirmed 2 benign leiomyomas and endometrial curettage. Six-month pelvic examination demonstrated continued apical support with point C at -6.

3. Discussion

Uterine inversions are typically categorized as obstetric, puerperal, or gynecologic nonpuerperal. Due to the rarity and nonspecific symptomatology of nonpuerperal inversions, diagnosis is often delayed. Patients frequently present with bleeding, discharge, pain, or symptomatic anemia. However, acute inversion patients may present with hypovolemic shock [3]. Physical exam often demonstrates a dark red, friable mass at the perineum, and differential diagnosis includes cervical, vaginal, or vulvar cancer. When presenting complaints and physical exam are not sufficient for diagnosis, imaging with MRI or ultrasound is indicated. Sagittal views will demonstrate a U-shaped uterine cavity with thickened fundus and axial views often demonstrate a "Bulls-eye" pattern [2]. This case did not require the additional imaging, and the acute nature of presentation necessitated prompt intervention.

An inversion staging system has been described in the literature, classifying this case as stage 4 inversion (Table 1) [1]. Systematic evaluation of an inversion should include biopsy of any mass if present with appropriate oncology referral if necessary. Patient age, fertility desires, desired route of surgical correction, manual reduction success, and morbidity of surgical options should all be considered and discussed with the patient.

Though hysterectomy is the most common surgical procedure performed for inversion, four surgical options for repositioning of the inverted fundus are described in the literature. Abdominal correction of the inverted fundus may be accomplished by a Haultain or Huntington technique, and vaginal correction of the inversion may be accomplished by a Kustner or Spinelli vaginal approach [3, 6].

This case allowed for a minimally invasive technique of correction, and, in our experience, is the first documented case of a nonpuerperal inversion with advanced stage uterine prolapse managed laparoscopically with robotic assistance. This surgical technique may be considered in management algorithms of nonpuerperal uterine eversion with advanced stage prolapse. Uterine preservation with hysteropexy may provide a less morbid surgical option when compared to hysterectomy.

References

[1] B. Rosa Silva, F. de Oliveira Meller, M. L. Uggioni et al., "Non-puerperal uterine inversion: a systematic review," *Gynecologic and Obstetric Investigation*, vol. 83, no. 5, pp. 428–436, 2018.

[2] R. Rocconi, W. K. Huh, and S. Chiang, "Postmenopausal uterine inversion associated with endometrial polyps," *Obstetrics and Gynecology*, vol. 102, no. 3, pp. 521–523, 2003.

[3] R. P. Herath, M. Patabendige, M. Rashid, and P. S. Wijesinghe, "Nonpuerperal uterine inversion: what the gynaecologists need to know?," *Obstetrics and Gynecology International*, vol. 2020, 12 pages, 2020.

[4] A. Kumari, A. Vidhyarthi, and K. M. Salini, "Chronic uterine inversion secondary to submucous fibroid: a rare case report," *International Journal of Scientific Study*, vol. 3, no. 11, pp. 302–304, 2016.

[5] A. Kouamé, S. V. Koffi, R. Adjoby et al., "Non-puerperal uterine inversion in a young woman: a case report," *Journal of the West African College of Surgeons*, vol. 5, no. 3, pp. 78–83, 2015.

[6] V. L. Handa and L. Van Le, *Te Linde's Operative Gynecology*, Lippincott Williams & Wilkins, Pennsylvania, 2019.

11

Diagnostic and Management Challenges of Caesarean Scar Ectopic Pregnancy in a Lower Middle Income Country

Kwaku Asah-Opoku [1,2,3,4] Nana Essuman Oduro,[2] Alim Swarray-Deen,[2] Kareem Mumuni,[1,2] Isaac Osei Koranteng,[2] Rita Catherine Senker,[2] Marcus Rijken,[3,4] and Kobinah Nkyekyer[1,2]

[1]*Department of Obstetrics and Gynecology, University of Ghana School of Medicine and Dentistry (UGSMD), Korle-Bu, Accra, Ghana*
[2]*Korle-Bu Teaching Hospital, Department of Obstetrics and Gynaecology, Korle-Bu, Accra, Ghana*
[3]*Department of Obstetrics and Gynaecology, University Medical Centre Utrecht, Utrecht University, Utrecht, Netherlands*
[4]*Julius Global Health, Julius Centre for Health Sciences and Primary Care, University Medical Centre Utrecht, Utrecht University, Utrecht, Netherlands*

Correspondence should be addressed to Kwaku Asah-Opoku; kasahopoku@yahoo.com

Academic Editor: Maria Grazia Porpora

Caesarean scar ectopic pregnancy is defined as the implantation of the blastocyst in a previous Caesarean scar. It is a rare type of ectopic pregnancy. The incidence is however rising due to the increasing rates of Caesarean sections as well as in-vitro fertilization embryo-transfer. It can be diagnosed early by ultrasound. This remains a challenge in lower middle income countries where the availability of high resolution ultrasound and the skill for such sonography may be lacking. Misdiagnosis or a delay in diagnosis often leads to poor treatment outcomes. We present a case of a gravida 3 para 2 + 0 who had laparotomy for a caesarean scar pregnancy and highlight the challenges associated with diagnosis and management of this rare ectopic pregnancy in a lower middle income country.

1. Introduction

Caesarean scar ectopic pregnancy or simply Caesarean scar pregnancy (CSP) refers to a gestational sac that is implanted wholly or partially within a previous Caesarean section (CS) scar. It was first reported in 1978 [1, 2]. Incidence rates of 1/1800–1/2500 pregnancies have been documented [3, 4]. Its incidence is increasing due to increasing rates of CS and in-vitro-fertilization embryo- transfer [5, 6]. Various mechanisms have been proposed as pathophysiology of the CSP but the main mechanism is the invasion of a microscopic tract within the CS scar by the blastocyst as it implants [7]. Fibrosis and poor wound healing are responsible for the formation of the defect in the wound [3]. High income countries have easy access to high resolution ultrasound and magnetic resonance imaging compared to lower middle income countries(LMICs) enabling prompt diagnosis and treatment of CSP in these high income countries.

2. Case Presentation

A 38-year-old gravida 3 para 2 presented with scanty vaginal bleeding and mild lower abdominal pain in early pregnancy. Her last menstrual period was two months prior to presentation. She conceived naturally and the pregnancy had been uneventful until her presentation. She had had two previous CS: the first was planned for primigravida breech presentation and the second was performed for fetal distress in a woman with previous CS. She had no significant medical history. On clinical examination, she looked generally well with normal general, cardiovascular, respiratory and abdominal findings. On vaginal examination, there was some scanty blood at vaginal introitus. A sterile speculum exams showed a normal looking cervix with scanty blood at the external cervical os. A bimanual examination showed an anteverted uterus which was bulky. The external cervical os was closed with no adnexal tenderness or cervical excitation

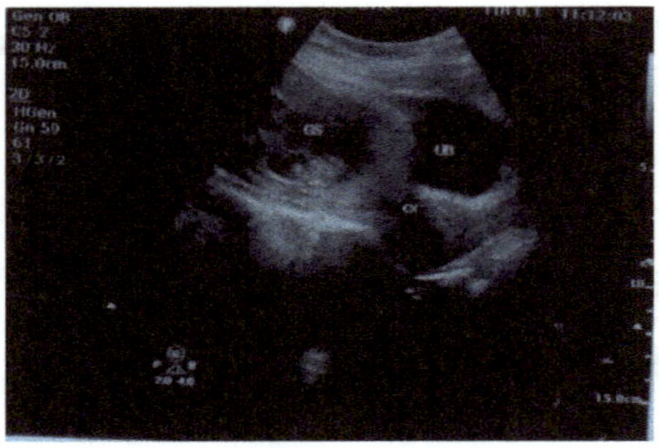

Figure 1: An empty endocervical canal and a gestational sac in the lower uterine segment with a ballooned out lower uterine segment, GS = Gestational sac, Cx = Cervix, UB = Urinary bladder.

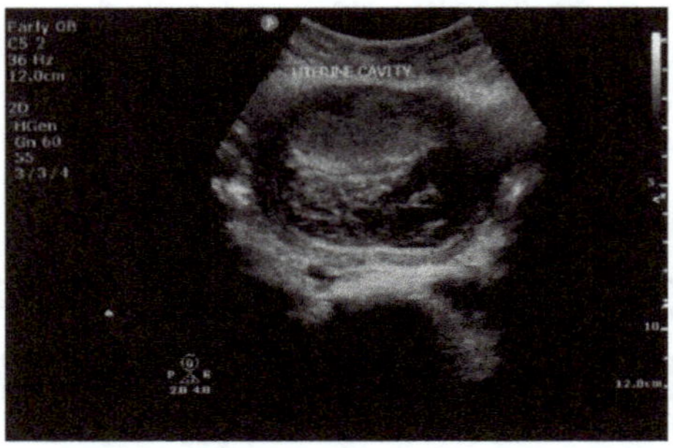

Figure 2: Uterine cavity with some clots.

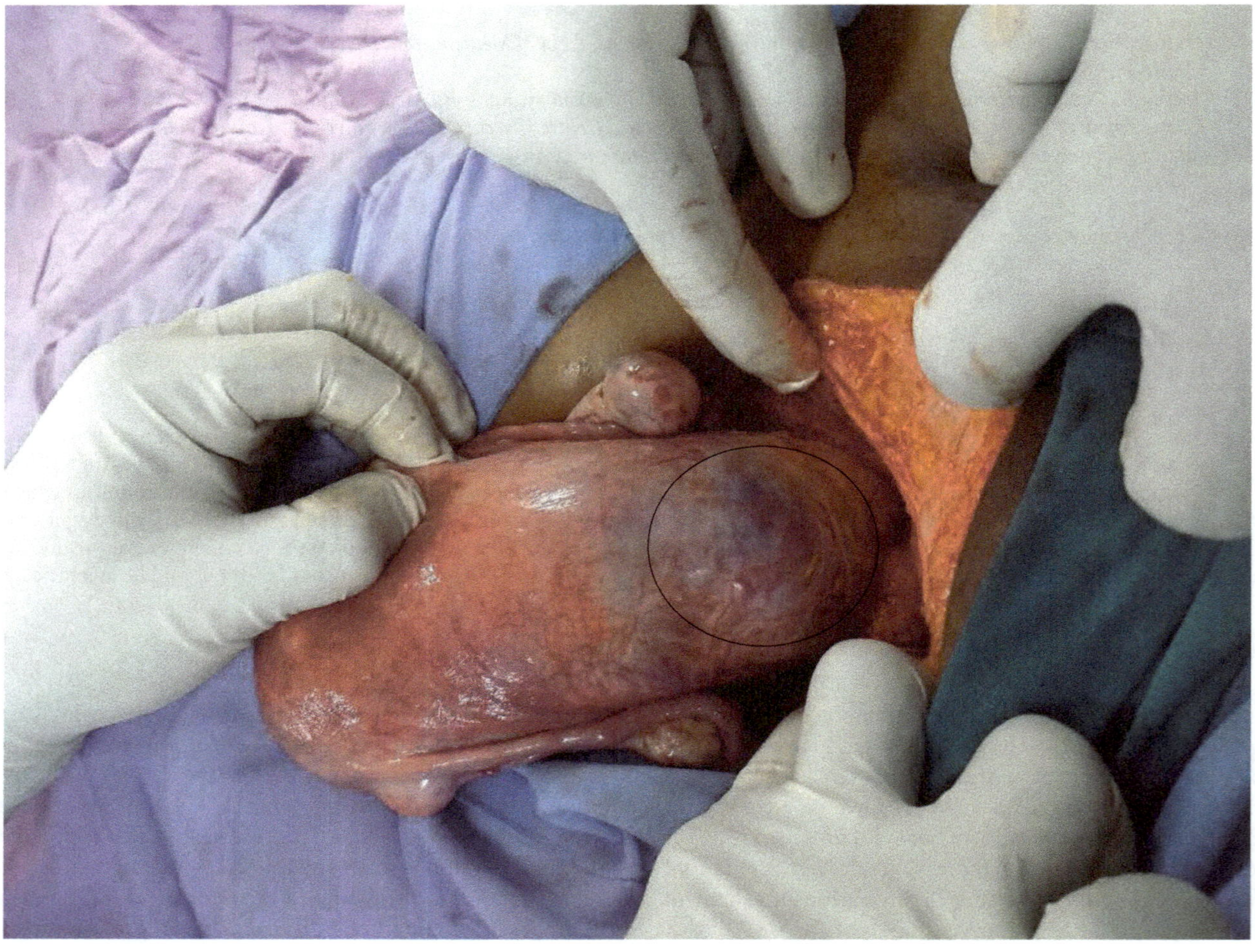

Figure 3: Thinned and ballooned out lower uterine segment.

tenderness. A urine pregnancy test was positive and therefore this patient was managed as a case of threatened abortion. An appointment for clinical review and pelvic ultrasound was scheduled at the outpatient department (OPD) the next day. The scan showed a singleton intrauterine pregnancy with a gestational age of 7 weeks 4 days. The bleeding per vaginam had subsided and therefore she was scheduled for review in a week. However, five days after this OPD visit, she presented to the gynaecology emergency room with repeat minimal bleeding per vaginam and mild lower abdominal pain. Her cervical os remained closed and a repeat pelvic ultrasound scan with an abdominal probe showed a bulky uterus with a gestational sac that appeared to be within the endocervical canal. A sonographic impression of cervical ectopic pregnancy was made. She was admitted and the laboratory investigations showed haemoglobin level of 12.6 g/dl, her WBC = 7.19×10^9 /L and platelet level 288×10^9/L. Her serum beta-HCG level was 105,000 mIU/ml. Her liver function tests and blood urea electrolytes and creatinine were normal. She had a repeat abdominal ultrasound scan 2 days into admission. This scan was done in combination with a transvaginal ultrasound. The findings were a bulky uterus with a gestational sac that

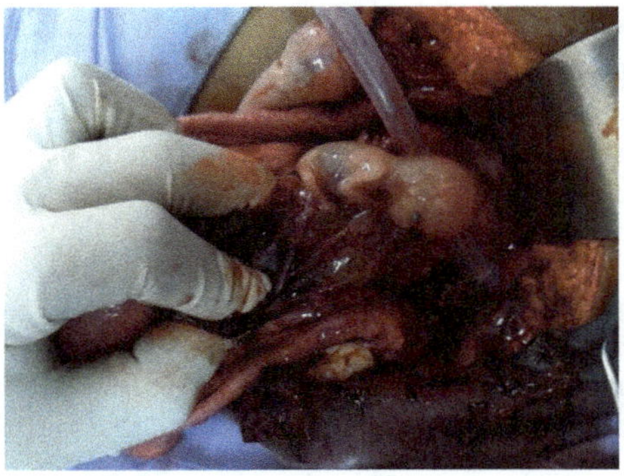

FIGURE 4: Conceptus and trophoblastic tissue after incision was made through the lower uterine segment.

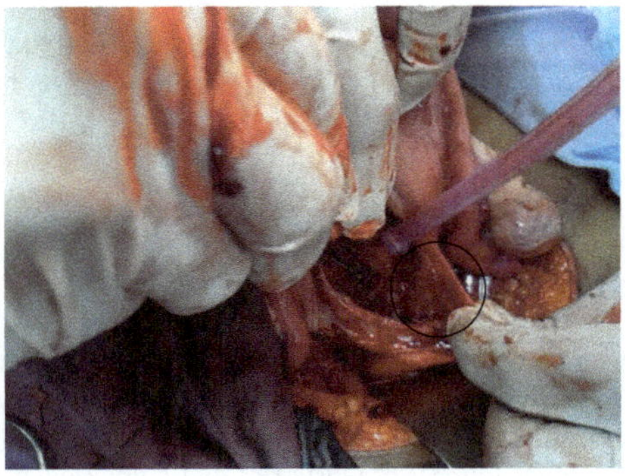

FIGURE 5: The thinned out Caesarean section scar and bleeding from the base of the trophoblastic tissue attachment to the previous Caesarean section scar.

appeared to be within the endocervical canal but on transvaginal interrogation, the gestational sac appeared to be at the upper part of the endocervix above the isthmus and in close proximity to the endometrial cavity. The chorionic tissue appeared to cover the internal os. No adnexal mass or pouch of Douglas mass was seen. The impression was a low implantation pregnancy likely to be a developing placenta praevia or a cervical pregnancy at 9 weeks. She was managed as a case of cervical ectopic pregnancy at this point and she received 50 mg of intramuscular methotrexate and had a repeat serum beta HCG done 3 days after, which showed a level of 106,730 mIU/ml. A repeat pelvic ultrasound showed a gestational sac containing single viable fetal pole in the lower segment of the uterus bulging into the bladder (Figure 1). The myometrial wall thickness between the gestational sac and the bladder was 2 mm. There was accumulation of hypoechoeic fluid in a lattice appearance suggestive of clots behind the gestational sac (Figure 2). The endocervical canal was empty (Figure 1). A sonographic diagnosis of unruptured Caesarean section scar ectopic was made. She was counselled for exploratory laparotomy same day and had dissection into the thinned out uterine wall through the Caesarean section scar, removal of the gestational sac and use of figure of eight stitches to secure haemostasis at the site of attachment of the gestational sac. The dissection invariably ended up as a hysterotomy which was repaired after evacuation of the conceptus (Figure 3). The findings were a fourteen week size uterus with a bulge in the lower portion (Figure 4). There was a gestational

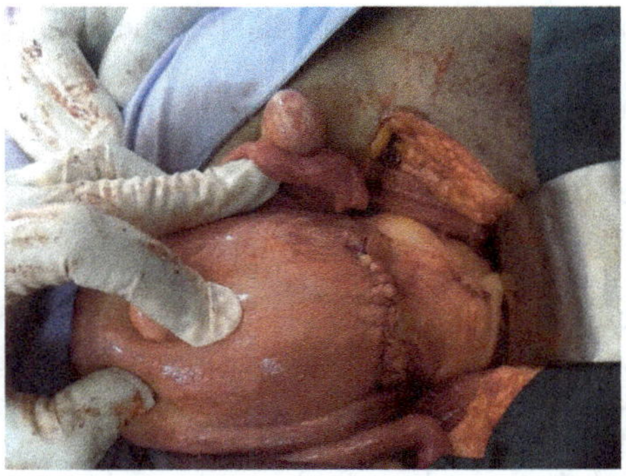

FIGURE 6: The hysterotomy wound repaired in two layers.

sac approximately one centimeter from the internal cervical os of the uterus embedded in the myometrial wall with retroplacental clots of approximately 400 ml (Figures 5 and 6). There was thinning out of the wall of the lower uterine segment (Figure 6). She had normal fallopian tubes and ovaries and the total blood loss was approximately 800 ml. Her recovery was uneventful and she was discharged home on the third postoperative day.

3. Discussion

CSP is one of the rarest types of ectopic pregnancy. It occurs when the blastocyst implants on the Caesarean scar [1].

Various risk factors have been identified as increasing the chances of a woman developing a CSP. The number of previous CS does not correlate with the risk for a CSP [8]. However, women who have had an elective CS for breech presentation in a previous pregnancy are the ones mostly at risk due to poor formation of the lower uterine segment [8]. This patient's first CS was on account of a breech presentation at term and put her at a higher risk. This history should raise a higher suspicion of a CSP as a cervical pregnancy has been found to be very uncommon in women with a previous CS [9].

Women with CSP often present with slight vaginal bleeding with mild abdominal discomfort [10] as was the case in this presentation. The diagnosis is usually made by a high resolution pelvic ultrasound, a transvaginal ultrasound or a magnetic resonance imaging technique. A combination of the transabdominal and transvaginal ultrasound scanning procedures have been shown to have a higher accuracy than the transabdominal or transvaginal ultrasound used alone [11]. CSP diagnosis with an ultrasound may pose some diagnostic challenges and a high index of suspicion is required to make an accurate diagnosis of CSP. It is not surprising therefore, that three different transabdominal ultrasound scans and a transvaginal ultrasound were done in this patient before the diagnosis of CSP was finally made. The sonographic criteria for CSP include an empty uterine cavity and closed and empty cervical canal, a gestational sac that is implanted in the previous CS scar, a gestational sac that fills the niche of the scar, a thin or absent myometrial layer between the gestational sac and the bladder, yolk sac, embryo and cardiac activity may or may not be present, evidence of functional trophoblastic circulation on colour flow Doppler and the negative 'sliding organs' sign [9]. The absence of myometrium between the gestational sac and the bladder and an empty uterine cavity as well as an empty cervical canal helps to distinguish cervical ectopic pregnancy from a CSP [12, 13]. There were challenges with accurate ultrasound diagnosis of the CSP in the earlier three ultrasound scans. CSP was not diagnosed in this patient with the earlier ultrasound scans mainly because of the low index of suspicion in the patient. The challenge with diagnosis of CSP could also be because of the fact that because it is rare, most of the Obstetricians and Gynaecologists and sonographers may not have encountered it previously in their ultrasound experience. Indeed the challenges of diagnosing CSP and misdiagnosis of CSP have been highlighted in previous publications [14, 15]. The final ultrasound however that was done in this patient showed the uterine cavity with some clots of blood (Figure 2) and an empty cervical canal (Figure 1), a gestational sac implanted in the previous CS scar with the gestational sac containing a single viable fetal pole in the lower segment bulging into the bladder(Figure 1). There was a thin myometrial wall thickness of 2 mm between the gestational sac and the bladder (Figure 1). Reduction in CS rates by reducing unnecessary CS will help to reduce the rates of CSP. In an era of increasing CS, emphasis should be made on the diagnosis of CSP in women with a history of CS during training and refresher courses in ultrasonography for Obstetrician Gynaecologists and sonographers.

There are various modalities for the management of CSP. These include expectant management, intramuscular or intralesional injection of methotrexate and surgical treatment. Surgical treatment is associated with reduced risk of uterine rupture and torrential bleeding from the CSP [16]. That was why it was employed for management of this patient. Expectant management of CSP has a high risk of uterine rupture and maternal death. With the thinned out myometrial tissue at the site of the previous CS scar, an attempt at dilatation and curettage or manual vacuum aspiration could have resulted in incomplete evacuation, bladder injury or uterine rupture along the previous CS scar and increased the morbidity and mortality associated with the management of this case. Laparoscopic and endoscopic management of CSP have been described [17] but the skill and equipment needed for it in our center were not available.

In future pregnancies, the risk of recurrence of CSP is higher [9]. There is also an increased risk of morbidly adherent placenta. There is the need to educate women at risk about the need to report early when pregnant. There is therefore the need for early ultrasound scan in the subsequent pregnancies to rule out recurrence [9]. This was communicated to the patient before she was discharged. Most reports have advocated a CS in the next pregnancy to reduce the risk of uterine rupture and to also enhance adequate closure of the incision in the lower uterine segment [9].

4. Conclusion

The diagnosis and management of CSP can be challenging in LMICs and a high index of suspicion is required to allow for early diagnosis and management to reduce the morbidities and mortalities associated with it. Transvaginal ultrasound scan is required in early pregnancy for women with a previous CS scar where the suspicion of CSP is high. Provision of high resolution ultrasound scans and training and refresher courses that highlight the diagnosis of CSP in a world with increasing rates of Caesarean sections will help in early diagnosis of CSP.

Consent

An informed consent to publish this patient's case report has been obtained from the patient and is available for the editor's perusal.

Acknowledgments

The authors are grateful to Dr. Lawrence Hasford for assisting in the ultrasound imaging of the patient and also to staff of the gynaecology wards and theatre of the Korle-Bu Teaching Hospital.

References

[1] A. Herman, Z. Weinraub, O. Avrech, R. Maymon, R. Ron-El, and Y. Bukovsky, "Follow up and outcome of isthmic pregnancy located in a previous caesarean section scar," *BJOG: An International Journal of Obstetrics and Gynaecology*, vol. 102, no. 10, pp. 839–841, 1995.

[2] J. Larsen and M. H. Solomon, "Pregnancy in a uterine scar sacculus—an unusual cause of postabortal haemorrhage," *South African Medical Journal*, vol. 53, no. 4, pp. 142–143, 1978.

[3] D. Jurkovic, K. Hillaby, B. Woelfer, A. Lawrence, R. Salim, and C. J Elson, "First-trimester diagnosis and management of pregnancies implanted into the lower uterine segment Cesarean section scar," *Ultrasound in Obstetrics and Gynecology*, vol. 21, no. 3, pp. 220–227, 2003.

[4] K.-M. Seow, L.-W. Huang, Y.H. Lin, M. Yan-Sheng, Y.-L. Tsai, and J.-L. Hwang, "Cesarean scar pregnancy: issues in management," *Ultrasound in Obstetrics and Gynecology*, vol. 23, no. 3, pp. 247–253, 2004.

[5] H.-Y. Chueh, P.-J. Cheng, C.-W. Wang, S.-W. Shaw, C.-L. Lee, and Y.-K. Soong, "Ectopic twin pregnancy in cesarean scar after in vitro fertilization/embryo transfer: case report," *Fertility and Sterility*, vol. 90, no. 5, pp. 2009–2011, 2009.

[6] M. A. Patel, "Scar ectopic pregnancy," *The Journal of Obstetrics and Gynecology of India*, vol. 65, no. 6, pp. 372–375, 2015.

[7] Z.-D. Qian, Q.-Y. Guo, and L.-L. Huang, "Identifying risk factors for recurrent cesarean scar pregnancy: a case-control study," *Fertility and Sterility*, vol. 102, no. 1, pp. 129–134.e1, 2014.

[8] M. A. Rotas, S. Haberman, and M. Levgur, "Cesarean Scar Ectopic Pregnancies," *Obstetrics & Gynecology*, vol. 107, no. 6, pp. 1373–1381, 2006.

[9] I. E. Timor-Tritsch, A. Monteagudo, and A. K. Agten, "Cesarean scar pregnancy diagnosis and management," *Contemporary Obstetrics and Gynecology*, vol. 60, pp. 16–24, 2015.

[10] Y. Zhang, Y. Gu, J.-M. Wang, and Y. Li, "Analysis of cases with cesarean scar pregnancy," *Journal of Obstetrics and Gynaecology Research*, vol. 39, no. 1, pp. 195–202, 2013.

[11] R. Maymon, R. Halperin, S. Mendlovic, D. Schneider, and A. Herman, "Ectopic pregnancies in a Caesarean scar: review

of the medical approach to an iatrogenic complication," *Human Reproduction Update*, vol. 10, no. 6, pp. 515–523, 2004.

[12] D. L. Fylstra, "Ectopic pregnancy not within the (distal) fallopian tube: etiology, diagnosis, and treatment," *American Journal of Obstetrics and Gynecology*, vol. 206, no. 4, pp. 289–299, 2012.

[13] B. Rizk, C. P. Holliday, S. Owens, and M. Abuzeid, "Cervical and Cesarean scar ectopic pregnancies: diagnosis and management," *Middle East Fertility Society Journal*, vol. 18, no. 2, pp. 67–73, 2013.

[14] B. Sujutha, S. Bharatmur, and S. Virmani, "Ruptured caesarian scar ectopic pregnancy," *Online Journal of Health & Allied Sciences*, vol. 16, pp. 3–5, 2017.

[15] S. Brancazio, I. Saramago, W. Goodnight, and K. McGinty, "Cesarean scar ectopic pregnancy: case report," *Radiology Case Reports*, vol. 14, no. 3, pp. 354–359, 2019.

[16] P. M. Jayaram, G. O. Okunoye, and J. Konje, "Caesarean scar ectopic pregnancy: diagnostic challenges and management options," *The Obstetrician & Gynaecologist*, vol. 19, no. 1, pp. 13–20, 2017.

[17] C.-J. Wang, A.-S. Chao, L.-T. Yuen, C.-W. Wang, Y.-K. Soong, and C.-L. Lee, "Endoscopic management of cesarean scar pregnancy," *Fertility and Sterility*, vol. 85, no. 2, pp. 494.e1–494.e4, 2006.

12

A Case of Cornelia de Lange Syndrome: Difficulty in Prenatal Diagnosis

Tadatsugu Kinjo, Keiko Mekaru, Miyuki Nakada, Hayase Nitta, Hitoshi Masamoto, and Yoichi Aoki

Department of Obstetrics and Gynecology, Graduate School of Medicine, University of the Ryukyus, 207 Uehara Nishihara, Okinawa 903-0215, Japan

Correspondence should be addressed to Yoichi Aoki; yoichi@med.u-ryukyu.ac.jp

Academic Editor: A. O. Awonuga

We report a case of Cornelia de Lange syndrome (CdLS) where prenatal diagnosis was not made even with major anomaly. A 33-year-old Japanese woman was referred to our institution at 23 weeks of gestation because of fetal forearm defect. Ultrasound examination revealed short forearms and short humeri and femurs (−2.1 SD). The fetal estimated body weight was 450 g (−1.3 SD). Fetal MRI at 26 weeks of gestation revealed short forearms and hypoplasty of hand fingers. Fetal growth restriction became evident thereafter, leading to intrauterine fetal death occurring at 29 weeks of gestation. A stillbirth baby was of 798 g in body weight and 33.0 cm in length. External examination showed a low hairline, synophrys, low-set ear, hypertrichosis, and smooth long philtrum with thin lips. The neck appeared short and broad. Finally, CdLS was diagnosed. The prenatal diagnosis might be possible as the arm findings were totally characteristic in a small fetus, regardless of whether an overhanging upper lip was identified. Because CdLS is a rare condition, it is important to consider its possibility as a part of differential diagnosis.

1. Introduction

The Cornelia de Lange syndrome (CdLS) was first reported by Vrolik in 1849 and Brachmann in 1916, followed by Cornelia de Lange in 1933, after whom the syndrome is named [1–3]. CdLS is a clinically variable disorder mainly characterized by distinctive facial features, growth restriction, hirsutism, psychomotor delay, intellectual disability, and malformations of the upper limbs [4]. The precise prevalence of the disease is unknown but is estimated to be 1–10:100,000 [5]. The diagnosis of CdLS is generally performed after birth, but the syndrome could be suspected during the second and third trimester of pregnancy by observing a wide range of features through ultrasound examination. However, a previous report showed that a routine prenatal ultrasonography failed to detect more than two-thirds of cases of CdLS with major malformations [5].

We report a case of CdLS where prenatal diagnosis was not made even with major anomaly.

2. Case Presentation

A 33-year-old Japanese woman, para 0-0-1-0, with no known family and past histories of the disease, was referred to our institution at 23 weeks of gestation because of fetal forearm defect as detected by ultrasound examination at 21 weeks and 5 days of gestation. Ultrasound examination (Figure 1) revealed short forearms of 7 mm and 9 mm and short humeri and femurs (−2.1 standard deviation, SD). The fetal estimated body weight was 450 g (−1.3 SD). Fetal MRI at 26 weeks of gestation revealed short forearms and hypoplasty of hand fingers (Figure 2). The serum analyses of the mother showed no TORCH syndrome, and the exposure of drugs as teratogen was denied. No other anomalies were found. However, fetal growth restriction (FGR) became evident thereafter, leading to intrauterine fetal death (IUFD) occurring at 29 weeks of gestation. A stillbirth baby was of 798 g in body weight and 33.0 cm in length. External examination showed a low hairline, synophrys, low-set ear, hypertrichosis, and smooth long philtrum with thin lips (Figure 3). The neck appeared

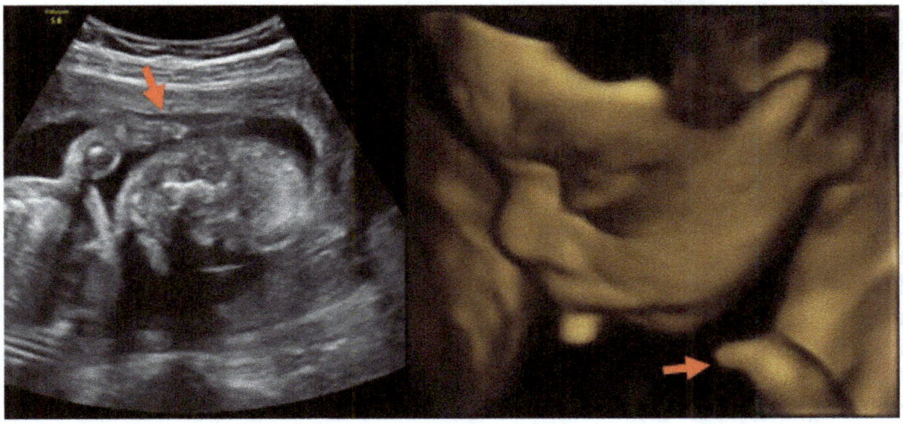

FIGURE 1: Two-dimensional (right) and three-dimensional (left) prenatal ultrasound images showing short forearms of 7 mm and 9 mm (arrows) and short humeri and femurs (−2.1 standard deviation, SD).

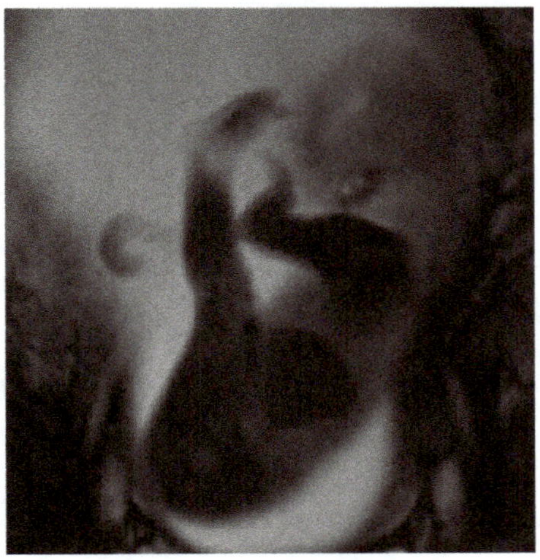

FIGURE 2: Fetal MRI at 26 weeks of gestation showing short forearms and hypoplasty of hand fingers.

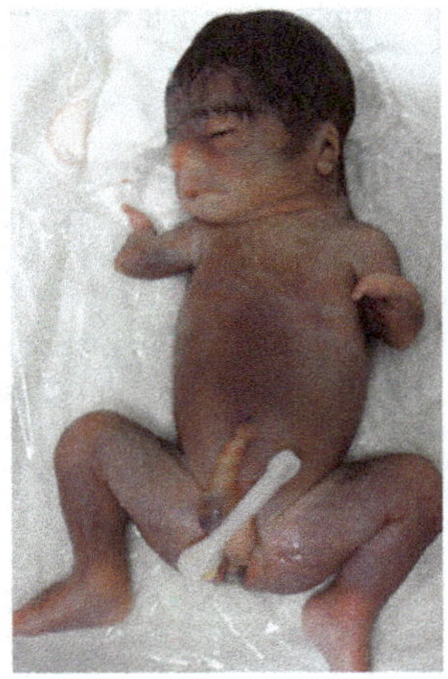

FIGURE 3: External examination showing a low hairline, synophrys, low-set ear, hypertrichosis, and smooth long philtrum with thin lips. The neck appears short and broad.

short and broad. Finally, CdLS was diagnosed. Autopsy and genetic and chromosomal analyses were declined.

3. Discussion

Because of a wide range of features of CdLS, its diagnosis is generally performed after birth, although it could be suspected by ultrasound examination during the second and third trimester of pregnancy. Indeed, CdLS diagnosis is still underperformed and extremely rare before birth. Avagliano et al. [6] proposed that following a sequence of detailed scans and examinations, CdLS-affected fetuses could be diagnosed in utero, when one or more characteristics, such as FGR, limb defects, facial abnormalities, diaphragmatic hernia, and heart diseases, are detected and confirmed by specific molecular diagnostic tests, such as Nipped-B-like protein (NIPBL), structural maintenance of chromosomes 1A (SMC1A), structural maintenance of chromosomes 3 (SMC3), human homolog of Schizosaccharomyces pombe radiation sensitive mutant 21 (RAD21), and histone deacetylase 8 (HDAC8) [7]. To date, maternal serum pregnancy associated placental protein-A (PAPP-A), which is a glycoprotein produced by the placenta, level is reported to be a reliable predictor of CdLS in the first and second trimester of pregnancy. It is not considered to be a specific marker, but a very low PAPP-A can also support this diagnosis [6]. PAPP-A was not done in our patient, because it is not routinely offered in Japan.

Although FGR is nearly always detected as was in our case, it is a nonspecific characteristic; therefore, other associated ultrasound findings should be detected for a more appropriate prenatal prediction of the syndrome [8]. Limb abnormalities, ranging from small fingers and hand abnormalities to complete absence of the upper limbs, are often detected in prenatal ultrasonography for CdLS [8]. A careful ultrasound examination of the arms in relation to FGR may lead to the early detection of the possible presence of CdLS. The affected babies present with the following facial characteristics, including a bulging forehead with frontal bossing, depressed nasal bridge, long bulging philtrum, and micrognathia. A three-dimensional and/or two-dimensional ultrasound scan may identify these findings [8, 9]. The prenatal detection associated with limb defects and FGR may significantly improve the early prenatal diagnosis of CdLS. Other malformations, such as diaphragmatic hernia, congenital heart diseases, and anatomical brain disorders, have been reported [6, 8], and ultrasound examination should be performed for a prognostic value.

In our case, FGR and upper limb abnormality were identified but not facial characteristics. Thus, the prenatal diagnosis of CdLS was not made even with major anomaly, but might be possible as the arm findings were totally characteristic in a small fetus, regardless of whether an overhanging upper lip was identified (profile photo not shown). Because CdLS is a rare condition, it is important to consider its possibility as a part of differential diagnosis. Possible diagnostic evidences should lead to tests that could provide an early diagnosis, at least in some cases, which is important in any rare disease.

References

[1] W. Vrolik, *Tabulae Ad Illustrandam Embryogenesin Hominis Et Mammalium Tam Naturalem Quam Abnormem*, Londonck, Amsterdam, 1849.

[2] W. Brachmann, "Ein fall von symmetrischer monodaktylie durch Ulnade- fekt, mit symmetrischer flughautbildung in den ellenbeugen, sowie anderen abnormitaten (zwerghaftogkeit, halsrippen, behaarung)," *Jarb Kinder Phys Erzie*, vol. 84, pp. 225–235, 1916.

[3] C. de Lange, "Sur un type nouveau de degenerescence (typus Amstelo- damensis)," *Arch Med Enfants*, vol. 36, pp. 713–719, 1933.

[4] L. Jackson, A. D. Kline, M. A. Barr, and S. Koch, "de Lange syndrome: A clinical review of 310 individuals," *American Journal of Medical Genetics*, vol. 47, no. 7, pp. 940–946, 1993.

[5] I. Barisic, V. Tokic, M. Loane et al., "Descriptive epidemiology of Cornelia de Lange syndrome in Europe," *American Journal of Medical Genetics Part A*, vol. 146A, no. 1, pp. 51–59, 2008.

[6] L. Avagliano, G. P. Bulfamante, and V. Massa, "Cornelia de Lange syndrome: To diagnose or not to diagnose in utero?" *Birth Defects Research Part A: Clinical and Molecular Teratology*, vol. 109, no. 10, pp. 771–777, 2017.

[7] M. A. Deardorff, S. E. Noon, and I. D. Krantz, "Cornelia de Lange Syndrome," in *Gen- eReviewsV® [Internet]*, R. A. Pagon, M. P. Adam, and H. H. Ardinger, Eds., pp. 1993–2017, University of Washington, Seattle, Wash, USA, 2016.

[8] D. M. Clark, I. Sherer, M. A. Deardorff et al., "Identification of a prenatal profile of Cornelia de Lange syndrome (CdLS): A review of 53 CdLS pregnancies," *American Journal of Medical Genetics Part A*, vol. 158, no. 8, pp. 1848–1856, 2012.

[9] W. Sepulveda, A. E. Wong, and V. Dezerega, "Brachmann-de Lange syndrome: Prenatal diagnosis with 2- and 3-dimensional sonography," *Journal of Ultrasound in Medicine*, vol. 28, no. 3, pp. 401–404, 2009.

13

A Case of Peritoneal Tuberculosis Mimicking Ovarian Cancer in a Young Female

Oriel Nissim,[1] F. Richard Ervin,[2] Susan E. Dorman,[1,2] and Deeksha Jandhyala[1]

[1]*Medical University of South Carolina, Charleston, South Carolina, USA*
[2]*South Carolina Department of Health and Environmental Control, South Carolina, USA*

Correspondence should be addressed to Susan E. Dorman; dorman@musc.edu

Academic Editor: Manvinder Singh

Background. Tuberculosis causes significant morbidity and mortality globally. Peritoneal tuberculosis can have a similar presentation to ovarian cancer. *Case.* We present a case of a 42-year-old female referred to gynecology oncology with imaging findings of enlarged right ovary, omental caking, and elevated CA-125 (1289 U/mL). A diagnostic laparoscopy revealed diffuse studding of intraperitoneal surfaces. Histopathological examination of omental and abdominal wall biopsies showed granulomas, but stains and cultures for mycobacteria were negative. Antimicrobial treatment for tuberculosis was initiated. Within eight weeks, there was clear clinical and radiographic improvement, consistent with a diagnosis of peritoneal tuberculosis. *Conclusion.* This case highlights the importance of including peritoneal tuberculosis in the differential diagnosis when evaluating for ovarian cancer in women with epidemiologic risk factors for tuberculosis.

1. Introduction

Tuberculosis is a leading cause of morbidity and mortality on a global level, with approximately 10 million incident cases and 1.3 million deaths annually [1]. Tuberculosis is relatively uncommon in the United States (2.7 case rate/100,000 population in 2019) and typically presents as a lung infection, although it can affect any organ system [2].

Here, we describe peritoneal tuberculosis in a young female from Brazil who presented with elevated CA-125 and radiological findings concerning for ovarian malignancy.

2. Case Presentation

A 42-year-old G0 female was referred to the gynecology oncology outpatient clinic for evaluation of symptoms and imaging findings concerning for ovarian cancer. She reported six months of abdominal discomfort and distension, night sweats, fever, and weight loss. Her previous gynecologic history included a ruptured ovarian cyst five years prior, but medical records were not available for review. She had no chronic medical conditions and did not take any medications. She had been born and lived in Brazil until moving to the U.S. three years prior to the current presentation. In Brazil, she had worked in a public health clinic that provided tuberculosis care; she had never been evaluated for *M. tuberculosis* infection or tuberculosis. On physical examination, she was generally well-appearing. The abdomen was distended but soft and nontender to palpation. External genitalia, vagina, and cervix had normal appearance; the uterus and cervix were deviated to the right on exam, and rectovaginal examination was normal. There was no thrush, peripheral lymphadenopathy, or lower extremity edema; heart and lung exams were normal.

CT with contrast of the abdomen and pelvis showed a moderate volume of free fluid throughout the abdomen with diffuse nodularity throughout the omentum, enlarged right retroperitoneal lymph nodes measuring 1.4 and 1.2 cm in the short axis diameter, and a bilobed right ovarian cyst measuring 6.5 cm at maximum diameter (Figure 1(a)). A transvaginal ultrasound showed a hypoechoic lesion with low-level internal reticular echoes within the right ovary, consistent with a hemorrhagic cyst (which resolved based on follow-up ultrasound examination); an 0.8 cm hypoechoic structure

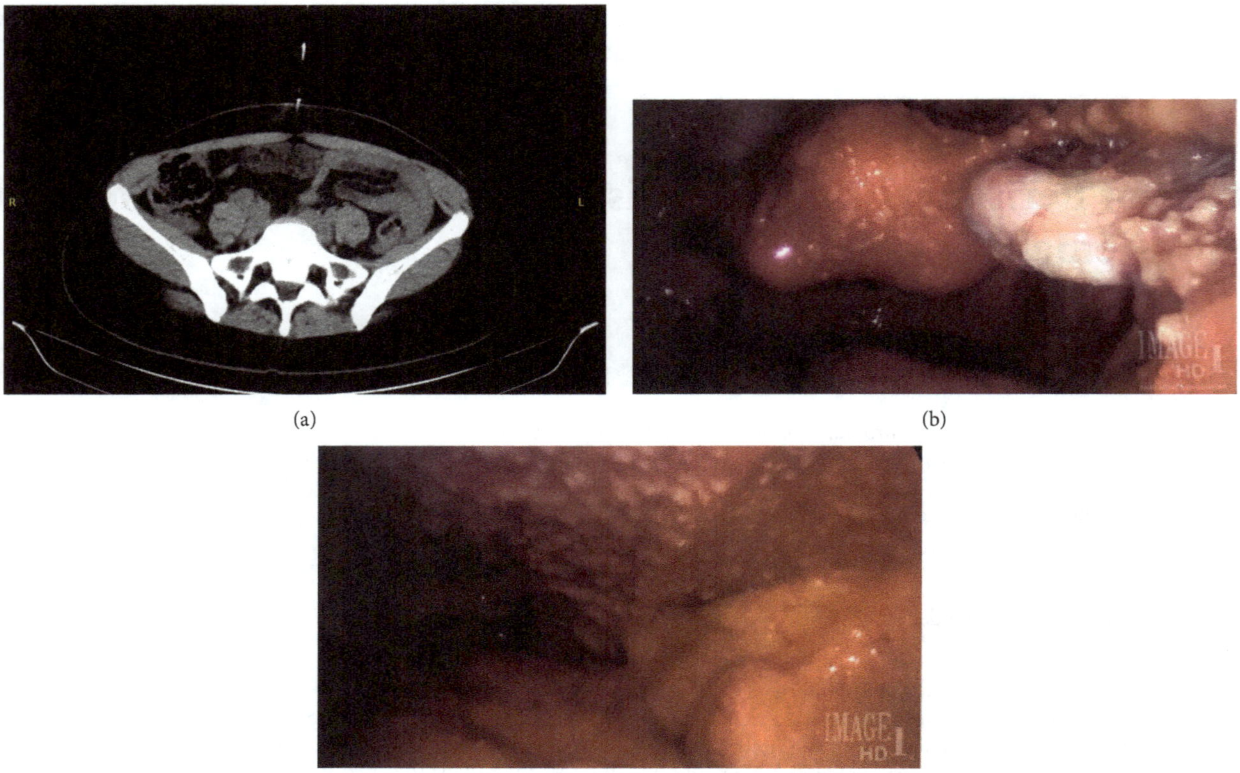

(a) (b) (c)

Figure 1: (a) Computed tomography (CT) imaging of the pelvis at the time of presentation and needle biopsy of omental caking. (b) Diagnostic laparoscopy showing innumerable tan, 1-2 mm nodules on the surface of the right ovary and uterus. (c) Diagnostic laparoscopy showing innumerable tan, 1-2 mm nodules on the anterior abdominal wall.

in the endometrium; and cystic structures throughout the myometrium. A test for antibodies to HIV-1 and HIV-2 was nonreactive. Complete blood count and metabolic panel were normal. Blood CA-125 level was 1289 U/mL (normal ≤ 38.1 U/mL).

Paracentesis was performed and showed rare benign mesothelial cells. Endometrial biopsy showed secretory endometrium without evidence of malignant cells. A CT-guided omental biopsy showed granulomas without evidence of neoplasm; mycobacterial and fungal stains and cultures were negative. Diagnostic laparoscopy was performed. Upon inspection, there was diffuse studding of intraperitoneal surfaces with 1-2 mm tan nodules, and the omentum was adherent to the anterior abdominal wall (Figures 1(b) and 1(c)). There was an enlarged uterus with multiple fibroids, and the ovaries were without masses. Pathology of the omental and abdominal wall biopsies showed benign fibroadipose tissue with necrotizing and nonnecrotizing granulomas but without acid fast bacilli seen on modified Ziehl-Neelsen staining; mycobacterial cultures using the Mycobacteria Growth Indicator Tube (MGIT) liquid culture system and Lowenstein-Jensen solid media were negative, and nucleic acid amplification testing was negative for *Mycobacterium tuberculosis*.

Due to unknown cause of intraperitoneal granulomas, she was referred to an infectious disease physician and to the local health department. CT of the chest showed a 4 mm left lower lobe nodule and biapical mild pleural parenchymal scarring. A tuberculin skin test showed 10 mm induration, and a blood QuantiFERON-TB Gold Plus interferon-gamma release assay (Qiagen) was positive. Due to concern for peritoneal tuberculosis, treatment was initiated with isoniazid, rifampin, pyrazinamide, and ethambutol. Within four weeks of treatment, the CA-125 had decreased to 74 U/mL, and she had substantial clinical improvement including resolution of fevers, reduction in abdominal discomfort, increased appetite, and weight gain. At eight weeks after tuberculosis treatment initiation, her abdominal pain was entirely resolved, weight had increased from 56.6 kg at presentation to 62.1 kg, and CT abdomen and pelvis showed resolution of omental caking, ascites, and lymphadenopathy. A clinical diagnosis of tuberculosis peritonitis was made, and standard tuberculosis treatment was administered for a total of 6 months.

3. Discussion

Tuberculosis is caused by the bacterium *Mycobacterium tuberculosis* and typically manifests as a pulmonary infection. However, tuberculosis can affect any organ system, and from 10 to 42% of all tuberculosis patients have disease outside the respiratory tract (so-called "extrapulmonary" tuberculosis) without or with pulmonary tuberculosis [3]. Peritoneal tuberculosis is uncommon, with most cases reported in countries with a high overall prevalence of tuberculosis including India and China [4, 5]. Tuberculous peritonitis is thought to arise most commonly from activation of latent foci of *M. tuberculosis* infection in the peritoneum and less commonly from direct spread from genitourinary sites or hematogenous spread of bacteria from active pulmonary lesions [6]. A high index of suspicion is required since tuberculous peritonitis can present insidiously and with a variety of systemic and organ-specific signs and symptoms that can mimic other conditions.

Our patient's presentation with radiographic imaging suggestive of ovarian carcinomatosis and elevated CA-125 levels is typical. CA-125, a mucin-type glycoprotein that is encoded by the MUC16 gene and associated with the cell membrane, is an imperfect biomarker for ovarian cancer due to shortcomings in sensitivity and specificity [7]. Elevated CA-125 levels can be observed in physiological (e.g., menstruation and pregnancy) and pathological conditions, particularly inflammatory diseases of the peritoneum including tuberculosis, endometriosis, pelvic inflammatory disease, adenomyosis, and peritoneal sarcoid [8].

Laparoscopy has emerged as an important tool for diagnosis of peritoneal tuberculosis as it permits direct visualization as well as biopsy of affected tissues [9, 10]. The characteristic laparoscopic visual finding is diffuse studding of the visceral and parietal peritoneum with tan nodules as in this patient; turbid ascites and adhesions can also be present. Although laparoscopy is important in diagnosing peritoneal tuberculosis, the visual view can be deceiving even to experienced clinicians, since laparoscopic features of tuberculosis can mimic those of disseminated abdominal malignancies such as can occur with ovarian cancer [11].

In this patient, an epidemiologic clue was her prior residence in Brazil and work there in a public health clinic that provided tuberculosis care. In addition, she had evidence of prior *M. tuberculosis* infection on chest CT scan, but no evidence of ongoing active pulmonary tuberculosis. The positive delayed-type hypersensitivity response to intradermal inoculation of purified protein derivative (tuberculin skin test) and elaboration of interferon-gamma by peripheral blood cells stimulated with *M. tuberculosis*-specific antigens (interferon-gamma release assay) also provided evidence of prior *M. tuberculosis* infection. Granulomas on histopathologic examination were strongly supportive of the diagnosis of tuberculosis peritonitis. While mycobacterial culture and nucleic acid amplification testing of affected lesions should be performed in order to obtain a definitive microbiological diagnosis and antimicrobial susceptibility information, the sensitivity of these assays is imperfect due to low bacterial burden and/or sampling error; histopathology remains the diagnostic gold standard [12, 13]. This patient had clinical, radiographic, and biomarker response to antituberculous therapy.

In sum, this report describes a woman with tuberculous peritonitis, an entity seen uncommonly in areas of low TB prevalence such as the United States. This case exemplifies the multidisciplinary effort needed to identify tuberculous peritonitis, an often-elusive diagnosis, and highlights the critical role that gynecologists play when this disease occurs in women.

Additional Points

Teaching Points. (i) Peritoneal tuberculosis typically presents with signs, symptoms, and imaging findings that can mimic those of ovarian cancer. (ii) Peritoneal tuberculosis can cause a markedly elevated CA-125. (iii) Peritoneal tuberculosis should be in the differential diagnosis when evaluating for ovarian cancer in women with epidemiological risk factors for tuberculosis infection. Biopsies should be sent for histopathology as well as mycobacterial cultures.

Consent

Written informed consent was obtained from the patient for publication of her condition and accompanying images. A copy of the written consent form is available from the corresponding author for review by the editor of this journal.

Acknowledgments

This work was supported in part by the National Institutes of Health (grant number K24AI104830 to SED).

References

[1] World Health Organization, "Global Health Observatory (GHO) data," 2021. https://www.who.int/gho/tb/epidemic/cases_deaths/en/.

[2] Centers for Disease Control and Prevention, "Tuberculosis (TB)," 2021 https://www.cdc.gov/tb/statistics/tbcases.htm.

[3] A. Zumla, M. Raviglione, R. Hafner, and C. F. von Reyn, "Tuberculosis," *The New England Journal of Medicine*, vol. 368, no. 8, pp. 745–755, 2013.

[4] A. Thomas, A. Sebastian, R. George et al., "Abdominal tuberculosis mimicking ovarian cancer: a diagnostic dilemma," *Journal of Obstetrics and Gynaecology of India*, vol. 70, no. 4, pp. 304–309, 2020.

[5] X. Xi, L. Shuang, W. Dan et al., "Diagnostic dilemma of abdominopelvic tuberculosis: a series of 20 cases," *Journal of Cancer Research and Clinical Oncology*, vol. 136, no. 12, pp. 1839–1844, 2010.

[6] U. Vaid and G. C. Kane, "Tuberculous peritonitis," *Microbiology Spectrum*, vol. 5, no. 1, 2017.

[7] Z. G. Dikmen, A. Colak, P. Dogan, S. Tuncer, and F. Akbiyik, "Diagnostic performances of CA125, HE4, and ROMA index in ovarian cancer," *European Journal of Gynaecological Oncology*, vol. 36, no. 4, pp. 457–462, 2015.

[8] F. Tahmasebi, R. Nath, N. Sokolovsky et al., "Incidental finding of raised CA125: a cause for concern?," *Critical Care Obstetrics*, vol. 5, no. 1, 2019.

[9] J. Hossain, A. K. Al-Aska, and I. Al-Mofleh, "Laparoscopy in tuberculous peritonitis," *Journal of the Royal Society of Medicine*, vol. 85, no. 2, pp. 89–91, 1992.

[10] S. McLaughlin, T. Jones, M. Pitcher, and P. Evans, "Laparoscopic diagnosis of abdominal tuberculosis," *ANZ Journal of Surgery*, vol. 68, no. 8, pp. 599–601, 1998.

[11] A. W. Meshikhes, "Pitfalls of diagnostic laparoscopy in abdominal tuberculosis," *Surgical Endoscopy*, vol. 24, no. 4, pp. 908–910, 2010.

[12] M. Bertlich, M. Paparoupa, H. Wechauf, A. Wittig, S. Linnemuller, and F. Schuppert, "The diagnostic challenge of abdominal tuberculosis in non-endemic countries: a case series from a tertiary hospital in Germany," *Clinical Case Reports*, vol. 9, no. 7, article e04524, 2021.

[13] R. Ahmad, M. Changeez, J. S. Khan et al., "Diagnostic accuracy of peritoneal fluid GeneXpert in the diagnosis of intestinal tuberculosis, keeping histopathology as the gold standard," *Cureus*, vol. 10, no. 10, article e3451, 2018.

14

Antenatal Indomethacin Treatment for Congenital Myotonic Dystrophy

Kyohei Yamaguchi, Hiroaki Tanaka, Fumi H. Furuhashi, Kayo Tanaka, Eiji Kondo, and Tomoaki Ikeda

Department of Obstetrics and Gynecology, Mie University, Mie, Japan

Correspondence should be addressed to Kyohei Yamaguchi; kyokyokyo330@gmail.com

Academic Editor: Kyousuke Takeuchi

Myotonic dystrophy is an autosomal-dominant disorder. Its congenital type is the most severe form, with respiratory failure that can be a life-threatening event after birth. There are no antenatal treatments that can improve neonatal outcomes of myotonic dystrophy. We treated a fetus with congenital myotonic dystrophy by administering indomethacin to the 31-year-old Japanese mother affected by myotonic dystrophy and polyhydramnios. We observed increased fetal breathing movement and a reduction of the amniotic fluid volume. The baby was born at 37 weeks and discharged from the neonatal intensive care unit with a favorable outcome. Indomethacin treatment is likely to improve fetal lung function and to control the amniotic fluid volume. This report emphasizes the importance of further investigations regarding the optimal management of congenital myotonic dystrophy.

1. Introduction

Myotonic dystrophy (DM) is a common autosomal-dominant systemic condition characterized by various symptoms including muscular weakness and atrophy, myotonia, cardiac conduction defects, temporal balding, mental retardation, and various endocrinopathies [1]. The incidence of DM is estimated to be 1 in 8,000 adults. Congenital myotonic dystrophy is the most severe form of DM. Genetically, DM is caused by the expansion of an unstable CTG sequence in the myotonic protein kinase (DMPK) gene at chromosome 19q13.3 [2]. The expansion is observed in parent to child transmission, which is called "anticipation." The anticipation is more frequent and critical when the inheritance occurs from the mothers rather than the fathers [3]. Respiratory failure is the most critical complication of congenital DM, resulting in a high mortality rate in the neonatal period [4]. There are no effective antenatal treatments for a fetus with congenital DM at this time.

We present the case of a fetus with congenital DM who we treated with antenatal indomethacin (which is thought to stimulate fetal breathing movement), with a favorable outcome. We hope this report will encourage further investigations into the optimal treatments for congenital DM.

2. Case Presentation

A 31-year-old primipara Japanese patient by natural conception with a history of miscarriage was referred to our department at 24 weeks of gestation because of polyhydramnios. The amniotic fluid index (AFI) was 32 cm, and there was no evidence of diabetes mellitus or fetal neurologic impairment. Ultrasound examinations showed decreased fetal body movement without any fetal structural anomalies.

At 28 weeks of gestation, blood sampling revealed that the patient's serum creatine phosphokinase (CPK) level was markedly high at 7136 U/L, accompanied by lower-body muscular pain. The physical and neurological examinations showed grip myotonia and percussion myotonia with hatchet face. The patient was diagnosed as having myotonic dystrophy based on electromyographic investigations. DNA testing at 30 weeks and 4 days of gestation revealed an expansion of 1100–1200 abnormal CTG repeats within the myotonin protein kinase gene. The patient's family history was not known.

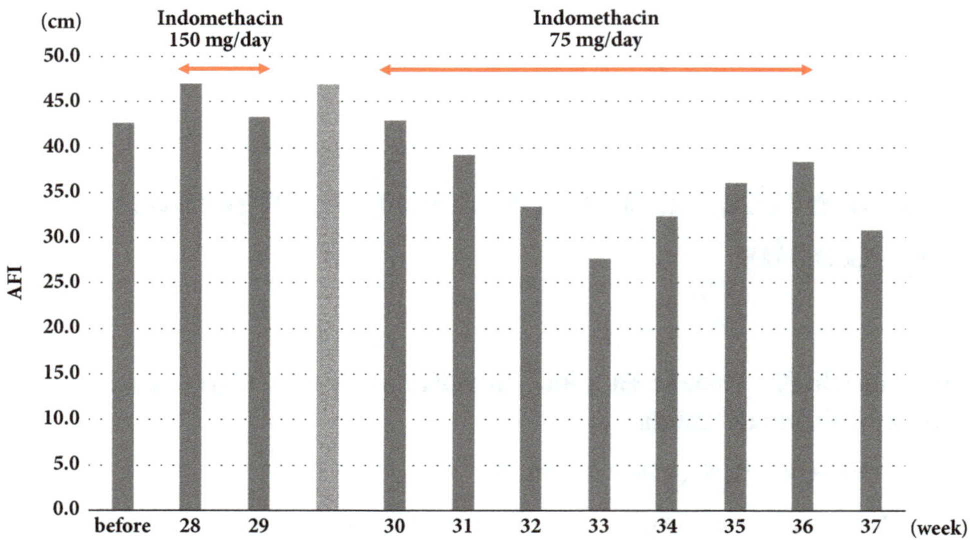

FIGURE 1: Amniotic fluid index (cm). The data are weekly averages. The data in the gray bar are corrected at 29 weeks and 6 days of gestation.

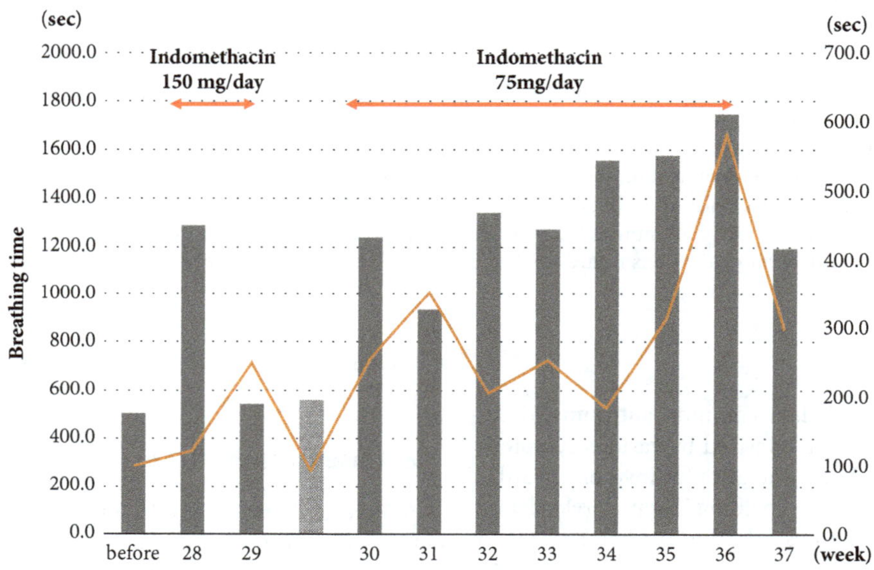

FIGURE 2: Breathing time (sec). The data are weekly averages. The left vertical scale is the total breathing time (shown in the black bar) in 30 min. The right vertical scale is each average breathing time (the orange line). The data in the gray bar are corrected at 29 weeks and 6 days of gestation.

We hypothesized that the prostaglandin inhibitor indomethacin could improve the fetus' lung function. A rectal 150 mg/day of indomethacin was administered to the mother from 28 weeks and 4 days of gestation, and weekly serum sampling and daily ultrasound examinations (at 2:00–3:00 pm) were performed. Fetal breathing movement lasting more than 30 seconds in 30 minutes was counted and total breathing time was measured. However, at 29 weeks and 4 days of gestation the indomethacin administration was stopped temporarily due to constriction of the fetal ductus arteriosus (0.6 mm dia.) [5] and severe tricuspid regurgitation. Thereafter, a rectal 75 mg/day of indomethacin was administered to the mother until 37 weeks of gestation, and the fetal ductal arteriosus returned to a normal value thereafter. The AFI had not increased through the course of the treatment (Figure 1), and no signs of threatened labor were observed. During the indomethacin treatment, a tendency for an increase in both the total breathing time and each average breathing time in 30-min ultrasonographic examinations was observed (Figure 2).

At 37 weeks and 6 days of gestation, we performed an elective cesarean with spinal anesthesia because of the abnormal fetal position. The patient required the support of biphasic positive airway pressure for 24 hr after the operation. The total blood loss was 1.8 L (including amniotic fluid), but the patient did not need any blood transfusion and there were no signs of uterine atony. The patient was discharged 7 days after the operation without any complications.

The female infant's body weight was 2838 g and the Apgar scores were 5 and 6 at 1 and 5 min, respectively. Umbilical cord blood gas studies showed normal values. The newborn was markedly hypotonic with weakness of breathing, and she required intubation for 2 days and oxygen support until day 9. The ductus arteriosus closed at day 23. A physiological examination showed distal dominant hypotonia and swallowing dysfunction, but no arrhythmia, endocrinopathies, cataracts, or sensory-neural hearing loss was observed. A genetic test was performed at day 10 confirming congenital DM by expansion of 1300–1450 abnormal CTG repeats. The baby was discharged from the hospital at day 49.

3. Discussion

Our patient's case provides two important clinical implications. The most striking finding is that an antenatal rectal 75 mg/day of indomethacin has the potential benefit of safely improving fetal breathing movement. Additionally, indomethacin may be a useful drug for preventing threatened preterm labor in patients with DM.

Fetal breathing movements play an important role in lung growth and maturation by the cyclic expansion and retraction of the pulmonary parenchyma. The lung dysfunction of congenital DM fetus comes from both defect of respiratory control system and respiratory muscle function. There is much evidence that prostaglandins (especially PGE2) are responsible for the inhibition of breathing activity, which is controlled mainly at the brainstem [6, 7], since the inhibition of prostaglandins by indomethacin stimulated continuous breathing movement in an animal fetal model [8]. One prospective, randomized, placebo-controlled clinical trial demonstrated that a single dosage of indomethacin (50 mg) increases fetal breathing movement [9]. Although fetal breathing movement becomes episodic and its amplitude deepens with maturation [10], the present case showed an apparent trend of the improvement of both the single-measurements' average and the 30-min total fetal breathing movement.

Indomethacin, a nonsteroidal anti-inflammatory medication that inhibits prostaglandin production, freely crosses the placenta and enters fetal circulation. It is widely used as a tocolytic drug generally limited to short courses of therapy (48–72 h) [11]. However, the optimal dose and course of indomethacin have not been established and remain controversial.

Constriction of the fetal ductus arteriosus is a well-recognized side effect of indomethacin, and tricuspid regurgitation is caused by elevated pressure in the right ventricular outflow tract, producing mild endocardial ischemia with papillary muscle dysfunction. However, these side effects are usually transient and reversible when indomethacin therapy is stopped at an adequate time before delivery. In the present case, the constriction of the fetal ductus arteriosus (0.6 mm dia.) [5] and severe tricuspid regurgitation at 29 weeks and 4 days were resolved after the total rectal indomethacin dose was reduced to 75 mg/day.

Idiopathic polyhydramnios is one of the important expressions of congenital DM that leads to threatened preterm labor. Physiologically, idiopathic polyhydramnios is considered a consequence of reduced or absent fetal swallowing associated with impaired pharyngo-esophageal motility. Unfortunately, there are no useful tocolytic agents for pregnant women with DM because of its side effects such as rhabdomyolysis [12] and maternal respiratory compromise; [13] therefore, indomethacin treatment is recommended instead.

Our present patient similarly presented polyhydramnios during the 3rd trimester as in previous studies [4, 14] and as we had expected, the amniotic fluid volume gradually decreased as a result of reduced fetal urine output without any signs of threatened preterm labor. However, the relative increase of amniotic fluid volume in the late preterm period was unclear, and presumably this reflects the complex mechanisms of the regulation of amniotic fluid volume in utero [15] and depressed swallowing of the affected fetus.

To the best of our knowledge, this is the first report of the indomethacin treatment of a fetus with congenital DM with the goal of ameliorating fetal lung function and controlling the amniotic fluid volume, which eventually helped prevent threatened preterm labor.

We conclude that indomethacin may be an appropriate therapeutic drug for a fetus with congenital DM, as long as careful monitoring and management are performed. Further studies are needed to establish the safe dose and optimal course for indomethacin administration to a fetus with congenital DM.

References

[1] P. S. Harper, "Myotonic disorders," *The Practitioner*, vol. 226, no. 1368, pp. 1065–1071, 1982.

[2] M. Mahadevan, C. Tsilfidis, L. Sabourin et al., "Myotonic dystrophy mutation: an unstable CTG repeat in the 3′ untranslated region of the gene," *Science*, vol. 255, no. 5049, pp. 1253–1255, 1992.

[3] A. L. De Munain, A. Blanco, J. I. Emparanza et al., "Anticipation in myotonic dystrophy: A parental-sex-related phenomenon," *Neuroepidemiology*, vol. 13, no. 1-2, pp. 75–78, 1994.

[4] M. Zaki, P. A. Boyd, L. Impey, A. Roberts, and P. Chamberlain, "Congenital myotonic dystrophy: Prenatal ultrasound findings and pregnancy outcome," *Ultrasound in Obstetrics & Gynecology*, vol. 29, no. 3, pp. 284–288, 2007.

[5] L. Pasquint, M. Mellander, A. Seale et al., "Z-scores of the fetal aortic isthmus and duct: An aid to assessing arch hypoplasia," *Ultrasound in Obstetrics & Gynecology*, vol. 29, no. 6, pp. 628–633, 2007.

[6] R. E. Alvaro, S. U. Hasan, S. Chemtob, M. Qurashi, S. Al-Saif, and H. Rigatto, "Prostaglandins are responsible for the inhibition of breathing observed with a placental extract in fetal sheep," *Respiratory Physiology & Neurobiology*, vol. 144, no. 1, pp. 35–44, 2004.

[7] A. Kelleman, Z. Binienda, X.-Y. Ding, L. Rittenhouse, M. Mitchell, and P. W. Nathanielsz, "Prostaglandin production in the umbilical and uterine circulations in pregnant sheep at 129-136 days gestation," *Journal of Developmental Physiology*, vol. 17, no. 2, pp. 63–67, 1992.

[8] A. H. Jansen, C. De Boeck, S. Ioffe, and V. Chernick, "Indomethacin-induced fetal breathing: mechanism and site of action," *Journal of Applied Physiology*, vol. 57, no. 2, pp. 360–365, 1984.

[9] M. Hallak, K. J. Moise, N. Lira, K. F. Dorman, E. O'Brian Smith, and D. B. Cotton, "The effect of tocolytic agents (indomethacin and terbutaline) on fetal breathing and body movements: A prospective, randomized, double-blind, placebo-controlled clinical trial," *American Journal of Obstetrics & Gynecology*, vol. 167, no. 4, pp. 1059–1063, 1992.

[10] M. Higuchi, H. Hirano, H. Takahashi, O. Mochizuki, M. Maki, and M. Hasegawa, "Human fetal breathing movements: Basic analysis and clinical relationship to fetal well-being (author's transl.)," *Acta Obstetrica Et Gynaecologica Japonica*, vol. 33, no. 5, pp. 597–606, 1981.

[11] "Practice bulletin No.171: management of preterm labor," *Obstetrics & Gynecology*, vol. 128, no. 4, pp. e155–e164, 2016.

[12] M. Ogoyama, H. Takahashi, Y. Kobayashi, R. Usui, and S. Matsubara, "Ritodrine-induced rhabdomyolysis, infantile myotonic dystrophy, and maternal myotonic dystrophy unveiled," *Journal of Obstetrics and Gynaecology Research*, vol. 43, no. 2, pp. 403–407, 2017.

[13] V. Catanzarite, D. Gambling, L. M. Bird, J. Honold, and E. Perkins, "Respiratory compromise after MgSO4 therapy for preterm labor in a woman with myotonic dystrophy: A case report," *Obstetrics, Gynaecology and Reproductive Medicine*, vol. 53, no. 3, pp. 220–222, 2008.

[14] S. Rudnik-Schöneborn and K. Zerres, "Outcome in pregnancies complicated by myotonic dystrophy: A study of 31 patients and review of the literature," *European Journal of Obstetrics & Gynecology and Reproductive Biology*, vol. 114, no. 1, pp. 44–53, 2004.

[15] R. A. Brace and C. Y. Cheung, "Regulation of amniotic fluid volume: evolving concepts," *Advances in Fetal and Neonatal Physiology*, vol. 814, pp. 49–68, 2014.

An Unexpected Case of Intrapartum Pneumomediastinum

Drishti Madhok,[1] **Vinayak Smith**,[2] **and Erik Gunderson**[1]

[1]*Bundaberg Base Hospital, 271 Bourbong St Bundaberg, QLD 4670, Australia*
[2]*Department of Obstetrics and Gynaecology, Monash University, 252 Clayton Road, 3168 VIC, Australia*

Correspondence should be addressed to Drishti Madhok; drishti.madhok@gmail.com

Academic Editor: Maria Grazia Porpora

The dyad of spontaneous pneumomediastinum and subcutaneous emphysema is collectively known as Hamman's syndrome. This rare complication is known to occur during the intrapartum period and its aetiology has been linked to the Valsalva maneuver in the second stage of labour. Nitrous oxide inhalation increases the risk. We present the case of a 21-year-old healthy woman who experienced these symptoms after nitrous oxide inhalation during the second stage of labour.

1. Introduction

Spontaneous pneumomediastinum is defined as free air in the mediastinum without any precipitating cause. Hamman was the first to describe the dyad of spontaneous pneumomediastinum in conjunction with subcutaneous emphysema in a labouring patient in 1939 [1]. Its incidence is now thought to be between 1 in 2000 and 1 in 100,000 deliveries [2]. Alveolar rupture leads to free air tracking through the mediastinum and then into the subcutaneous tissues [1]. We report a case of a 21-year-old healthy nulliparous female who had a normal vaginal birth followed by the presence of Hamman's syndrome 3.5 hours into her postpartum period.

2. Case Report

A 21-year-old healthy nulliparous female presented to a regional hospital in Australia in spontaneous labour at 39 weeks and 4 days of gestation. Her pregnancy was otherwise uncomplicated and she had no medical and surgical history of note.

The patient presented to the hospital with a cervical dilation of 4 cm. Her first stage of labour lasted 1 hr and 45 minutes and her second stage lasted 1 hr and 16 minutes, respectively. Analgesic treatment in the first stage included nitrogen oxide as required and 10 mg of intramuscular morphine. Analgesic used in the second stage was only nitrous oxide as required. An episiotomy was performed at delivery. She delivered a live born infant weighing 3690 g with APGAR scores of 9 and 10. The 3rd stage lasted 15 minutes with delivery of an intact placenta.

After delivery, she further requested nitrous oxide and had 10 mls of 1.0% lignocaine infiltrated into the perineum for an episiotomy repair.

Approximately 2 hours postpartum, the patient started complaining of sudden onset dyspnea and lower chest tightness. Her GCS was 15 at this time and her vital signs were oxygen saturation >95% on room air with a respiratory rate of 18 breaths per minute, pulse of 85 beats per minute, BP 130/78, and a temperature 37.2°C.

Physical examination at the time revealed swelling in the neck and jaw line and palpable crepitus in the anterior chest wall, neck, and jaw, consistent with subcutaneous emphysema.

Initial management included observation and pulse oximetry, as she was clinically stable and able to have a conversation without increase in chest pain or decrease in oxygen saturation.

Subsequently a chest X-ray (CXR) was obtained which demonstrated pneumomediastinum with air tracking superiorly into the pericardiac spaces (Figure 1). Following telephone consultation with a cardiothoracic team at our major tertiary referral center, a computed tomography (CT) contrast study was ordered as recommended. CT contrast reconfirmed pneumomediastinum and subcutaneous emphysema and ruled out esophageal injury (Figure 2). It

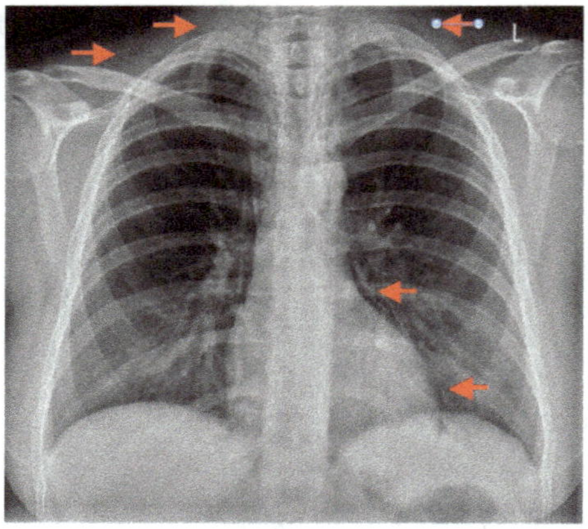

FIGURE 1: CXR confirmed the presence of free air in the pleural spaces and pneumomediastinum.

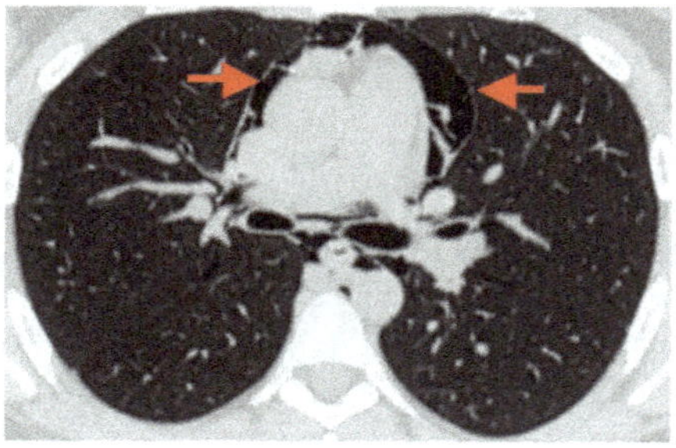

FIGURE 2: CT scan reconfirmed pneumomediastinum and subcutaneous emphysema and ruled out esophageal injury.

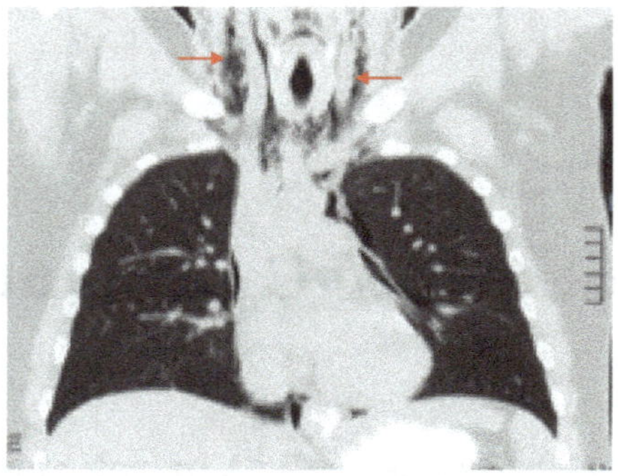

FIGURE 3: CT chest demonstrating extension of air in the cervical region.

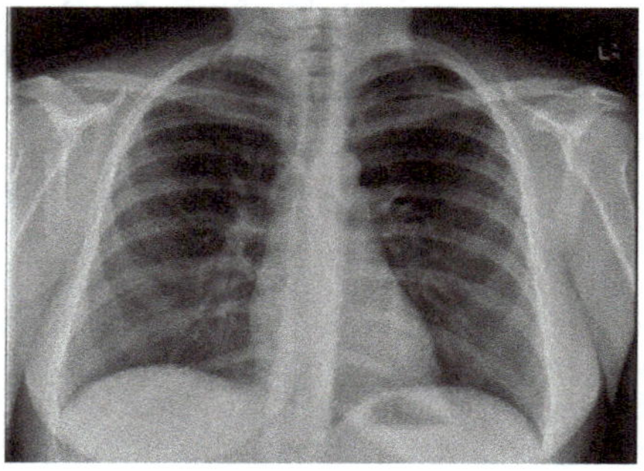

FIGURE 4: Normal CXR-resolution of free air in pleural spaces and pneumomediastinum.

also demonstrated extension of air in the cervical region (Figure 3).

The findings were once again discussed with the cardiothoracic team who advised expectant management due to the stability of the patient's clinical state.

Her postnatal course was uncomplicated thereafter and she only requested routine oral postpartum analgesia such as Panadol and Ibuprofen. Subcutaneous crepitus receded and became minimal by postpartum day 2 for the remainder of her hospital stay. She remained clinically stable and all observations were within normal limits. She was observed for 48 hours postpartum and was discharged on day 2 with the extended midwifery service. A repeat CXR done 2 weeks postpartum was normal and showed resolution of all findings (Figure 4).

3. Discussion

Hamman's syndrome is a rare complication of labour with a prevalence between 1:2000 and 1:100,000 deliveries [1]. Risk factors associated with it include nulliparous patients, prolonged second stage of labour, and any conditions that increase intrathoracic pressure such as coughing or heavy lifting [1]. There have been several documented cases [3–6] over the past 80 years.

3.1. Pathophysiology. The underlying pathophysiology of Hamman's syndrome is likely secondary to the Macklin effect [7]. In their experimental model, Macklin et al. proved that a rise in intra-alveolar pressure leads to terminal alveolar rupture which then allows alveolar air to pass through the perivascular interstitial tissue towards the hilum [7, 8]. The air remains trapped subsequently amongst the mediastinal structures but may eventually leak into the surrounding soft tissues [7, 9]. The air escape into the surrounding structures is facilitated through the fascial planes of the hilum, neck, and diaphragm around the aorta and oesophagus and pleural cavities [7, 8]. It is this air escape which causes the clinical signs of subcutaneous emphysema.

3.1.1. Valsalva Maneuver. The Valsalva maneuver is thought to be contributory due to the increase in intrathoracic pressure it generates. There can be a repetitive and continuous rise in intrathoracic pressure with active pushing in the second stage of labour. There has been a demonstrable association between the length of Valsalva and risk of spontaneous pneumomediastinum [1, 3, 7, 10].

3.1.2. Nitrous Oxide Utilization. Nitrous oxide utilization has been demonstrated as a causative mechanism of spontaneous pneumomediastinum during anaesthesia. It has a lower absorption into blood than the nitrogen component of air due to its lower blood: gas solubility index. This can potentiate abnormal extrapulmonary air spaces within the pulmonary parenchyma [11]. Therefore, contrary to the norm where air filled cavities decrease in size and eventually resolve, nitrogen oxide would tend to expand these cavities potentially leading to primary alveolar rupture or exacerbation of symptoms [12]. Once alveolar rupture occurs, continued use of nitrous oxide will lead to rapid gas dissection along the fascial tissue planes [12].

3.2. Clinical Presentation

3.2.1. Symptoms. Commonly reported symptoms include [1, 5, 8]

(a) substernal pain/chest tightness due to distension of mediastinal space with air [1, 8]

(b) dysphagia due to the tracking of air into the laryngeal and pharyngeal tissue spaces [1, 8, 13]

(c) dysphonia due to the tracking of air into the laryngeal and pharyngeal tissue spaces [1, 1, 8]

(d) dyspnea due to increased air in the mediastinum which can result in pleural and diaphragmatic irritation [1, 8]

3.2.2. Signs [1, 5, 8]. The signs include

(a) subcutaneous and retroperitoneal emphysema due to infiltration of air into the tissues [1, 8]

(b) obliteration of cardiac dullness or altered sounds over the heart due to distension of mediastinal space with air [1, 8]

(c) evidence of increased mediastinal pressure, cyanosis, and engorged veins: rising mediastinal pressure causing obstruction of blood flow to the heart (therefore, the peripheral veins become distended resulting in cyanosis and dyspnea) [1, 8]

(d) pneumothorax which is diagnosed clinically by shortness of breath and hypoxia and confirmed by CXR [8]

3.2.3. Differential Diagnosis. When faced with a clinical presentation of Hamman's syndrome, the following differentials should be considered as well.

(a) Boerhaave's syndrome—spontaneous rupture of the esophagus—is precipitated by increased pressure and presenting with chest pain, dyspnea, pneumomediastinum, and emphysema. Unlike Hamman's syndrome, those who have Boerhaave's syndrome are not clinically stable and require immediate intervention [9, 10].

(b) Pericarditis: the sounds over the heart when air infiltrates the mediastinum consist of crackles/bubbles. They are accentuated in systole and when sitting up as opposed to lying down. This can mimic the "scratching" of pericarditis especially when in conjunction with sternal pain [1, 8].

(c) Myocardial infarction: when air tracks into the mediastinum the pain is usually beneath the sternum and can radiate over the chest and shoulders occasionally down the arms similar to angina [1, 8].

(d) Pulmonary embolus: when air tracks into the mediastinum it can also cause shortness of breath and chest pain also seen in pulmonary embolus [1, 4, 8, 9].

3.3. Management. Spontaneous pneumomediastinum is commonly a benign condition that can be treated conservatively [3–6, 9]. Bed rest, analgesia, and observation to prevent any other secondary complication are adequate [5]. Increasing inspired oxygen via nasal prongs or face mask will resolve any remaining alveolar distension. Symptomatic care can be managed similar to that of the bends from deep sea diving.

4. Conclusion

This case report documents the occurrence of Hamman's syndrome in an otherwise healthy 21-year-old patient. As a very rare complication of labour, we wish to add to the available literature. Commonly thought to occur as a result of alveolar barotrauma, this case highlights the interaction of Valsalva pushing and nitrous oxide use. Diagnosis is usually established via physical exam and routine CXR and/or CT. It is usually a benign condition that resolves spontaneously without significant morbidity.

References

[1] L. Hamman, "Mediastinal emphysema the frank billings lecture," *Journal of the American Medical Association*, vol. 128, no. 1, pp. 1–6, 1945.

[2] K. Vasileios, P. Konstantinos, L. Geirge, B. Sofia et al., "Pneumomediastinum," *Journal of Thoracic Disease*, vol. 7, Suppl. 1, pp. 44–49, 2015.

[3] E. M. Karson, D. Saltzman, and M. R. Davis, "Pneumomediastinum in pregnancy: two case reports and a review of the literature, pathophysiology, and management," *Obstetrics & Gynecology*, vol. 64, no. 3, pp. 39–43, 1984.

[4] S. R. Reeder, "Subcutaneous emphysema, pneumomediastinum, and pneumothorax in labor and delivery," *American Journal of Obstetrics & Gynecology*, vol. 154, no. 3, pp. 487–489, 1986.

[5] M. Unlu, P. Cimen, and E. Oner, "An unusual cause of cough: hammans syndrome," *International Journal of Scientific Study*, vol. 3, no. 6, pp. 214–216, 2015.

[6] G. Kosmak, "The occurrence of subcutaneous emphysema in labour," *Bull Lying-In Hosp NY*, vol. 3, no. 76, 1925.

[7] M. T. Macklin and C. C. Macklin, "Malignant interstitial emphysema as an important occult complication in many respiratory diseases and other conditions: an interpretation of the clinical literature in the light of laboratory experiment," *Medicine*, pp. 281–314, 1944.

[8] L. S. Gaspar, "Hamman's syndrome: Pneumomediastinum and subcutaneous emphysema occurring in labour," *International Journal of Obstetric Anesthesia*, vol. 6, no. 1, pp. 55–58, 1997.

[9] G. J. Koullias, D. P. Korkolis, X. J. Wang, and G. L. Hammond, "Current assessment and management of spontaneous pneumomediastinum: experience in 24 adult patients," *European Journal of Cardio-Thoracic Surgery*, vol. 25, no. 5, pp. 852–855, 2004.

[10] S. Kelly, S. Hughes, S. Nixon, and S. Paterson-Brown, "Spontaneous pneumomediastinum (Hamman's syndrome)," *Journal of the Royal Colleges of Surgeons of Edinburgh and Ireland*, vol. 8, no. 2, pp. 63–66, 2010.

[11] E. S. Munson, "Transfer of nitrous oxide into body air cavities," *British Journal of Anaesthesia*, vol. 46, no. 3, pp. 202–208, 1974.

[12] T. J. Poulton, L. W. Haldeman, and E. S. Munson, "Nitrous oxide administration in the presence of subcutaneous emphysema: an experimental model," *Canadian Anaesthetists' Society Journal*, vol. 29, no. 5, pp. 435–438, 1982.

A Case of Type I Sirenomelia Complicated by Severe Oligohydramnios in the First Trimester

Atsushi Yoshida, Asumi Okumura, Masahiro Nakao, and Ryo Suzuki

Department of Obstetrics and Gynecology, Sakakibara Heart Institute, Fuchu, Tokyo, Japan

Correspondence should be addressed to Atsushi Yoshida; yoshida.atsushi@nifty.ne.jp

Academic Editor: Maria Grazia Porpora

Sirenomelia is a very rare congenital anomaly. Type I is the mildest type, and the long bone structures are all normally present with only soft tissue fusion. We experienced a case of type I sirenomelia complicated by severe oligohydramnios. Because of severe oligohydramnios, ultrasonographic images were not very clear. The associated findings with sirenomelia (single umbilical artery and bilateral renal agenesis) were helpful for the prenatal diagnosis of this disease. Detailed sonographic examination of the fetus was thought to be necessary for the accurate prenatal diagnosis of sirenomelia.

1. Introduction

Sirenomelia is a very rare congenital anomaly, and its incidence is reported to be 0.8 to 1 case per 100,000 births [1]. Sirenomelia is characterized by various kinds of fusions of the lower extremities and usually complicated by dysgenesis or agenesis of the kidneys, ureters, and urinary bladder. In most cases, it is also associated with single umbilical arteries. Because of the dysgenesis of the urinary system, sirenomelia is usually complicated by severe oligohydramnios in the second and third trimesters of gestation. Oligohydramnios may cause poor visualization in the ultrasonographic images, and it is not easy to make a diagnosis of sirenomelia in the second and third trimesters. Therefore, it is very difficult to diagnose sirenomelia with oligohydramnios, especially in cases with the normal number of long bones. We experienced a case of type I sirenomelia complicated by severe oligohydramnios at 13 weeks of gestation. We consider that this is the first report on type I sirenomelia with severe oligohydramnios diagnosed in the first trimester.

2. Case Presentation

The patient was a 22-year-old nulliparous Japanese woman. Her medical and family histories were noncontributory. She had no previous history of smoking, habitual alcohol drinking, or drug abuse. She was referred to our hospital for fetal anatomical evaluation because of severe oligohydramnios at 13 weeks and 6 days of gestation. The gestational age was calculated from the first day of her last menstrual period. At her 10 weeks and 6 days' visit to the previous clinic, the crown-rump length of the fetus was 34.7 mm and no remarkable abnormalities of amniotic fluid volume were recorded. However, at 13 weeks and 4 days of gestation, a remarkable decrease in the amniotic fluid volume was found. At the first visit to our hospital, we carried out an antenatal ultrasonographic scan and a single live fetus was noted. The crown-rump length, biparietal diameter, and nuchal translucency of the fetus were 66.1 mm, 23.6 mm, and 2.1 mm, respectively. Because of severe oligohydramnios (Figure 1), ultrasonographic images were not very clear, and no clear 3D images were obtained. As far as we could check, no structural abnormalities were found in the fetal cranium, brain, upper extremities, thorax, and heart. However, the lower extremities remained in the fixed extension, but all long bones were visible (Figure 2). The lower extremities stayed in the same position, and no individual movements of the two legs were seen, which suggested the fusion of the two lower extremities. Color Doppler ultrasound revealed a single umbilical artery (Figure 3). Neither kidneys nor the urinary bladder was

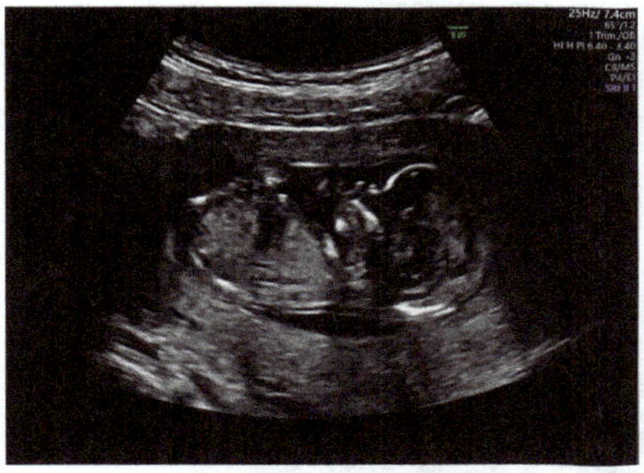

Figure 1: Gray-scale ultrasonography at the 13 weeks of gestation. Severe oligohydramnios was noted.

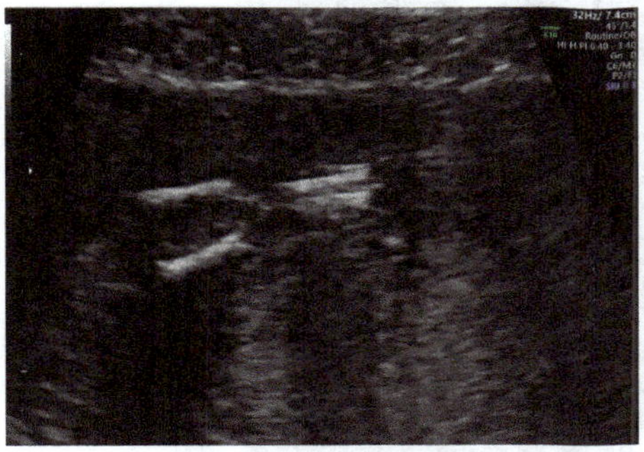

Figure 2: Gray-scale ultrasonography at the 14 weeks of gestation. Two femurs, two tibiae, and two fibulae were visualized.

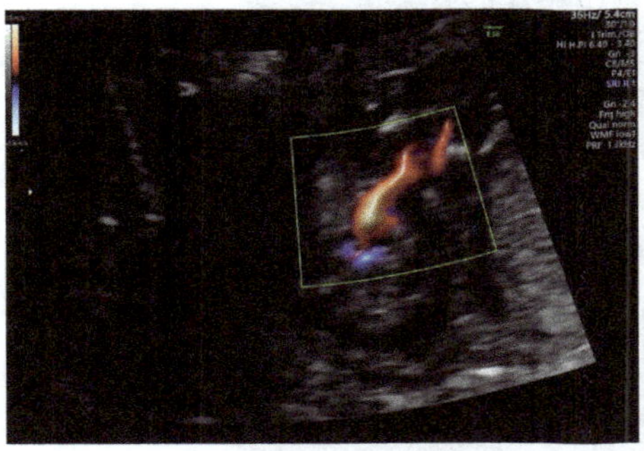

Figure 3: Color Doppler ultrasonography at the 13 weeks of gestation. A single umbilical artery was seen.

visualized. Therefore, the diagnosis of type I sirenomelia was made prenatally.

The couple was informed about the findings and the suspected poor prognosis of the fetus. They then opted to have a termination of pregnancy, which was performed at 15 weeks and 1 day of gestation. On the postnatal examination, the baby weighed 60 grams and the external examination revealed the fusion of both lower extremities (Figure 4). The external genitalia and anal structures of the baby were ambiguous. Postmortem imaging studies with the radiography and CT scans revealed a single lower limb containing two femurs, two tibiae, and two fibulae, and none of them were fused (Figure 5(a)). Agenesis of the lower lumbar and sacral spines was also noted (Figure 5(b)).

A 75 g oral glucose tolerance test (OGTT) was performed 2 days postpartum, which showed a mildly impaired glucose

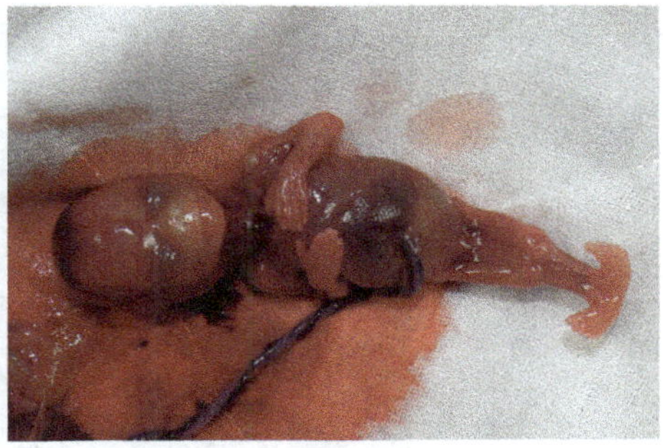

Figure 4: Macroscopic image of the delivered baby. A fused single lower extremity was noted.

tolerance pattern of the mother (Figure 6(a)). At 17 weeks postpartum, another OGTT was carried out and the blood glucose levels were in the normal range (Figure 6(b)).

3. Discussion

Stocker and Heifetz classified sirenomelia into 7 types by the degree of fusion of lower extremities' bones (Figure 7) [2]. Type I is the mildest type, and the long bone structures are all normally present with only soft tissue fusion. We found no clear-cut data of the prenatal diagnostic rate by Stocker and Heifetz's classifications of sirenomelia, but Langer and colleagues reported that the difficulty of prenatal diagnosis depends on the shape of the lower extremity (the symelia apus, unipus, or dipus), and the dipus type is the most difficult to make a prenatal diagnosis [3]. Therefore, it is suspected that type I sirenomelia by Stocker and Heifetz's classifications is the least easy to make a prenatal diagnosis. In other types, the abnormality in the number of long bones may be a great help for the diagnosis of sirenomelia. In type I sirenomelia, however, it may be difficult to make a diagnosis by prenatal ultrasonography only with the abnormality in fetal soft tissue.

To detect the soft tissue abnormalities, 3D images of ultrasound are thought to be useful, but it is difficult to obtain clear 3D images in cases with anhydramnios or severe oligohydramnios. Langer and colleagues reported that it is difficult to make a prenatal diagnosis of this disease when complicated by severe oligohydramnios [3]. As far as we could check, we found no previous reports of type I sirenomelia with severe oligohydramnios diagnosed in the first trimester. In our case, we could not obtain clear 3D images of the fetus because of severe oligohydramnios. Some authors proposed to carry out amnioinfusion to obtain clearer ultrasound images when the case is complicated by severe oligohydramnios [4, 5]. However, we think that this invasive procedure is not necessary when the baby's prognosis is thought to be poor, and actually, in this case, we did not perform amnioinfusion.

The associated findings with sirenomelia may be helpful for the prenatal diagnosis of this disease. Table 1 shows the common complications of sirenomelia [6]. In our case, agenesis of the lower lumbar and sacral spines and the presence of the single umbilical artery were noted. Bilateral renal agenesis was also suspected. These abnormalities have been suspected

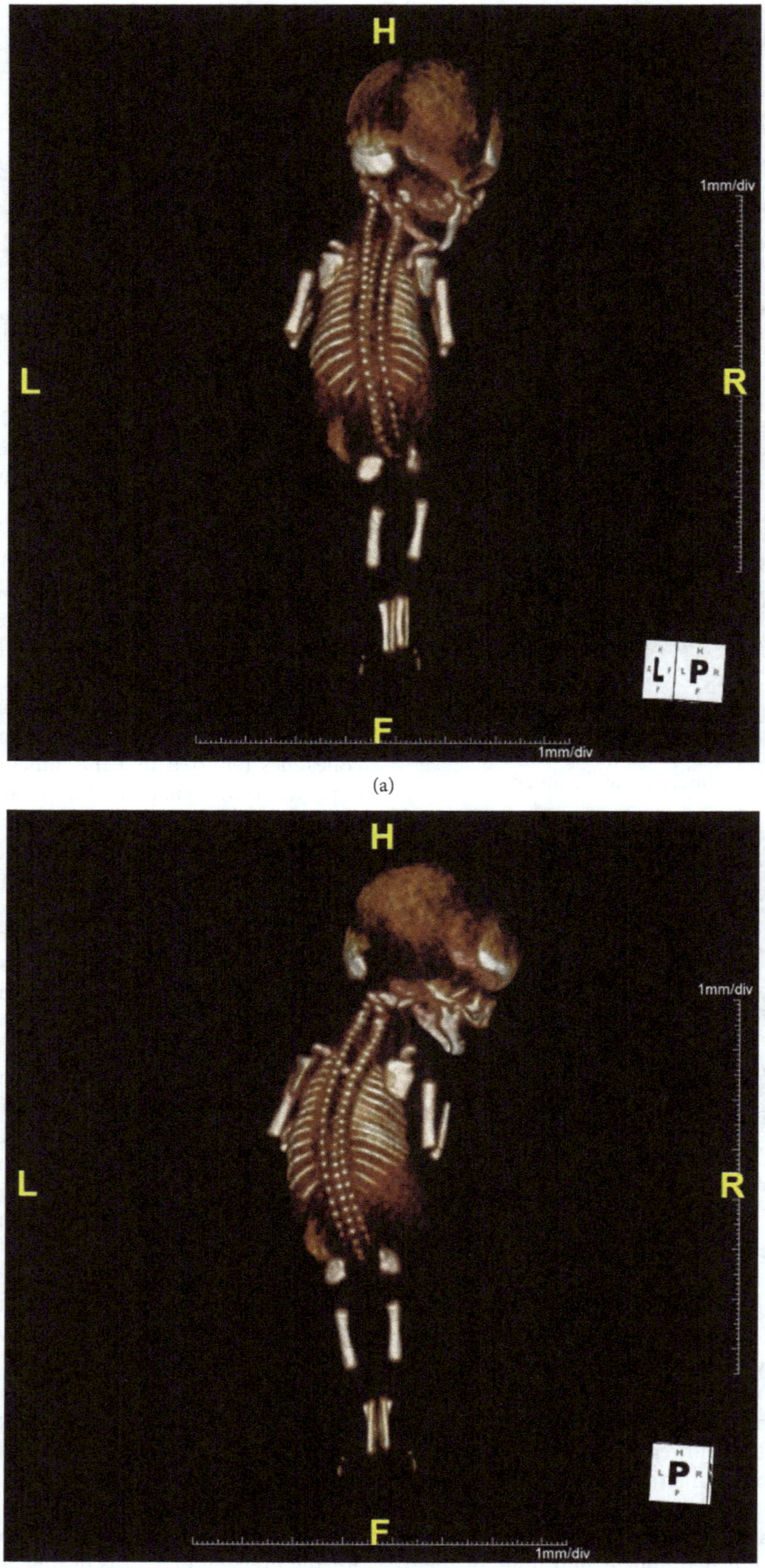

(a)

(b)

FIGURE 5: Postmortem CT images of the delivered baby. Two femurs, two tibiae, and two fibulae were contained in the single lower limb, and none of them was fused (a). Agenesis of lower lumbar and sacral spines was noted (b).

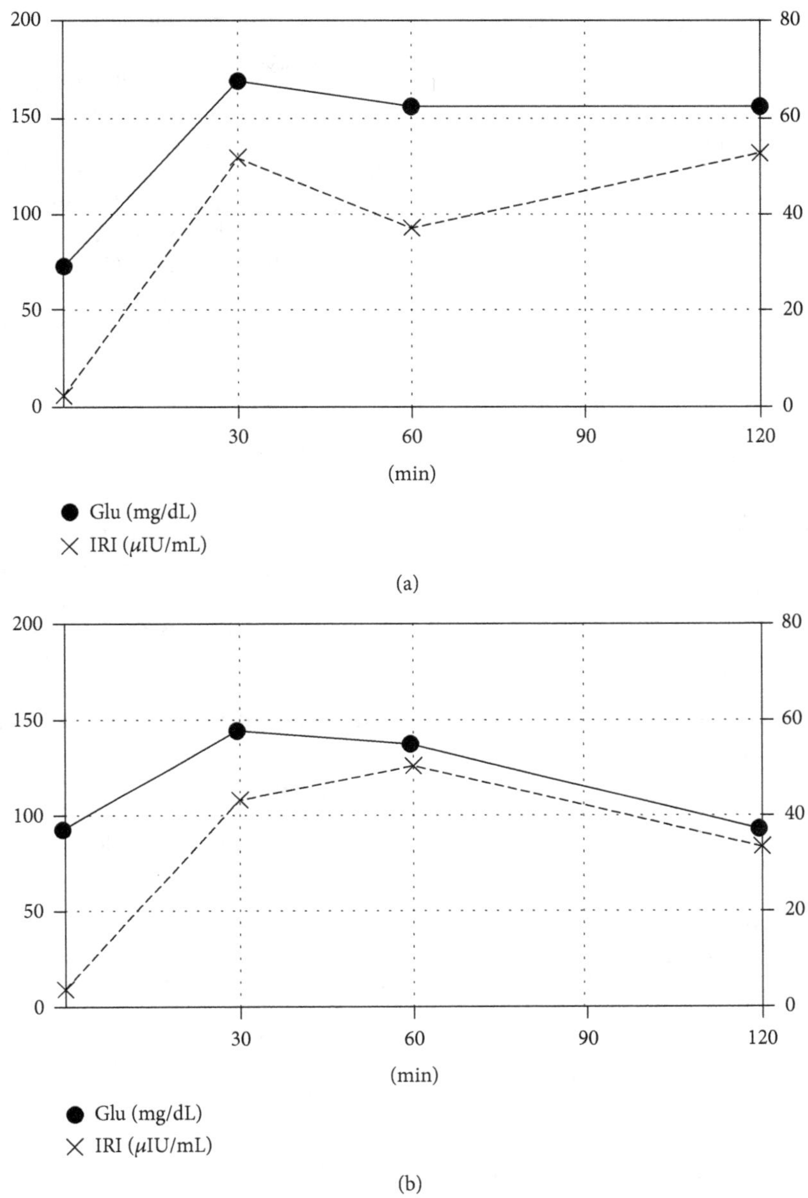

FIGURE 6: Results of the 75 g oral glucose tolerance test. (a) Two days postpartum: HOMA − R = 0.47, QUICKI = 0.44, MI = 9.38, DI = 4.81, and II = 0.51. (b) Seventeen weeks postpartum: HOMA − R = 0.82, QUICKI = 0.40, MI = 8.02, DI = 6.08, and II = 0.76. HOMA-R: homeostasis model assessment insulin resistance; QUICKI: quantitative insulin-sensitivity check index; MI: Matsuda index; DI: disposition index; II: insulinogenic index.

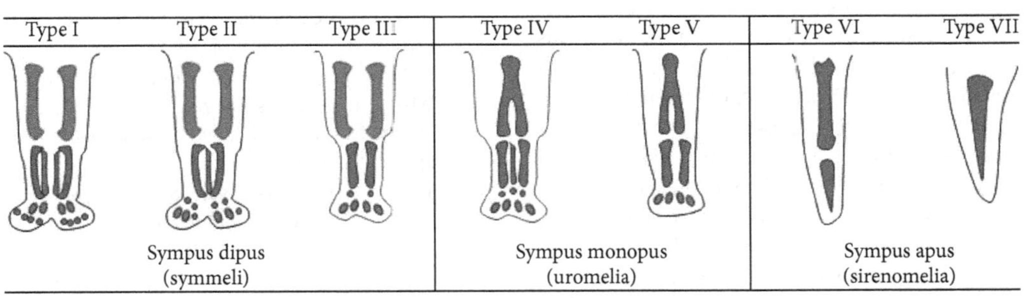

FIGURE 7: Classification of sirenomelia by Stocker and Heifetz [2]. Type I: all bones of thigh and lower leg present; type II: fused fibula; type III: fibula absent; type IV: partially fused femur, fused fibula; type V: partially fused femur, fibula absent; type VI: fused femur, fused tibia; type VII: fused femur, tibia absent.

Table 1: Possible associated abnormalities with sirenomelia.

Urogenital
Renal agenesis
Multicystic dysplastic kidneys (rare)
Genital ambiguity/absence of external genitalia
Müllerian anomalies
Cloacal abnormalities
Gastrointestinal tract
Anorectal atresia
Sacral agenesis
Skeletal
Neural tube defects
Lumbosacral dysgenesis/agenesis
Sacral agenesis
Varying degrees of limb reduction, soft tissue fusion of lower extremities, single lower extremity
Hypoplasia/aplasia of pelvic girdle
Complex fusion of feet (sympodia)
Absent feet
Radial ray abnormalities
Phocomelia
Rotational abnormalities of lower limbs
Hip dislocation
Others
Single umbilical artery (virtually always present) Vestigial tail
Cardiac system anomalies (less common)
Central nervous system anomalies (less common)

*Listed based on Reference [6].

by prenatal ultrasound, and they were great help to diagnose sirenomelia.

As we described above, sirenomelia is often associated with agenesis or dysgenesis of bilateral kidneys. Even in the first trimester, it is possible to identify both kidneys with careful ultrasound examination, but recognizing oligohydramnios as a consequence of renal agenesis or dysgenesis in the second trimester is much easier. It is reported that usually, the onset of renal oligohydramnios starts after 16 weeks of gestation when amniotic fluid production is primarily renal in origin [7]. Therefore, the suspicion of renal agenesis before 15 weeks is sometimes challenging. Several cases with renal oligohydramnios before 15 weeks have been reported. Klaassen and colleagues reviewed 21 cases of renal oligohydramnios and reported that one of the 21 cases was detected at 14 weeks of gestation [8]. Ceylan and colleagues reported a case of sirenomelia diagnosed at 12 weeks of gestation [9], and they said that their case was complicated by oligohydramnios. However, they reported that they could obtain 3D ultrasound images of the fetus, which means that oligohydramnios in their case was not very severe. In our case, the cause of severe oligohydramnios at 13 weeks of gestation was not clear. It is said that the primary site of amniotic fluid production before 14 weeks of gestation is the amnion, but in our case, no pathological findings of the amnion were reported in the histopathological examination.

The causes of malformation in sirenomelia remain unknown, but it is reported that maternal diabetes mellitus is one of the possible causative factors of sirenomelia [10]. In our case, OGTTs were carried out 2 days and 17 weeks postpartum. The OGTT done after 2 days postpartum revealed a mildly impaired glucose tolerance pattern of the mother. However, the OGTT result after 17 weeks was normal. Therefore, we think that sirenomelia in our case was not directly caused by glucose intolerance. The mother had no other risk factors, and in this case, the etiology of sirenomelia remained unclear.

4. Conclusion

We experienced a case of type I sirenomelia complicated by severe oligohydramnios. Prenatal diagnosis of sirenomelia with severe oligohydramnios may be difficult, especially in type I sirenomelia in which all long bones are visible. The associated findings with sirenomelia may be helpful for the prenatal diagnosis of this disease. Detailed sonographic examination of the fetus was thought to be necessary for the prenatal diagnosis of sirenomelia.

Disclosure

The summary of this article was presented at the 29th World Congress on Ultrasound in Obstetrics and Gynecology (ISUOG 2019, Berlin).

Acknowledgments

The authors would like to thank Professor Emeritus Mitsunao Kobayashi of the National Defense Medical College for supporting them.

References

[1] B. Kallen, E. E. Castilla, P. A. Lancaster et al., "The cyclops and the mermaid: an epidemiological study of two types of rare malformation," *Journal of Medical Genetics*, vol. 29, no. 1, pp. 30–35, 1992.

[2] J. T. Stocker and S. A. Heifetz, "Sirenomelia. A morphological study of 33 cases and review of the literature," *Perspectives in Pediatric Pathology*, vol. 10, pp. 7–50, 1987.

[3] B. Langer, C. Stoll, R. Nicolau, B. Gasser, and G. Schlaeder, "Sirenomelia and situs inversus: case report and review of the literature," *Fetal Diagnosis and Therapy*, vol. 11, no. 1, pp. 79–84, 1996.

[4] M. C. Haeusler, G. Ryan, S. C. Robson, S. Lipitz, and C. H. Rodeck, "The use of saline solution as a contrast medium in suspected diaphragmatic hernia and renal agenesis," *American Journal of Obstetrics and Gynecology*, vol. 168, no. 5, pp. 1486–1492, 1993.

[5] A. Adra, D. Cordero, A. Mejides, S. Yasin, F. Salman, and M. J. O'Sullivan, "Caudal regression syndrome: etiopathogenesis, prenatal diagnosis, and perinatal management," *Obstetrical & Gynecological Survey*, vol. 49, no. 7, pp. 508–516, 1994.

[6] J. L. B. Byrne, *Sirenomelia. Diagnostic Imaging Obstetrics*, Elsevier, Basel, Switzerland, Third edition, 2016.

[7] A. Abuhamad and R. Chaoui, "The fetal nrogenital system," in *First Trimester Ultrasound Diagnosis of Fetal Abnormalities*, pp. 255–280, 218 Wolster Kluwer, 2017.

[8] I. Klaassen, T. J. Neuhaus, D. E. Mueller-Wiefel, J. Markus, and M. J. Kemper, "Antenatal oligohydramnios of renal origin: long_term outcome," *Nephrology Dialysis Transplantation*, vol. 22, no. 2, pp. 432–439, 2007.

[9] Y. Ceylan, Y. Doğan, S. Ö. Özdemir, and G. Yücesoy, "Prenatal diagnosis of sirenomelia in the first trimester: a case report," *Journal of Turkish Society of Obstetric and Gynecology*, vol. 13, no. 1, pp. 50–52, 2016.

[10] M. Valenzano, R. Paoletti, A. Rossi, D. Farinini, G. Garlaschi, and E. Fulcheri, "Sirenomelia. Pathological features, antenatal ultrasonographic clues and a review of current embryogenic theories," *Human Reproduction Update*, vol. 5, no. 1, pp. 82–86, 1999.

17

Delayed Interval Delivery in Preterm Premature Rupture of Membranes in Dichorionic Triamniotic Triplets: Ethical Considerations for Maternal Health Case Report

Ali Hosiani[1] **James Brown,**[2] **and Indika T. Alahakoon**[2]

[1]*Department of Obstetrics & Gynaecology, Blacktown Hospital, Blacktown, New South Wales, Australia*
[2]*Department of Maternal Foetal Medicine, Westmead Hospital, Westmead, New South Wales, Australia*

Correspondence should be addressed to Ali Hosiani; ali.hosiani@health.nsw.gov.au

Academic Editor: Giovanni Monni

Background. Although there are numerous studies on delayed interval delivery in twins, this study is one of few reporting on preterm premature rupture of membranes in triplets and even fewer on dichorionic triamniotic triplet twins. The case presented here highlights the important interplay between informed consent and patient autonomy. *Case Presentation.* A 37-year-old woman gravida 1, para 0 with a dichorionic triamniotic triplet pregnancy experienced preterm premature rupture of membranes of the singleton triplet at 15 weeks and six days of gestation. Delayed interval delivery was offered to the parents, who chose to continue the pregnancy while acknowledging the risks for maternal and foetal health. The patient was treated with prophylactic intravenous antibiotics and discharged on oral antibiotics after an eight-day admission. Two days after being discharged, she was readmitted with clinical signs of chorioamnionitis. Within six hours, the preterm premature rupture of membranes singleton was delivered. Three days later, she again presented to the hospital with preterm premature rupture of membranes of one of the dichorionic twins. After discussion with the maternal foetal medicine team, the parents chose to terminate the pregnancy. Delayed interval delivery was not successful in this patient, and it is unclear at which gestational age it is too early to offer expectant management. *Conclusions.* The case affirmed the very poor foetal survival rate when the first delivery occurs at under 20 weeks' gestation. A standardised management of delayed interval delivery should be established to assist with consistent parental counselling.

1. Introduction

Multiple pregnancies carry greater risks to maternal and foetal health than singleton pregnancies [1]. These risks include miscarriage, preterm premature rupture of membranes (PPROM), and preterm birth. PPROM complicates 3% of all pregnancies and is associated with up to 30% of preterm births [2]. Up to 36% of twin and 28% of triplet pregnancies are affected by PPROM before 28 weeks of gestation [3, 4]. The incidence of PPROM has increased in the past decade, primarily due to the increased use of assisted reproductive technologies [5].

2. Case Presentation

A 37-year-old woman (gravida 1, para 0) became pregnant with dichorionic triamniotic (DCTA) triplets following the transfer of two fresh embryos. She underwent in vitro fertilisation (IVF) due to a history of grade 4 endometriosis. The patient's treatment for endometriosis had included multiple laparoscopic surgeries: a left salpingectomy, a small bowel resection, and a stent insertion for a left ureteric stricture. An early dating scan at eight weeks and two days of gestation confirmed that foetus A was a singleton while foetuses B and C were diamniotic twins. The foetal biometry of triplet B was smaller by four days compared to the other two foetuses. Her antenatal serology was unremarkable except for subclinical hypothyroidism and vitamin D deficiency. She was managed in a tertiary maternal foetal medicine unit from 12 weeks' gestation.

The patient was counselled about the foetal and maternal risks of a triplet pregnancy and was given the option of selective foetal reduction. An early structural scan at 12 weeks' gestation was unremarkable. After the scan, she continued to take early pregnancy progesterone pessaries (200 mg nocte) and aspirin (150 mg daily), in addition to pregnancy multivitamins.

At 15 weeks and 6 days of gestation, the patient presented to hospital with spontaneous PPROM of the singleton pregnancy. She was admitted and commenced on intravenous ampicillin and gentamicin. The couple were extensively counselled about the poor prognosis of her pregnancy with PPROM at such early gestation and the possible poor maternal sequala if she developed chorioamnionitis. Given her history of infertility, they decided to continue with conservative management. After an eight-day admission, the patient was sent home on oral phenoxymethylpenicillin. The patient's progress was monitored by measuring her inflammatory markers weekly (as an outpatient) and her temperature daily, and the foetal heart rate was monitored regularly.

Two days after discharge, at 17 weeks and 3 days of gestation, she represented to the emergency department with increased vaginal spotting and discharge. She was tachycardic, and her inflammatory markers were increased. She was diagnosed with chorioamnionitis. After multiple vasovagal episodes, a speculum revealed an open cervix with a foot in the vagina. The foetus was delivered manually, with the placenta left in situ, and the umbilical cord was clamped and left in the vaginal vault.

Ultrasound assessment at this stage showed a viable monochorionic diamniotic (MCDA) twin pregnancy with foetus B estimated to weigh in the 7th centile and foetus C on the 16th centile. Although there was some disparity in growth, no evidence of twin-to-twin transfusion syndrome was observed. The patient was again managed as an outpatient and monitored for signs of chorioamnionitis. Rotating antibiotics were commenced, alternating between erythromycin 500 mg BD and clindamycin 300 mg BD to reduce the risk of antimicrobial resistance.

At 18 weeks and three days of gestation, the patient represented with PPROM of one MCDA twin. Despite initial intravenous antibiotic therapy, the patient had ongoing signs of sepsis: febrile, hypotensive, and tachycardic. The parents were counselled about the worsening maternal condition secondary to chorioamnionitis. This was the fourth and final counselling session for the pregnancy, and they chose to proceed with induction of labour at 18 weeks and three days of gestation. The partner was always supportive of the patient's decisions. The delivery was uneventful.

Histopathology of the two separate placental discs revealed necrotising chorioamnionitis, a sign of maternal inflammatory response. No foetal response was observed in all three umbilical cords.

The patient was followed up in the preconception clinic four months after the delivery of her remaining twins. She was keen to try another cycle of IVF using her stored frozen embryos. It was recommended that she only have one embryo transferred in future, to avoid the complications she experienced in her previous pregnancy. The patient was advised that the outcome of her previous pregnancy was likely due to the multiple embryo transfer and resulting triplet pregnancy.

3. Discussion

This study illustrates a rare case of failed DID in a DCTA pregnancy affected by PPROM in the second trimester. The patient's willingness to persevere despite potential severe maternal morbidity reflects a highly valued pregnancy after a long-standing history of complicated primary infertility. The events raise important questions about the ethics of avoidable maternal sequelae in pregnancies unlikely to result in a good long-term outcome.

3.1. Maternal Morbidity and Delayed Interval Delivery. Maternal morbidity is common with DID. Up to half of the documented patients suffer intrauterine infections leading to fulminant maternal sepsis [5, 6].

A systematic review conducted by Cheung et al. included three cases of DCTA triplets [1]. The study concluded that DID is associated with improved perinatal outcomes for those second twins/triplet pregnancies when the first twin is delivered between 20 and 29 weeks [1]. A prospective cohort study reported on one DCTA triplet pregnancy, which was delayed by only five days. However, the mean delay in all the triplet pregnancies was 18 days in comparison to 19 days in twins [3]. There were 12 triplet pregnancies in the cohort study, among which seven triplets were born before 25 weeks. None of the initial foetuses survived, and only two remaining triplets from the same pregnancy survived with a DID of 118 days [1]. However, these patients had received tocolysis as part of their DID protocol.

Our patient was 15 weeks and six days of gestation when she experienced PPROM of the singleton triplet. This rupture occurred in the previable period. The literature indicates that for DID to be considered, the following conditions should not be present: nonreassuring foetal status, congenital abnormalities, rupture of membranes of the remaining foetus, chorioamnionitis, and/or severe haemorrhage, which is a sign of placental abruption [3]. This case did not have any of these conditions initially and was, therefore, deemed appropriate for DID.

3.2. Patient Factors and Decision-Making in Delayed Interval Delivery. Despite the patient being at previable gestation and the literature reporting survival of the remaining foetuses to be as low as 29% [1], other factors were considered in the decision-making process. The patient was a primiparous woman with an IVF pregnancy and a significant history of endometriosis requiring multiple laparoscopic procedures to correct her pathology. These factors undoubtedly influenced the parents' decision to continue the pregnancy despite extensive counselling on the maternal risks. There are documented cases of similar situations where one or more of the babies has reached viability.

Wooldridge et al. reported on a trichorionic triamniotic pregnancy of a 27-year-old woman who experienced a miscarriage of one triplet at home. The patient was given a rescue cerclage and treated with antibiotics and daily progesterone suppositories until delivery. She delivered two babies at 31 weeks' gestation. The babies were in good condition but required ventilatory support for 72 hours. There were no specific maternal complications [7].

Ghorbani and Moghadam reported on a PPROM and delivery of a foetus in a triplet pregnancy despite a cerclage being performed early in the pregnancy. The placenta did not expel spontaneously and was left in situ. The patient was discharged following administration of prophylactic antibiotics and tocolysis. She subsequently gave birth via caesarean section at 33 weeks and four days of gestation to two babies with good agars but who required admission to the neonatal intensive care unit [8].

Therefore, it appears the choice to offer conservative management throughout the pregnancy was appropriately informed by the published literature. The woman and her partner were counselled at many stages of the pregnancy and given the opportunity to think of their options and ask questions. The partner was always very supportive of the patient's decisions and actively involved in the discussions.

3.3. Antibiotic Choice in Delayed Interval Delivery. After the delivery of the singleton triplet, the patient was treated with the same antibiotics mentioned above. There is no published recommended routine antibiotic regimen, duration, or route, but most clinicians have opted for administration of prophylactic therapy [5, 6, 9, 10]. Most of the antibiotics of choice were the same as those typically used for PPROM, as it is believed that the cause and route of infections are essentially the same [5].

When the patient was stepped down to rotating erythromycin and clindamycin, this was an improvised approach followed in the absence of standard protocols for antimicrobials in DID. Our centre used rotating antibiotics as a standard treatment for PPROM, which was done to prevent antibiotic resistance [11].

3.4. Delayed Interval Delivery and Cervical Cerclage. A cervical cerclage was not performed in this case as an ultrasound showed the cervix to be long and closed. The idea behind cerclage in DID is that it can only stabilise the cervix but minimise exposure of the foetal membranes to vaginal bacteria [12]. Some authors have opted for routine cervical cerclage [5], while others have not [5, 12–14]. The idea of cerclage is controversial without cervical incompetence as some suggest that the actual procedure puts the patient at risk of further infection and can contribute to the rupture of membranes of the remaining foetus [15]. As there is no consensus or adequate evidence on the application of cervical cerclage, it is difficult to determine if having performed it routinely in the patient, who did not show evidence of cervical incompetence and was on progesterone, would have resulted in an alternative outcome. However, it was an appropriate decision to not perform cervical cerclage when the patient presented with PPROM of one MCDA twin only seven days after delivering the first triplet.

A study on obstetric DID with and without cerclage in twin and triplet pregnancies found that cerclage may provide a longer interval. However, there is no consensus on the best treatment protocol, and each case should be evaluated individually [16].

4. Conclusion

Although there are numerous studies on PPROM in twins, this study is one of few reporting on PPROM in triplets and even fewer on DCTA twins. None of the triplets survived, and the delay was short-lived, lasting seven days, limited by the reoccurrence of PPROM in the remaining triplet. The case affirmed the very poor foetal survival rate (29%) when the first delivery occurs at under 20 weeks' gestation.

The case presented here highlights the important interplay between informed consent and patient autonomy. Throughout the pregnancy, the patient was included in therapeutic discussions and, ultimately, chose the course of action that she thought was best for her and her pregnancy.

Abbreviations

PPROM:	Preterm premature rupture of membranes
DID:	Delayed interval delivery
DCTA triplets:	Dichorionic triamniotic
MCDA:	Monochorionic diamniotic
IVF:	In vitro fertilisation.

Consent

The patient has provided us with written informed consent for their personal and clinical details along with any images to be published in this study.

Authors' Contributions

AH was involved in the care of the patient and put together the manuscript. IA was involved in the care of the patient and contributed in editing the manuscript. JB was involved in the care of the patient and contributed in editing the manuscript.

References

[1] K. W. Cheung, M. T. Y. Seto, W. Wang, C. W. S. Lai, M. D. Kilby, and E. H. Y. Ng, "Effect of delayed interval delivery of remaining fetus(es) in multiple pregnancies on survival: a systematic review and meta-analysis," *American Journal of Obstetrics and Gynecology*, vol. 222, no. 4, pp. 306–319.e18, 2020.

[2] G. Abou El Senoun, T. Dowswell, and H. Mousa, "Planned home versus hospital care for preterm prelabour rupture of the membranes (PPROM) prior to 37 weeks' gestation," *Cochrane Database of Systematic Reviews*, vol. 14, 2014.

[3] B. Arabin and J. van Eyck, "Delayed-interval delivery in twin and triplet pregnancies: 17 years of experience in 1 perinatal center," *American Journal of Obstetrics and Gynecology*, vol. 200, no. 2, pp. 154.e1–154.e8, 2009.

[4] T. Pakrashi and E. A. Defranco, "The relative proportion of preterm births complicated by premature rupture of membranes in multifetal gestations: a population-based study," *American Journal of Perinatology*, vol. 30, no. 1, pp. 69–74, 2013.

[5] C. A. S. de Frias, A. Queiros, and H. T. F. Simoes, "Delayed-interval delivery in dichorionic twin pregnancies: a case report of 154 latency days," *Revista Brasileira de Ginecologia e Obstetrícia*, vol. 42, no. 1, pp. 61–64, 2020.

[6] S. Cao, L. Walter, G. J. Valenzuela, and K. Roloff, "Delayed-interval delivery of twin gestation via cesarean section: a case report," *American Journal of Case Reports*, vol. 20, pp. 739–742, 2019.

[7] R. J. Wooldridge, E. A. Oliver, and T. Singh, "Delayed interval delivery in a triplet gestation," *BML Case Reports*, vol. 2012, no. nov22 2, p. bcr2012007232, 2012.

[8] M. Ghorbani and S. Moghadam, "A triplet pregnancy with spontaneous delivery of a fetus at gestational age of 20 weeks and pregnancy continuation of two other fetuses until week 33," *Global Journal of Health Science*, vol. 8, no. 2, pp. 88–92, 2015.

[9] M. I. Raposo, M. Cardoso, M. Ormonde, S. Stokreef, L. Correia, and A. Pereira, "Obstetric management of delayed-interval delivery," *Case Reports in Women's Health*, vol. 16, pp. 11–13, 2017.

[10] X. Q. Zheng, J. Y. Yan, R. L. Xu, X. C. Wang, L. Y. Li, and Z. Lin, "An analysis of the maternal and infant outcomes in the delayed interval delivery of twins," *Taiwanese Journal of Obstetrics & Gynecology*, vol. 59, no. 3, pp. 361–365, 2020.

[11] R. E. Beardmore and R. Pena-Miller, "Rotating antibiotics selects optimally against antibiotic resistance, in theory," *Mathematical Biosciences and Engineering*, vol. 7, no. 3, pp. 527–552, 2010.

[12] M. Benito Vielba, C. De Bonrostro Torralba, V. Pallares Arnal, and R. Herrero Serrano, "Delayed-interval delivery in twin pregnancies: report of three cases and literature review," *Journal of Maternal-Fetal & Neonatal Medicine*, vol. 32, no. 2, pp. 351–355, 2019.

[13] M. Kaneko, Y. Kawagoe, J. Oonishi, N. Yamada, H. Sameshima, and T. Ikenoue, "Case report and review of delayed-interval delivery for dichorionic, diamniotic twins with normal development," *The Journal of Obstetrics and Gynaecology Research*, vol. 38, no. 4, pp. 741–744, 2012.

[14] F. Magdaleno-Dans, S. Lopez-Magallon, M. Sancha-Naranjo, M. De la Calle, and J. L. Bartha, "Asynchronous twin births. Case report and obstetric management review," *Ginecología y Obstetricia de México*, vol. 84, no. 1, pp. 53–59, 2016.

[15] M. Cozzolino, V. Seravalli, G. Masini, L. Pasquini, and M. Di Tommaso, "Delayed-interval delivery in dichorionic twin pregnancies: a single-center experience," *The Ochsner Journal*, vol. 15, no. 3, pp. 248–250, 2015.

[16] E. Doger, Y. Cakiroglu, Y. Ceylan, E. Kole, S. Ozkan, and E. Caliskan, "Obstetric and neonatal outcomes of delayed interval delivery in cerclage and non-cerclage cases: an analysis of 20 multiple pregnancies," *The Journal of Obstetrics and Gynaecology Research*, vol. 40, no. 7, pp. 1853–1861, 2014.

18

A Case of Maternal Sepsis and Fetal Demise Associated with *Streptococcus pseudoporcinus*

Stephanie L. Pierce ,[1] Dena R. Shibib,[2,3] Denise Robison,[4] and Rodney K. Edwards[1]

[1]*Department of Obstetrics and Gynecology, College of Medicine, University of Oklahoma Health Sciences Center, Oklahoma City, OK, USA*
[2]*Department of Pathology, College of Medicine, University of Oklahoma Health Sciences Center, Oklahoma City, OK, USA*
[3]*Department of Pathology, Oklahoma City VA Health Care System, Oklahoma City, OK, USA*
[4]*OU Medicine Microbiology Laboratory, Oklahoma City, OK, USA*

Correspondence should be addressed to Stephanie L. Pierce; stephanieboespierce@gmail.com

Academic Editor: Edi Vaisbuch

Streptococcus pseudoporcinus has recently been described in relation to its colonization of the female genitourinary tract. Since prior reports have linked *S. pseudoporcinus* only with minor morbidities, the organism previously has not been considered to be a cause of serious puerperal infections. A 41-year-old gravida 2, para 1-0-0-1 presented with abdominal pain and intrauterine fetal demise. A beta hemolytic *Streptococcus* was isolated from her placenta, endometrium, urine, and two blood culture sets. The isolate was a *Streptococcus pseudoporcinus*, which colonizes the female genital tract and can resemble *Streptococcus agalactiae*. This case demonstrates that *S. pseudoporcinus* is a potential cause of severe maternal and fetal morbidity and mortality.

1. Introduction

Puerperal infection (e.g., chorioamnionitis, endometritis, or cesarean wound infection) is an important cause of maternal morbidity and mortality. Some of the most common organisms implicated in puerperal infection are *Escherichia coli*, other Enterobacteriaceae, *Staphylococcus aureus*, group A *Streptococcus*, and *Streptococcus agalactiae* (aka group B *Streptococcus*) [1]. Another member of the *Streptococcus* species, *Streptococcus pseudoporcinus*, recently has been found to colonize the female genitourinary tract [2, 3]. *S. pseudoporcinus* is noted to have biochemical characteristics similar to those of *S. agalactiae* and is therefore difficult to differentiate from *S. agalactiae* by traditional biochemical means [3]. As such, it is thought that the incidence of *S. pseudoporcinus* is likely underestimated due to misclassification as *S. agalactiae*. Prior case reports have linked *S. pseudoporcinus* with clinical infections including pyometra in a postmenopausal woman [4]. However, to our knowledge there have been no reports of major obstetric morbidity associated with this organism. Here, we discuss the case of a patient who presented with sepsis and fetal demise secondary to systemic infection with *S. pseudoporcinus*.

2. Case

A 41-year-old gravida 2, para 1-0-0-1 with no prenatal care presented to the Emergency Department (ED) with abdominal pain and was found to have a singleton fetal demise, ultrasound biometry consistent with 34 weeks gestational age. She had a past medical history significant for chronic hypertension. Her first pregnancy was uncomplicated and resulted in a term cesarean delivery of a liveborn infant. Upon presentation she was found to be in labor, with ruptured membranes and cervical dilation of 7 centimeters. Her exam was also notable for tachycardia and leakage of purulent fluid from the cervical os. She was afebrile, and labs were significant for a white blood cell count of 29,000 per mL and a serum lactate of 2.4 mmol/L. She received one dose each of intravenous piperacillin/tazobactam and cefazolin in the ED. Intravenous ampicillin and gentamicin were initiated in labor and delivery for a diagnosis of chorioamnionitis. She was also diagnosed with preeclampsia with severe features, and intravenous magnesium for seizure prophylaxis was administered.

Her labor progressed without augmentation, and she underwent spontaneous vaginal delivery of a stillborn infant. The patient declined autopsy and genetic testing for the infant.

After delivery, examination of the infant revealed no gross morphologic abnormalities. Placental pathology showed evidence of acute necrotizing chorioamnionitis and acute umbilical vasculitis, as well as mild decidual vasculopathy, consistent with maternal hypertension.

A beta hemolytic *Streptococcus* was isolated from the patient's urine, placenta, endometrium, and two blood culture sets. Lancefield grouping for *Streptococcus* groups A, B, C, F, and G were negative (Streptex, Remel, Lenexa, KS). Biochemical studies included a positive pyrrolidonyl aminopeptidase (PYR) test and a negative catalase reaction. The isolates were resistant to optochin. API (API 20 Strep, BioMerieux, Durham, NC) identification revealed *Streptococcus agalactiae* (biotype number 3063214) with 99.8% confidence at 24 hours. Identification of all isolates by matrix-associated laser desorption/ionization time-of-flight (MALDI-ToF; Bruker Daltronics, Billerica, MA) yielded *Streptococcus pseudoporcinus*, using the research use only (RUO) database (version 3.2.12.2) with log scores for each specimen ranging from 1.86 to 2.07. A blood culture isolate sent to a reference laboratory for bacterial 16S rRNA sequencing confirmed the identification of *Streptococcus pseudoporcinus*, with 100% identity of the first 467 base pairs of the 16S sequence to *Streptococcus pseudoporcinus* LQ 940–04. Isolates from the blood and placenta tested susceptible to ampicillin, clindamycin, erythromycin, penicillin, and vancomycin.

The patient recovered well in the postpartum period, remaining afebrile with normal vital signs and a normal serum lactate. On postpartum day 3, she was transitioned from intravenous ampicillin and gentamicin to oral amoxicillin. She left against medical advice on postpartum day 4. Written informed consent permitting the use of the patient's case for education and publication was obtained during her hospital stay.

3. Discussion

S. pseudoporcinus was first reported as a separate species in 2006, based on phenotypic analysis and gene sequencing of isolates that originated from the female genitourinary tract and were previously classified as *Streptococcus porcinus*. *S. porcinus* was first described in 1984 as mostly originating from swine [2]. Both species bear great resemblance to *S. agalactiae*, though *S. pseudoporcinus* typically demonstrates a wider zone of beta hemolysis. *S. porcinus* and *S. pseudoporcinus* may cross react with group B antisera, although some isolates do not [3]. Notably, in this case our isolates did not react with the Streptex group B reagents. In 2012, a review of 97 isolates previously identified as *S. porcinus* was performed using gene sequencing as well as conventional biochemical testing. It was found that 19 isolates were *S. porcinus*, while the remaining 78 isolates were actually *S. pseudoporcinus* [5]. Based on these and other similar findings, *S. pseudoporcinus* should be suspected in isolates that are phenotypically similar to *S. agalactiae* but demonstrate a wider zone of beta-hemolysis.

The similarity of *S. pseudoporcinus* to *S. agalactiae* raises concern that *S. pseudoporcinus* may be underreported. One study examining the prevalence of *S. pseudoporcinus* detected the organism in 1.6% of vaginorectal cultures screening for group B *Streptococcus* (GBS) [6]. It is therefore likely that some proportion of *S. pseudoporcinus* is misclassified as *S. agalactiae*, particularly in cultures of the female reproductive tract obtained specifically for the purpose of determining whether the patient is colonized with *S. agalactiae*.

Previous reports have demonstrated clinical infections associated with *S. pseudoporcinus* [4, 7, 8], but to our knowledge there have been no reports of this organism in association with severe obstetric morbidity. One recent report describes a patient with a vaginorectal culture at 39 weeks that grew a beta-hemolytic organism that was identified as *S. pseudoporcinus*, however there were no associated adverse maternal or neonatal outcomes in that pregnancy [9]. In addition, a study by Gaudreau et al. found that of 15 women colonized with *S. pseudoporcinus*, three patients developed chorioamnionitis, and two of those had preterm deliveries [10]. Furthermore, Grundy and colleagues recently demonstrated an increased risk of PPROM and preterm labor in a cohort of patients colonized with *S. pseudoporcinus* compared to those colonized with GBS [6]. However, one cannot conclude from these studies that the organism was the causative agent in those adverse outcomes. In contrast to the previous reports, our case demonstrates an instance of significant maternal morbidity (sepsis) and fetal demise in the setting of systemic maternal (and likely fetal) *S. pseudoporcinus* infection. Interestingly, Martin et al. previously reported a case of fetal demise associated with *S. porcinus* [11], however this was prior to the identification of *S. pseudoporcinus* as a separate organism in 2006. Therefore, it is possible the organism in that case may have been misidentified at the time as *S. porcinus*.

Currently there are no clinical guidelines that recommend screening or prophylaxis for *S. pseudoporcinus* in pregnancy. In a study of the incidence and epidemiology of *S. pseudoporcinus* [3], Stoner et al. conclude that there is a need to identify *S. pseudoporcinus* separately from *S. agalactiae* in order to avoid the unnecessary administration of antibiotics in pregnancy. However in light of our case which demonstrates significant morbidity related to *S. pseudoporcinus* infection in pregnancy, if this organism were misidentified as *S. agalactiae* and a patient received unnecessary intrapartum antibiotic prophylaxis, prophylaxis would pose minimal increased risk to the patient and could theoretically prevent some cases of puerperal infection caused by *S. pseudoporcinus*. If this organism is found to be the cause of morbidity in other cases, then this may have implications for screening and treatment guidelines in pregnancy.

The clinical necessity of specifically testing for *S. pseudoporcinus* in vaginorectal samples is questionable, since it remains unclear whether serious obstetric morbidity related to this organism occurs frequently enough to justify routine testing and because misclassification as *S. agalactiae* may occur. Although the exact clinical significance of *S. pseudoporcinus* remains to be seen, our case demonstrates that it is a potential cause of serious puerperal infection. If there are other reports of puerperal infections with this organism, its significance and prevalence in genital tract flora might warrant further investigation.

Acknowledgments

The authors thank the OU Medicine Microbiology Laboratory for their assistance.

References

[1] J. van Dillen, J. Zwart, J. Schutte, and J. van Roosmalen, "Maternal sepsis: epidemiology, etiology, and outcome," *Current Opinion in Infectious Diseases*, vol. 23, no. 3, pp. 249–254, 2010.

[2] S. Bekal, C. Gaudreau, R. A. Laurence, E. Simoneau, and L. Raynal, "*Streptococcus pseudoporcinus* sp. nov., a novel species isolated from the genitourinary tract of women," *Journal of Clinical Microbiology*, vol. 44, no. 7, pp. 2584–2589, 2006.

[3] K. A. Stoner, L. K. Rabe, M. N. Austin, L. A. Meyn, and S. L. Hillier, "Incidence and epidemiology of *Streptococcus pseudoporcinus*," *Journal of Clinical Microbiology*, vol. 49, no. 3, pp. 883–886, 2011.

[4] D. Ratna Harika, J. Sreenivasa Rao, and C. R. Setty, "A case of postmenopausal pyometra caused by *Streptococcus pseudoporcinus* – case report," *Journal of Medical and Dental Science Research*, vol. 3, no. 12, pp. 17–18, 2017.

[5] P. L. Shewmaker, A. G. Steigerwalt, A. M. Whitney et al., "Evaluation of methods for the identification and determination of the taxonomic status of strains belonging to the *Streptococcus porcinus-Streptococcus pseudoporcinus* complex isolated from animal, human, and dairy sources," *Journal of Clinical Microbiology*, vol. 50, no. 11, pp. 3591–3597, 2012.

[6] M. Grundy, N. Suwantarat, M. Rubin et al., "Differentiating *Streptococcus pseudoporcinus* from GBS: could this have implications in pregnancy?," *American Journal of Obstetrics and Gynecology*, vol. 220, no. 5, pp. 490.e1–490.e7, 2019.

[7] S. D. Mahlen and J. E. Clarridge, "Thumb infection caused by *Streptococcus pseudoporcinus*," *Journal of Clinical Microbiology*, vol. 47, no. 9, pp. 3041–3042, 2009.

[8] S. Sawamura, D. Niimori, and H. Inh, "A case of leg cellulitis caused by multidrug-resistant *Streptococcus pseudoporcinus*," *Intractable & Rare Diseases Research*, vol. 7, no. 4, pp. 280–282, 2018.

[9] J. C. Gullett, L. F. Westblade, D. A. Green, S. Whittier, and E. M. Burd, "The brief case: too beta to be a "B"," *Journal of Clinical Microbiology*, vol. 55, no. 6, pp. 1604–1607, 2017.

[10] C. Gaudreau, E. Simoneau, O. Labrecque et al., "Epidemiological, biochemical and antimicrobial susceptibility characteristics of *Streptococcus pseudoporcinus* isolated in Quebec, Canada, from 1997 to 2006," *Journal of Medical Microbiology*, vol. 56, no. 12, pp. 1620–1624, 2007.

[11] C. Martin, V. Fermeaux, J. L. Eyraud, and Y. Aubard, "*Streptococcus porcinus* as a cause of spontaneous preterm human stillbirth," *Journal of Clinical Microbiology*, vol. 42, no. 9, pp. 4396–4398, 2004.

19

A Successful Pregnancy in a Hemihysterectomized Patient–A Case Report

Sofia Jovina Domingues[1] **and Luísa Pinto**[2]

[1]*Centro Hospitalar de Setúbal, Setúbal, Portugal*
[2]*Centro Hospitalar e Universitário Lisboa Norte, Lisbon, Portugal*

Correspondence should be addressed to Sofia Jovina Domingues; sofia.domingues@chs.min-saude.pt

Academic Editor: Seung-Yup Ku

Introduction. Didelphys uterus, two separate uterine horns or a double uterus with two separate cervices, is one of several congenital uterine anomalies (CUA), accounting for 5% of CUA. CUA could be associated with dysmenorrhea, pelvic pain, and decreased fertility. During pregnancy, it has been associated with higher risk of miscarriage, preterm birth, malpresentation, and fetal growth restriction. There still is insufficient evidence on the efficacy and safety of surgical interventions in CUA, including hemihysterectomy, in what improvement of reproductive performance is concerned. *Objective.* The aim of the present case report is to review the literature and complement information on pregnancy outcomes after hemihysterectomy, contributing to a better counseling of women planning a pregnancy under these circumstances. *Case Presentation.* This paper case reports a successful pregnancy in a woman previously submitted to a hemihysterectomy and removal of a vaginal septum by hysteroscopy, due to a symptomatic didelphys uterus. An ipsilateral renal agenesis was also present. A cesarean was performed at 38 weeks' gestation and a healthy baby was born. *Discussion.* This paper reports an exceptional clinical situation, with only 9 cases described in the last 6 decades. As in previously reported cases, a cesarean was performed at term, resulting in a live childbirth. In these cases, a higher live birth rate and a lower incidence of preterm deliveries was found, comparing with uterine didelphys pregnancies. *Conclusion.* Understanding both the exact nature of a uterine anomaly before a surgical treatment and the prognosis for a future pregnancy after the intervention are of paramount importance for precise counseling of future parents.

1. Introduction

Congenital uterine anomalies (CUA) resulted from abnormal formation, differentiation, and/or fusion of the Müllerian or paramesonephric ducts during fetal life [1]. Coexisting renal, ureteral, and bladder anomalies are present in up to 40% of these patients [2]. There is no universally accepted classification system for CUA, but it seems that the classifications from the American Fertility Society (AFS) and from the European Society of Human Reproduction and Embryology/European Society for Gynecological Endoscopy (ESHRE/ESGE) have been the most widely accepted [3]. The prevalence of CUA in the general population varies from 0.06 to 38%. Most CUA are asymptomatic but they can be associated with adverse pregnancy outcomes [3]. Using AFS classification, didelphys uterus accounts for 5% of CUA and results from the lack of fusion of the paired Mullerian ducts, which should occur between the 6th and the 11th week of gestation [1]. The phenotype is that of two separate uterine horns or a double uterus with two separate cervices. Each uterine horn is linked to one fallopian tube and ovary [4]. A longitudinal vaginal septum is present in 75% of cases [1]. There still is insufficient evidence on the efficacy and safety of surgical interventions in CUA, in what improvement of reproductive performance is concerned. Surgical correction of CUA should be decided on an individual basis, depending on clinical symptoms, type of anomaly, and reproductive project.

We report a successful pregnancy in a woman previously submitted to surgical treatment for a didelphys uterus and a right-obstructed hemivagina (hemihysterectomy and hysteroscopic removal of a vaginal septum). There are only 9 cases in the literature describing pregnancy outcomes after a hemihysterectomy. The main purpose of this case report is to review the literature and complement information on pregnancy outcomes after hemihysterectomy and consequently contribute to a better counseling of women/couples planning a pregnancy under these circumstances. Patient consent for this report was obtained.

2. Case Presentation

A 25-year-old woman was referred to our maternal-fetal outpatient clinic at 20 weeks' gestation, due to a clinical history of CUA submitted to a surgical intervention 11 years before. Menarche occurred at the age of 11 and since then, she complained of severe dysmenorrhea, pelvic pain, and heavy menstrual bleeding. Pain did not decrease with the use of estroprogestative pill, anti-inflammatory drugs, or other pain killers. At 13 years of age, a gynecological appointment revealed normal stature and normal external genitalia, but gynecological examination was hampered by the presence of an intact hymen. Additional investigation with abdominal ultrasound showed two separate uterine cavities, and a single left kidney. Based on the suspicion of a CUA, at the age of 14, the patient underwent a diagnostic laparoscopy–which revealed a double uterus–and a diagnostic hysteroscopy which identified a longitudinal vaginal septum and a right-obstructed hemivagina. The laparoscopic approach was converted to open surgery and a supracervical right hemihysterectomy was performed. At the same operative time a hysteroscopic resection of the vaginal septum was undertaken and two uterine cervices were visualized. One year later, an abdominal ultrasound revealed an anteverted uterus with mild left laterality and normal dimensions ($98 \times 26 \times 45$ mm, longitudinal, anteroposterior, and transversal axes). At the age of 17 she initiated sexual life with no complaints and 5 years later she got pregnant and had a spontaneous abortion at 7 weeks' gestation for which no surgical treatment was needed.

Regarding current pregnancy, no fetal or maternal relevant complications occurred. Pregnancy surveillance was done according to department protocols, including obstetrical ultrasounds in every trimester of gestation. Route of delivery was discussed with the patient and given the previous uterine surgery, an elective cesarean was scheduled to week 39. However, gestational hypertension at 38 weeks' gestation led to the decision to terminate the pregnancy. An uneventful cesarean resulted in a male newborn, 3170 g, Apgar index 9/10 at 1 and 5 minutes, respectively. Immediately after the cesarean, normal blood pressure was restored and no other meaningful clinical events occurred.

3. Discussion

We describe a successful pregnancy in a woman previously submitted to a right hemihysterectomy due to the diagnosis of didelphys uterus.

The precise incidence of CUA in the general population is not known since most CUA are asymptomatic, they are diagnosed by different techniques and classified using different classification systems [3]. Accurate evaluation of the internal and external contours of the uterus is crucial in making the diagnosis and classifying CUA correctly. In the past, as reported in our case, the gold standard was a combination of laparoscopy and hysteroscopy. Currently, 3D transvaginal sonography (TVS) is considered the gold standard for the assessment of CUA, correctly classifying the different types of uterine anomalies [4]. Magnetic resonance imaging (MRI) of the pelvis has a high sensitivity and specificity for the diagnosis of CUA and is helpful in delineating the endometrium, detecting uterine horns and also in defining renal anatomy. MRI is not routinely recommended in women with a suspected CUA but it seems useful for those with unconfirmed diagnosis on 3D ultrasound, with suspected complex anomalies or who decline or are distressed by internal examinations [4].

Didelphys uterus can be suspected when two endometrial cavities are visualized in the transverse plane of conventional 2D ultrasound and 3D ultrasound, associated with a clinical demonstration of two cervices and/or two vaginas on speculum examination, can confirm the diagnosis [4].

CUA may be associated with congenital renal anomalies, mostly unilateral renal agenesis, as described in this paper, because of their closely related embryonic origin. Therefore, a urinary tract ultrasound, an MRI, or an intravenous pyelogram should be recommended [5].

CUA can be associated with adverse pregnancy outcomes. A recent systematic review and meta-analysis showed that didelphys uterus was not associated with an increased incidence of infertility or miscarriage, but it was mainly associated with a higher risk of preterm delivery, preterm premature rupture of membranes, fetal malpresentation, cesarean, fetal growth restriction, and small for gestational age [3]. Regarding the higher risk of cesarean in this CUA, Cwiertnia et al. demonstrated that the decision to perform cesarean depends on several factors, including fetal presentation, patient preference, and vaginal septum features [6].

However, there is a lack of evidence on improved reproductive outcomes after surgical interventions for CUA. The goal of CUA management is to correct anatomical distortions associated with obstructive anomalies in order to relieve symptoms, thereby improving quality of life, and to avoid long-term health and reproductive adverse consequences. In nonobstructive anomalies, the objective is to improve reproductive outcomes in infertile women or in women who have experienced recurrent miscarriages [4].

In our report, there was a suspicion of CUA on abdominal ultrasound (TVS was not performed due to the presence of an intact hymen) and then a hysteroscopy and a laparoscopy were performed. Given the severe pain, suggesting an obstructive anomaly, a hemihysterectomy and removal of a vaginal septum were performed, aiming to improve the quality of life. After surgical treatment, the symptoms are resolved.

Nine cases of pregnant women after hemihysterectomy have been reported since 1947 (Table 1). In these cases, most

Table 1: Pregnancy outcomes after hemihysterectomy (adapted from Kai et al. [7]).

Author (year)	Patient (n)	Pregnancies	Abortions	Preterm delivery	Term delivery	Type of delivery	Live births	Uterine rupture
Smith et al. [8]	1	1	0	0	1	Cesarean	1	0
Thelwall-Jone (1976) [9]	2	3	0	1	2	Cesarean	3[a]	0
Phillips [10]	1	1	1	0	0	Cesarean	0	0
Candiani et al. [11]	2	2	1	1	0	Cesarean	1	0
Berhan et al. [12]	1	1	0	0	1	Vaginal	1	0
Kai et al. [7]	1	2	0	2	0	Cesarean	2	0
Present case	1	1	0	0	1	Cesarean	1	0
TOTAL	9	11	2	4	4	—	9	0

[a] One singleton pregnancy and one twin pregnancy.

clinicians decided for a cesarean section, 82% of pregnancies resulted in live births and 37% in preterm deliveries.

A previous study including 114 pregnant patients with didelphys uterus showed a 56% live birth rate and 43% preterm delivery rate [13]. More recently, preterm delivery rates in women with didelphys uterus have been described as higher than post-hemihysterectomy surgery (66.7% vs. 44.4%) [14].

Although the reduced number of pregnancies after hemihysterectomy reported in literature, our case adds and corroborates information about pregnancy management after a hemihysterectomy, showing an adequate live birth. Regarding to preterm delivery rate, it should be interpreted individually with caution, because there are several factors to contribute it, such as a multiple pregnancy.

The strength of our case report relies on accurate description of hemihysterectomy and pregnancy outcomes after surgery, contributing to our knowledge on this subject. Prospective long-term studies in hemihysterectomized women should be carried out, to better assess pregnancy outcomes.

4. Conclusion

The decision to perform a surgery, such as a hemihysterectomy, at a young stage of life in order to improve quality of life must be considered, taking into account the risks and benefits, in the short and long term.

Understanding the exact nature of the uterine anomaly before a surgical treatment and explaining to the patient the prognosis of a future pregnancy is of paramount importance for precise counseling and adequacy of expectations. We report the case of a successful pregnancy after a hemihysterectomy; however, it is important to be aware of the possible different clinical implication for specific types of uterine anomalies and surgeries.

Authors' Contributions

All authors have contributed sufficiently in this work to warrant authorship and take public responsibility for it. Both authors followed and managed the patient. SD collected the data and drafted the manuscript. LP revised the manuscript.

References

[1] R. N. Troiano and S. M. McCarthy, "Mullerian duct anomalies: imaging and clinical issues," *Radiology*, vol. 233, no. 1, pp. 19–34, 2004.

[2] M. A. Hall-Craggs, A. Kirkham, and S. M. Creighton, "Renal and urological abnormalities occurring with Mullerian anomalies," *Journal of Pediatric Urology*, vol. 9, no. 1, pp. 27–32, 2013.

[3] M. A. Kim, H. S. Kim, and Y. H. Kim, "Reproductive, obstetric and neonatal outcomes in women with congenital uterine anomalies: a systematic review and meta-analysis," *Journal of clinical medicine*, vol. 10, no. 21, p. 4797, 2021.

[4] M. A. Akhtar, S. H. Saravelos, T. C. Li, K. Jayaprakasan, and Royal College of Obstetricians and Gynaecologists, "Reproductive implications and management of congenital uterine anomalies," *BJOG : An International Journal of Obstetrics and Gynaecology*, vol. 127, no. 5, pp. e1–e13, 2020.

[5] P. K. Heinonen, "Distribution of female genital tract anomalies in two classifications," *European Journal of Obstetrics, Gynecology, and Reproductive Biology*, vol. 206, pp. 141–146, 2016.

[6] A. Ćwiertnia, D. Borzyszkowska, A. Golara et al., "The impact of uterus didelphys on fertility and pregnancy," *International Journal of Environmental Research and Public Health*, vol. 19, no. 17, p. 10571, 2022.

[7] K. Kai, Y. Kawano, M. Yano et al., "Two cesarean deliveries after hemi-hysterectomy due to gestational trophoblastic neoplasia," *Taiwanese Journal of Obstetrics & Gynecology*, vol. 57, no. 2, pp. 315–318, 2018, PMID: 29673680.

[8] W. P. Smith, "Cesarean section seven years after hemihysterectomy in a bicornate uterus," *American Journal of Surgery*, vol. 74, no. 6, pp. 856–859, 1947.

[9] H. Thelwall-Jones, "Pregnancy after hemihysterectomy: Two case reports," *American Journal of Obstetrics and Gynecology*, vol. 125, no. 8, pp. 1156-1157, 1976.

[10] W. D. Phillips, "Twin pregnancy (intrauterine and cervical) after hemihysterectomy: Case reports," *American Journal of Obstetrics and Gynecology*, vol. 130, no. 5, pp. 603-604, 1978.

[11] G. B. Candiani, L. Fedele, and M. Candiani, "Double uterus, blind hemivagina, and ipsilateral renal agenesis: 36 cases and

long-term follow-up," *Obstetrics and Gynecology*, vol. 90, no. 1, pp. 26–32, 1997.

[12] Y. Berhan and L. Yusuf, "Viable pregnancies in women with different mullerian duct anomalies," *Ethiopian Medical Journal*, vol. 44, p. 291e9, 2006.

[13] G. F. Grimbizis, M. Camus, B. C. Tarlatzis, J. N. Bontis, and P. Devroey, "Clinical implications of uterine malformations and hysteroscopic treatment results," *Human Reproduction Update*, vol. 7, no. 2, pp. 161–174, 2001.

[14] E. Zambrotta, L. M. Di Gregorio, F. Di Guardo et al., "Congenital uterine anomalies and perinatal outcomes: a retrospective single-center cohort study," *Clinical and Experimental Obstetrics & Gynecology*, vol. 48, no. 1, pp. 160–163, 2021.

Severe Vitamin B12 Deficiency in Pregnancy Mimicking HELLP Syndrome

Shravya Govindappagari,[1] Michelle Nguyen,[2] Megha Gupta,[3] Ramy M. Hanna,[4] and Richard M. Burwick[1,5]

[1]*Department of Obstetrics and Gynecology, Division of Maternal-Fetal Medicine, Cedars-Sinai Medical Center, Los Angeles, CA, USA*
[2]*Department of Obstetrics and Gynecology, Adventist Health White Memorial, Los Angeles, CA, USA*
[3]*Department of Obstetrics and Gynecology, Division of Maternal-Fetal Medicine, University of Texas Health Science Center at Houston, Houston, TX, USA*
[4]*Department of Medicine, Division of Nephrology, UCLA David Geffen School of Medicine, Los Angeles, CA, USA*
[5]*Department of Obstetrics and Gynecology, UCLA David Geffen School of Medicine, Los Angeles, CA, USA*

Correspondence should be addressed to Richard M. Burwick; richard.burwick@cshs.org

Academic Editor: Yossef Ezra

Severe vitamin B12 deficiency may present with hematologic abnormalities that mimic thrombotic microangiopathy disorders such as hemolysis, elevated liver enzymes, and low platelet count (HELLP) syndrome. We report a patient diagnosed with severe vitamin B12 deficiency, following termination of pregnancy for suspected preeclampsia and HELLP syndrome at 21 weeks' gestation. When hemolysis and thrombocytopenia persisted after delivery, testing was performed to rule out other etiologies of thrombotic microangiopathy, including atypical hemolytic uremic syndrome, thrombotic thrombocytopenic purpura, and vitamin B12 deficiency. This work-up revealed undetectable vitamin B12 levels and presence of intrinsic factor antibodies, consistent with pernicious anemia. Parenteral B12 supplementation was initiated, with subsequent improvement in hematologic parameters. Our case emphasizes the importance of screening for B12 deficiency in pregnancy, especially in at-risk women with unexplained anemia or thrombocytopenia. Moreover, providers should consider B12 deficiency and pernicious anemia in the differential diagnosis of pregnancy-associated thrombotic microangiopathy.

1. Introduction

Mild vitamin B12 deficiency is common in pregnancy and due to increased fetal demand over gestation, 38% of women have low B12 levels by the time of delivery [1]. Early recognition is critical because low B12 levels in pregnancy have been associated with neural tube defects, preterm birth, and low neonatal birthweight [2, 3]. Heightened suspicion is warranted in women with risk factors for B12 deficiency, including obesity, prior bariatric surgery, inflammatory bowel disease, Helicobacter pylori infection, use of metformin or proton pump inhibitors, and certain vegan diets. Severe B12 deficiency may also result from pernicious anemia, which is caused by intrinsic factor blocking antibodies that interfere with B12 absorption.

In pregnancy, B12 deficiency may go unrecognized if anemia is mistakenly attributed to other causes such as iron deficiency or physiologic hemodilution. When severe B12 deficiency goes untreated, it can have profound effects, including severe anemia, peripheral neuropathy, cognitive decline, and a variety of neuropsychiatric manifestations. It may also manifest with microangiopathic hemolytic anemia and thrombocytopenia, mimicking other thrombotic microangiopathy (TMA) disorders such as atypical hemolytic uremic syndrome (aHUS), hemolysis, elevated liver enzymes, low platelet count (HELLP) syndrome, and thrombotic thrombocytopenic purpura (TTP) [4–6]. When TMA occurs in pregnancy, it is critical that B12 deficiency be ruled out because the treatment approach (B12 supplementation) varies greatly from other TMA disorders.

Table 1: Laboratory or treatment measures before and after delivery.

Laboratory or Treatment Measure*	Initial evaluation 21+4/7 weeks gestation	Prior to delivery 21+5/7 weeks gestation	PPD 1	PPD 2	PPD 3	PPD4	PPD5
Hemoglobin (g/dl)	11.0	9.7	8.4	9.0	9.5	8.8	9.3
Platelet Count (k/μl)	66	93	90	103	133	112	175
Lactate dehydrogenase (U/L)	985	872	706	n/a	n/a	n/a	404
Alanine transaminase (U/L)	20	14	24	12	12	13	15
Aspartate transaminase (U/L)	40	30	20	19	15	19	19
Creatinine (mg/dl)	0.7	0.9	0.9	0.6	0.8	0.8	0.8
Haptoglobin (mg/dl)	<8	n/a	<8	<8	n/a	n/a	n/a
Vitamin B12 (ρg/ml)	n/a	n/a	<146	n/a	n/a	n/a	n/a
Vitamin B12 supplementation (subcutaneous injection)	n/a	n/a	1000 mcg	1000 mcg	1000 mcg	1000 mcg	1000 mcg

PPD: postpartum day; n/a: not available.
* Normal ranges: Hemoglobin (11.6-15.4 g/dl); Platelet count (150-450 k/μl); Lactate dehydrogenase (125-220); Alanine transaminase (0-55 U/L); Aspartate transaminase (5-34 U/L); Creatinine (0.6-1.1 mg/dl); Haptoglobin (30-200 mg/dl); Vitamin B12 (213-816 ρg/ml).

Here, we report the case of a patient diagnosed with pernicious anemia, following pregnancy termination for suspected preeclampsia and HELLP syndrome at 21 weeks' gestation.

2. Case Presentation

A 40-year-old multiparous African American woman at 21 weeks' 4-day gestation, with known chronic hypertension, was transferred to our medical center for management of hypertensive emergency. Prior to transfer, the patient had marked blood pressure elevation (peak 192/129 mmHg) and laboratory evaluation notable for hemoglobin 11.0 g/dl, platelet count 66 k/μl, alanine transaminase (ALT) 20 U/L, aspartate transaminase (AST) 40 U/L, and creatinine 0.7 mg/dl (Table 1 for laboratory trends and reference range). Urine dipstick detected 4+ protein, 4+ blood, and +nitrites, and urine drug screen was positive for methamphetamines and marijuana. Intravenous ceftriaxone was given empirically for urinary tract infection.

On arrival to our medical center, blood pressure peaked at 205/114 mmHg and laboratory findings were like those noted above. In addition, lactate dehydrogenase (LDH) level was 985 U/L, with haptoglobin <8 mg/dl and 3 schistocytes per high power field on peripheral smear. Urine protein/creatinine ratio was 2.61 mg/mg (normal <0.3 mg/mg). Estimated fetal weight by ultrasound was 451g, which was appropriate for her gestational age. We suspect that methamphetamine use precipitated her hypertensive crisis, but the clinical picture and laboratory findings were concerning for severe preeclampsia and HELLP syndrome. Due to her previable gestational age and the life-threatening nature of her condition, termination of pregnancy was recommended, and she agreed. Magnesium sulfate was initiated for seizure prophylaxis, and she was managed in the intensive care unit on an intravenous nicardipine drip. Within 12 hours of her first misoprostol dose for labor induction, she had a precipitous vaginal delivery of a nonviable female neonate. Pathology examination of the placenta revealed decidual arteriopathy and accelerated villous maturation, which are findings reflective of severe hypertension and placental hypoxia.

Following delivery, severe hypertension (≥160/110 mmHg) persisted throughout the postpartum period despite triple agent antihypertensive therapy. On postpartum day 5, she continued to have severe range blood pressures, but declined inpatient stay and was discharged home on an oral regimen of chlorthalidone (50mg daily), amlodipine (10mg daily), and telmisartan (80mg daily). During her postpartum course in the hospital, patient had a work-up for secondary causes of hypertension. She had maternal echo showing mild left ventricular hypertrophy, but normal left ventricular ejection fraction (69%) and no evidence of aortic coarctation. She had normal renal artery Dopplers, ruling out renal artery stenosis. Serum aldosterone/renin ratio was normal, ruling out primary aldosteronism. She did not complete a 24-hour urine collection to measure total metanephrines and therefore pheochromocytoma was not formally ruled out. We suspect that methamphetamine use precipitated her hypertensive emergency, but blood pressures remained severe despite 7 days of inpatient observation and drug cessation.

TMA also persisted despite termination of pregnancy and drug cessation. On postpartum day 1 laboratory values were as follows: hemoglobin 8.4 g/dl, platelet count 90 k/μl, LDH 706 U/L, haptoglobin <8 mg/dl, 2-3 schistocytes per high power field on smear, and reticulocyte count 4.6% (normal 0.5-2.0%). Her reticulocyte production index was noted to be suboptimal at 2.1% (normal >3.0%), after adjustment for low hematocrit (30.5%) [1]. Considering that the patient's liver enzymes remained normal after delivery despite ongoing hemolysis and thrombocytopenia, the diagnosis of HELLP syndrome was questioned. Alternative TMA etiologies were considered, including aHUS, TTP, and vitamin B12 deficiency. Serum creatinine peaked at 0.9 mg/dl and aHUS genetic panel was negative for disease-associated complement gene variants (Machaon Diagnostics), making a diagnosis of aHUS less likely. ADAMTS13 activity was

75% (normal >67%), making a diagnosis of TTP less likely. Meanwhile, vitamin B12 level was undetectable <146 ρg/ml (normal 213-816 ρg/ml) and intrinsic factor blocking antibodies were positive, consistent with pernicious anemia. Mean corpuscular volume was paradoxically low at 75.3 FL (normal 80-100 FL), and other causes of anemia were ruled out with normal iron panel, hemoglobin electrophoresis, and folate level.

Following diagnosis of pernicious anemia, the patient was started on subcutaneous B12 injections at a dose of 1000 mcg daily. She received 5 injections of vitamin B12 during her postpartum hospital stay. While blood pressures remained severely elevated on the day of discharge (postpartum day 5), laboratory parameters showed signs of improvement: Hemoglobin 9.5 g/dl, platelet count 175 k/μl, and LDH 404 U/L (Table 1 for laboratory trends). The patient was discharged home with a plan for continued B12 supplementation and close outpatient follow up. At 2 weeks postpartum the patient had normal blood pressure (127/82) and was clinically well, but she declined additional laboratory testing.

3. Discussion

In pregnancy, TMA is most often secondary to preeclampsia or HELLP syndrome [7]. However, our case emphasizes the need to consider other etiologies in the differential diagnosis of TMA. It is critical to rule out TTP, aHUS, and B12 deficiency, because these disorders have established, nondelivery approaches to treatment. TTP is best treated with plasma exchange, aHUS with complement blockade, and B12 deficiency with B12 supplementation. For preeclampsia and HELLP syndrome, delivery is the only definitive treatment. Therefore, if delivery does not lead to TMA resolution, other etiologies should be carefully evaluated. TTP is less likely with a normal ADAMTS13 activity level, while the diagnosis of aHUS is less likely without renal failure or complement gene mutation. Vitamin B12 deficiency is initially considered with a low B12 level, but should be confirmed by metabolite testing (homocysteine, methylmalonic acid levels) or antibody testing (intrinsic factor blocking antibody, parietal cell antibody). In our case, positive intrinsic factor antibodies confirmed the diagnosis of pernicious anemia.

Providers may not immediately recognize B12 deficiency as a life-threatening condition, but it should be noted that pernicious anemia was fatal before B12 treatments were available. Vitamin B12 plays a critical role in DNA synthesis, and hematopoietic precursor cells are highly sensitive to abnormal DNA synthesis caused by B12 deficiency. While mild anemia, leukopenia, and thrombocytopenia are common, approximately 10% of patients with B12 deficiency develop life-threatening hematologic manifestations [8]. When erythropoiesis becomes ineffective, there is premature death of precursor red blood cells in the bone marrow, prior to their release in circulation. Cytoskeletal fragility predisposes to erythrocyte fragmentation, and laboratory findings of hemolysis include elevated LDH and low haptoglobin [4, 5]. This has been termed intramedullary hemolysis or pseudo-TMA and is also associated with low reticulocyte count or low reticulocyte production index. In the adult population, it is estimated that TMA accounts for 2-3% of the hematologic disorders related to B12 deficiency [8]. In addition, pernicious anemia accounts for most of these TMA cases, whereas TMA is less common with B12 deficiency secondary to malabsorption [4, 5].

In real-world practice, cases are complex with overlapping features, and we recognize that our case was no exception. Our patient had a positive urine drug screen for methamphetamines, and this likely precipitated her hypertensive crisis. The patient was also pregnant, and her clinical picture was worrisome for preeclampsia and HELLP syndrome. In this scenario, the safest and most prudent option is expedited delivery. However, it is worth noting that our patient had undiagnosed and untreated B12 deficiency, which may have contributed to her clinical picture. She did not have peripheral neuropathy or neuropsychiatric manifestations of B12 deficiency, but hematologic abnormalities can occur in the absence of neurologic abnormalities [9]. Considering the association between pernicious anemia and TMA, it is possible that severe B12 deficiency led directly to her hemolysis and thrombocytopenia. While termination of pregnancy may have been unavoidable, we want to emphasize the importance of recognizing and treating pernicious anemia. In our case, we suspect that B12 supplementation not only helped to improve laboratory parameters in the short-term, but also improved her long-term prognosis.

Our case emphasizes the importance of screening for B12 deficiency in pregnancy, especially in at-risk women with unexplained anemia or thrombocytopenia. Moreover, providers should consider B12 deficiency and pernicious anemia in the differential diagnosis of pregnancy-associated TMA.

References

[1] C. E. Visentin, S. P. Masih, L. Plumptre, T. H. Schroder, K. J. Sohn, A. Ly et al., "Low serum vitamin B-12 concentrations are prevalent in a cohort of pregnant canadian," *The Journal of Nutrition*, vol. 146, no. 5, pp. 1035–1042, 2016.

[2] E. Peker, N. Demir, O. Tuncer et al., "The levels of vitamin B12, folate and homocysteine in mothers and their babies with neural tube defects," *The Journal of Maternal-Fetal & Neonatal Medicine*, vol. 29, no. 18, pp. 1–5, 2015.

[3] T. Rogne, M. J. Tielemans, M. F. Chong et al., "Associations of maternal vitamin b12 concentration in pregnancy with the risks of preterm birth and low birth weight: a systematic review and meta-analysis of individual participant data," *American Journal of Epidemiology*, vol. 185, no. 3, pp. 212–223, 2017.

[4] P. N. Tran and M. Tran, "Cobalamin deficiency presenting with thrombotic microangiopathy (TMA) features: a systematic review," *Transfusion and Apheresis Science*, vol. 57, no. 1, pp. 102–106, 2018.

[5] N. Noël, G. Maigné, G. Tertian et al., "Hemolysis and schistocytosis in the emergency department: consider pseudothrombotic microangiopathy related to vitamin B12 deficiency," *QJM: An International Journal of Medicine*, vol. 106, no. 11, Article ID hct142, pp. 1017–1022, 2013.

[6] S. C. Hartong, E. A. Steegers, and W. Visser, "Hemolysis, elevated liver enzymes and low platelets during pregnancy due

to vitamin B12 and folate deficiencies," *European Journal of Obstetrics & Gynecology and Reproductive Biology*, vol. 131, no. 2, pp. 241-242, 2007.

[7] M. Gupta, B. Feinberg, and R. Burwick, "Thrombotic microangiopathies of pregnancy: Differential diagnosis," *Pregnancy Hypertension: An International Journal of Women's Cardiovascular Health*, vol. 12, pp. 29–34, 2018.

[8] E. Andrès, S. Affenberger, J. Zimmer et al., "Current hematological findings in cobalamin deficiency. A study of 201 consecutive patients with documented cobalamin deficiency," *Clinical & Laboratory Haematology*, vol. 28, no. 1, pp. 50–56, 2006.

[9] M. J. Shipton and J. Thachil, "Vitamin B12 deficiency - A 21st century perspective," *Clinical Medicine*, vol. 15, no. 2, pp. 145–150, 2015.

21

Association of Beta-Thalassaemia and Hypogonadotropic Hypogonadism

Angela Vidal and Carolin Dhakal

Department of Obstetrics and Gynecology, Lucerne Cantonal Hospital, Switzerland

Correspondence should be addressed to Angela Vidal; vidalgutierrez.angelamaria@gmail.com

Academic Editor: Manvinder Singh

Thalassaemic syndromes are among the most common haemoglobinopathies and are associated with high morbidity and mortality. Because of the various treatments, a secondary endocrinopathy due to iron overload—haemosiderosis—can occur, causing hypopituitarism leading to hypogonadotropic hypogonadism (HH) and infertility. We present a case of secondary amenorrhoea in a patient with beta-thalassaemia and a history of multiple therapies in her adolescence, such as multiple transfusions, chemotherapy, and allogeneic bone marrow transplantation, who presented with HH and premature ovarian insufficiency.

1. Background

The global incidence of haemoglobinopathy is 7%. Thalassa syndrome is one of the most common haemoglobinopathies associated with high morbidity and mortality rates [1]. Beta-thalassaemia is a severe haematological disease that results in reduced haemoglobin synthesis due to a genetic component [2]. Patients without transfusions experience massive erythroid expansion and severe haemolytic anaemia. Iron overload is a consequence of frequent blood transfusions, which is the most important treatment modality for thalassaemia major. Such treatment is the cause of secondary endocrinopathy due to iron overload, haemosiderosis, causing hypopituitarism, which leads to hypogonadotropic hypogonadism (HH). Other possible causes of hypogonadism in beta-thalassaemia major are liver disorders, chronic hypoxia, diabetes mellitus, and zinc deficiency [3, 4].

The quality of life of thalassaemic patients is affected by the need for chronic transfusions, lifelong iron chelation therapy, and related complications. Allogeneic haematopoietic stem cell transplantation (allo-HSCT) is a potentially curative treatment for transfusion-dependent patients without iron-related complications, especially at a young age. In some cases, bone marrow transplants are not sex-matched [5, 6].

Beta-thalassaemia major and its possible treatments may cause premature ovarian insufficiency (POI). POI is one of the leading causes of infertility in women worldwide. POI is defined as the presence of amenorrhoea for at least four consecutive months in women under 40 years of age and twice elevated follicle – stimulating hormone (FSH) levels > 25 IU/L according to the European Society for Human Reproduction and Embryology (ESHRE) guideline 2015 [7]. POI affects 1%–1.2% of the general population, and pregnancy with POI is rare (<1 : 9200). The following are the causes of POI: prior ovarian surgery, chemotherapy or radiation therapy, personal or family history of autoimmune diseases, family history of POI (fragile X premutation), or other genetic reasons [7, 8].

We present a case of secondary amenorrhoea in a patient with beta-thalassaemia and a history of multiple therapies in her adolescence, such as multiple transfusions, chemotherapy, and allogeneic bone marrow transplantation, presenting with HH and POI.

We discuss possible fertility problems after different treatments due to beta-thalassaemia.

1.1. Case Report. A 38-year-old woman was referred to our clinic with a 5-year history of amenorrhoea and infertility. Important diagnoses in her medical history are a beta-thalassaemia major since childhood and treatment with periodic blood transfusions to maintain adequate haemoglobin levels. From the age of 10 years, she was diagnosed with restrictive heart disease and treated with digoxin. She was also diagnosed with fibrosis of the liver, siderosis, and fibrosis of the pancreas. At the age of 19 years, she underwent a bone marrow transplant, at which time she underwent pretreatment with fludarabine, busulfan, and cyclophosphamide for 15 days as adjuvant chemotherapy. Her human leukocyte antigen- (HLA-) identical donor was her brother.

Her menarche was at 13 years of age. She had a regular menstrual cycle until she was 15 years old. Functional hypothalamic amenorrhoea was suspected due to the patient's medical history. Other possible causes of functional hypothalamic amenorrhoea, such as eating disorders, excessive exercise, and stress, were ruled out.

The laboratory test results showed reduced levels of FSH (1.06 IU/L), luteinizing hormone (LH) (<0.3 IU/L), oestradiol (>18.4 pmol/L), and antimullerian *hormone* (AMH) (<0.007 pmol/L). A gonadotropin-releasing *hormone* (GnRH)/luteinizing *hormone*-releasing *hormone* (LHRH) test was performed with a 0.1 mg synthetic LHRH bolus administered intravenously. Serum samples were extracted for gonadotropin measurements at 0 min (FSH 1.03 IU/L and LH < 0.3 IU/L) and 30 min after LHRH administration (FSH 1.15 IU/L and LH 0.57 IU/L). Even after LHRH stimulation, the pituitary response was subnormal, consistent with HH. A stimulation test with human menopausal gonadotropin 225 IE was performed without any detectable response.

Peak levels of growth hormone and cortisol with the insulin tolerance test were 11.6 ng/mL and 26.3 μg/dL, respectively. Magnetic resonance imaging (MRI) findings showed a decrease in the intensity of the pituitary gland signal on T2-weighted and size images (Figure 1).

Based on the above characteristics, the patient was diagnosed with secondary amenorrhoea and POI.

The patient was referred to a fertility centre abroad for oocyte donation, as this treatment option is not permitted in Switzerland. She became pregnant through oocyte donation.

The pregnancy and delivery ensued without complications. A primary caesarean section was performed due to maternal risk of complications during delivery. The patient delivered a boy with a normal weight of 3180 g, with normal pH and Apgar scores. Six weeks postpartum after cessation of voluntary breastfeeding, she was started on hormone replacement therapy with oestradiol and norethisterone because of persistent amenorrhoea due to POI. *Hormone replacement* therapy was recommended until the onset of normal menopause at 51 years of age.

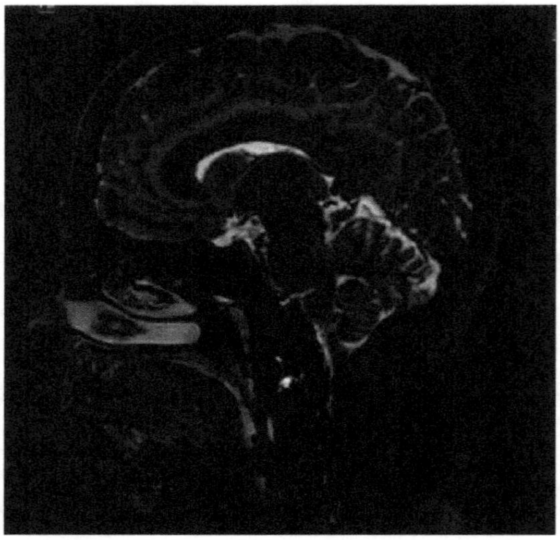

FIGURE 1: MRI of the pituitary gland, which is rather small for age and sex but without evidence of focal abnormalities.

2. Discussion

The differential diagnosis in patients with secondary amenorrhoea diagnosed with beta thalassaemia and after receiving various treatments is of great relevance due to the possible management and treatment depending on the aetiology. Here, we describe the possible causes:

(i) Primary ovarian insufficiency (POI)

POI is condition that affects 1 in 100 women under the age of 40 years (1%), 1 in 1000 women under the age of 30 years (0.1%), and 1 in 10,000 women under the age of 20 years (0.01%) [7, 9]. According to the ESHRE, POI is a clinical syndrome defined by the loss of ovarian activity before the age of 40 years. POI is characterised by menstrual disturbance (amenorrhoea) with increased gonadotropins and low oestradiol levels [7].

Although the exact cause is unknown in most cases, some of the causes of POI have been identified, including genetic disorders (such as fragile X syndrome and Turner syndrome, where genetic testing should be performed), autoimmune diseases (such as thyroiditis and Addison's disease), and iatrogenic causes (such as chemotherapy or other gonadotoxic treatments) [7, 8].

As a consequence of allogeneic bone marrow transplantation, it must be taken into account when carrying out genetic tests to ensure that the DNA mutations detected come from the patient's native DNA; therefore, the most suitable and reliable biological sample for DNA isolation must be obtained, and fibroblast culture is recommended [10].

(ii) Hypothalamic and pituitary causes

Functional hypothalamic amenorrhoea. Functional hypothalamic amenorrhoea is a chronic anovulation disorder caused by suppression of the hypothalamic–pituitary axis due to body weight loss, eating disorders, excessive exercise, stress, or iron overload and may result in infertility or loss of bone density [11].

(iii) Other central nervous system causes

Secondary amenorrhoea may be caused by damage to the hypothalamic–pituitary axis due to inflammation, ischemia, infiltration, infection, iron overload, or trauma. Disorders affecting pubertal development, such as gonadotropin-releasing hormone deficiency and constitutional delay, may cause secondary amenorrhoea [12].

Beta-thalassaemia is a severe transfusion-dependent anaemia that causes infertility due to iron deposition in the endocrine organs, especially after overtransfusion. This deposition is a major cause of POI. Most patients are infertile due to HH and require assisted reproductive techniques. Studies have been conducted in female patients with beta-thalassaemia to investigate the hypothalamic–pituitary–ovarian axis [13–15]. In the thalassaemic group, basal and peak posttest levels of GnRH and other reproductive hormones were significantly lower than those in the control group. Iron-induced effects play a central role in the pathogenesis of decreased reproductive capacity.

There are different treatment approaches for individuals with different types of beta-thalassaemia, including bone marrow transplantation, blood transfusion, and chelation. The choice of treatment depends on the patient's age, severity of symptoms, and response to treatment. Blood transfusion is the main treatment for individuals with moderate to severe thalassaemia [16].

Frequent blood transfusions can cause infertility in adolescents. Infertility is often due to HH, which is a consequence of transfusion haemosiderosis. Excessive deposition of iron and oxidative iron compounds occurs with blood transfusion, leading to dysfunction of the female reproductive axis [17].

Bone marrow and blood transplantation are also used for the treatment of beta-thalassaemia. Bone marrow and blood transplantation allow the replacement of defective stem cells with healthy stem cells from a compatible donor. Thus, this is the most effective treatment method. However, it is difficult to find a good donor match for a small number of patients with severe thalassaemia.

Thirty to eighty percent of patients with transfusion-dependent thalassaemia show long-term ovulatory dysfunction and hypogonadism. Iron chelation therapy is also a mode of treatment for beta-thalassaemia [18, 19]. This treatment approach is mainly due to regular blood transfusion [13]. Regular blood transfusion leads to excessive accumulation of iron in the body, causing iron overload. Iron overload can cause infertility and damage to the liver and heart.

HSCT is a well-established and often the only curative treatment for severe haematological diseases. Therefore, the number of stem cell transplantations for nonmalignant diseases has continuously increased over the last decades and has led to an overall improvement in the survival of patients with congenital and acquired nonmalignant diseases [20, 21].

There is already much information in the literature on fertility preservation in patients with cancer. However, there are other pathologies, such as haematological nonmalignant diseases, where there are no clear clinical guidelines for fertility preservation [20, 22].

All prepubertal and postpubertal patients should be counselled on the options for fertility preservation measures that may be appropriate for them. Counselling should include information on the risk of diminished fertility—as a result of the intended treatment in relation to disease, age, previous therapy, and other comorbidities. The concept of fertility preservation is an integral part of treatment. During counselling, the possibility of inheritance of the underlying disease and possible pregnancy complications should be addressed [20].

Various fertility preservation options are available, such as oocyte cryopreservation, embryo cryopreservation, ovarian tissue transplantation, or ovarian function suppression by GnRH-analogues [21].

A 2019 publication describes the best methods to assess ovarian reserve after chemotherapy or total body irradiation, such as dynamic levels of FSH and oestradiol. It should be noted that antral follicle count and AMH levels are menstrual cycle-independent markers of ovarian reserve. In the case of beta-thalassaemia with haemosiderosis due to multiple transfusions, there may be iron-induced damage to the pituitary gland and/or ovarian tissue [23].

Currently, there are several nongonadotoxic therapeutic approaches that may open up a new pathway for beta-thalassaemia, such as preservation of hormonal function and fertility [24].

Future treatments for beta-thalassaemia depend on the benefit/risk/cost ratio of conventional transfusion, iron chelation, allogeneic bone marrow transplantation, and gene therapy, as well as the availability of these treatments in different health systems.

Gene therapy is still at an early stage of development, but several clinical studies have demonstrated the principle of sustained clinical efficacy with low toxicity in a number of patients [24].

Until such therapies are established, there is a high risk of POI due to the various beta-thalassaemia therapies; therefore, a detailed assessment of fertility preservation in adolescents and young adults should be undertaken if a multidisciplinary approach is adopted.

In our clinical case, the cause of POI would be the absence of fertility treatment prior to cyclophosphamide exposure.

The incidence of temporary amenorrhoea or early menopause following chemotherapy or radiotherapy varies with age, existing ovarian reserve, type of chemotherapy, and cumulative chemotherapy dose. Cyclophosphamide causes progressive and irreversible damage to oocytes in a dose-dependent manner. Chemotherapy with alkylating agents, such as cyclophosphamide, is associated with the highest risk of amenorrhoea [24].

In our case report, genetic testing (karyotype and fragile X syndrome) was performed to rule out genetic causes of POI. The karyotype revealed a 46,XY karyotype due to the bone marrow transplant of her HLA-identical brother. The XX karyotype was not verified. Quantitative fluorescent PCR analysis was performed, which resulted in a mixture of the two karyotypes. Low levels of gonadotrophins may obscure a POI in patients with severe beta-thalassaemia major. Due to the undetected ovarian reserve, a diagnosis of POI was made.

In conclusion, the main cause of infertility in patients with beta-thalassaemia major is HH. Endocrine complications occur due to iron overload secondary to frequent blood transfusions and bone marrow transplantation (resulting in hypergonadotropic hypogonadism). The treatment of infertility in patients with thalassaemia involves thorough counselling and fertility preservation before therapy. Nongonadotoxic alternative therapies, such as gene therapy, may be a safe alternative for such patients.

Consent

Written informed consent was obtained from the patient for the publication of this case report and its accompanying images. Patient anonymity was maintained.

References

[1] M. Nourollahpour Shiadeh, E. Cassinerio, M. Modarres, A. Zareiyan, Z. Hamzehgardeshi, and Z. Behboodi Moghadam, "Reproductive health issues in female patients with beta-thalassaemia major: a narrative literature review," *Journal of Obstetrics and Gynaecology*, vol. 40, no. 7, pp. 902–911, 2020.

[2] A. Agarwal, S. Gupta, and R. K. Sharma, "Role of oxidative stress in female reproduction," *Reproductive Biology and Endocrinology*, vol. 3, no. 1, p. 28, 2005.

[3] P. Roussou, N. J. Tsagarakis, D. Kountouras, S. Livadas, and E. Diamanti-Kandarakis, "Beta-thalassemia major and female fertility: the role of iron and iron-induced oxidative stress," *Anemia*, vol. 2013, Article ID 617204, 2013.

[4] J. P. S. Chern, K.-H. Lin, W.-Y. Tsai et al., "Hypogonadotropic hypogonadism and hematologic phenotype in patients with transfusion-dependent beta-thalassemia," *Journal of Pediatric Hematology/Oncology*, vol. 25, no. 11, pp. 880–884, 2003.

[5] G. Lucarelli, A. Isgrò, P. Sodani, and J. Gaziev, "Hematopoietic stem cell transplantation in thalassemia and sickle cell anemia," *Cold Spring Harbor Perspectives in Medicine*, vol. 2, no. 5, 2012.

[6] A. Makis, E. Voskaridou, I. Papassotiriou, and E. Hatzimichael, "Novel therapeutic advances in β-thalassemia," *Biology*, vol. 10, no. 6, p. 546, 2021.

[7] European Society for Human Reproduction and Embryology (ESHRE) Guideline Group on POI, L. Webber, M. Davies et al., "ESHRE Guideline: management of women with premature ovarian insufficiency," *Hum Reprod*, vol. 31, pp. 926–937, 2016.

[8] J. S. E. Laven, "Primary ovarian insufficiency," *Seminars in Reproductive Medicine*, vol. 34, no. 4, pp. 230–234, 2016.

[9] K. Maclaran, E. Horner, and N. Panay, "Premature ovarian failure: long-term sequelae," *Menopause International*, vol. 16, no. 1, pp. 38–41, 2010.

[10] U. Boehm, P.-M. Bouloux, M. T. Dattani et al., "Expert consensus document: European Consensus Statement on congenital hypogonadotropic hypogonadism–pathogenesis, diagnosis and treatment," *Nature Reviews Endocrinology*, vol. 11, pp. 547–564, 2015.

[11] A. Capozzi, G. Scambia, A. Pontecorvi, and S. Lello, "Hyperprolactinemia: pathophysiology and therapeutic approach," *Gynecological Endocrinology*, vol. 31, no. 7, pp. 506–510, 2015.

[12] D. A. Klein, J. E. Emerick, J. E. Sylvester, and K. S. Vogt, "Disorders of puberty: an approach to diagnosis and management," *American Family Physician*, vol. 96, no. 9, pp. 590–599, 2017.

[13] E. Khandros and J. L. Kwiatkowski, "Beta thalassemia: monitoring and new treatment approaches," *Hematology/Oncology Clinics of North America*, vol. 33, no. 3, pp. 339–353, 2019.

[14] C. Hershko, "Pathogenesis and management of iron toxicity in thalassemia," *Annals of the New York Academy of Sciences*, vol. 1202, no. 1, pp. 1–9, 2010.

[15] V. De Sanctis, A. T. Soliman, M. A. Yassin et al., "Hypogonadism in male thalassemia major patients: pathophysiology, diagnosis and treatment," *Acta Bio-Medica*, vol. 89, no. 2-S, pp. 6–15, 2018.

[16] E. Fibach and E. A. Rachmilewitz, "Pathophysiology and treatment of patients with beta-thalassemia - an update," *F1000Res*, vol. 6, p. 2156, 2017.

[17] A. Albu, C. G. Barbu, L. Antonie, F. Vladareanu, and S. Fica, "Risk factors associated with hypogonadism in β-thalassemia major patients: predictors for a frequent complication of a rare disease," *Postgraduate Medicine*, vol. 126, no. 5, pp. 121–127, 2014.

[18] K. T. Carlberg, S. T. Singer, and E. P. Vichinsky, "Fertility and pregnancy in women with transfusion-dependent thalassemia," *Hematology/Oncology Clinics of North America*, vol. 32, no. 2, pp. 297–315, 2018.

[19] E. B. Fung, P. R. Harmatz, P. D. K. Lee et al., "Increased prevalence of iron-overload associated endocrinopathy in thalassaemia versus sickle-cell disease," *British Journal of Haematology*, vol. 135, no. 4, pp. 574–582, 2006.

[20] E. M. Mobley, G. L. Ryan, A. E. Sparks, V. Monga, and W. W. Terry, "Factors impacting fertility preservation in adolescents and Young adults with cancer: a retrospective study," *Journal of Adolescent and Young Adult Oncology*, vol. 9, no. 2, pp. 208–221, 2020.

[21] N. Sänger, A. Jarisch, F. Ochsendorf et al., "Fertility preservation in prepubertal und pubertal children and adolescents," *Klinische Pädiatrie*, 2018.

[22] A. N. Schüring, T. Fehm, K. Behringer et al., "Practical recommendations for fertility preservation in women by the FertiPROTEKT network. Part I: indications for fertility preservation," *Archives of gynecology and obstetrics*, vol. 297, no. 1, pp. 241–255, 2018.

[23] F. Tomao, P. Vici, and S. Tomao, "Fertility preservation and reproductive health in patients undergoing hematopoietic stem cell transplantation," *Biology of Blood and Marrow Transplantation*, vol. 25, no. 12, pp. e389–e390, 2019.

[24] E. de Dreuzy, K. Bhukhai, P. Leboulch, and E. Payen, "Current and future alternative therapies for beta-thalassemia major," *Biomedical Journal*, vol. 39, no. 1, pp. 24–38, 2016.

22

Symptomatic Clitoral Neuroma within an Epidermal Inclusion Cyst at the Site of Prior Female Genital Cutting

Dani Zoorob,[1] **Kristrun Kristinsdottir**,[1] **Thomas Klein**,[1] **and Sonyoung Seo-Patel**[2]

[1] *University of Toledo, Department of Obstetrics and Gynecology Academic Offices, 2142 N. Cove Blvd., Toledo, OH 43606, USA*
[2] *ProMedica Health System, Women's Services, 2142 N. Cove Blvd., Toledo, OH 43606, USA*

Correspondence should be addressed to Dani Zoorob; dzobgyn@gmail.com

Academic Editor: Kyousuke Takeuchi

Background. Clitoral neuromas occurring after female genital mutilation/cutting (FGM/C) can vary in presentation and may require surgical management. *Case.* A 39-year-old East African female with a history of FGM/C presented during pregnancy with a progressively enlarging mass and worsening periclitoral pain. Postpartum surgical excision restored cosmesis and resolved the discomfort with pathology confirming the presence of a neuroma within the epidermal inclusion cyst. *Conclusion.* We present the first published case of a symptomatic clitoral neuroma within an epidermal inclusion cyst. This unique pathology demonstrates that complications of female genital cutting can present in complex and varied ways. Considering the prevalence of FGM/C and increasing rates of emigration from countries in which FGM/C is performed, complex clitoral neuromas are an important long-term complication which providers in Africa or internationally must be aware of.

1. Introduction

Female genital mutilation/cutting (FGM/C) is sociocultural practice defined by the World Health Organization as the "partial or total removal of the external female genitalia or other injury to the female genital organs for nonmedical reasons" [1]. It is most commonly performed in parts of Africa, the Middle East, and Asia and frequently before the age of fifteen by a community leader. Analgesia is often not utilized, resulting in severe acute pain [1–3].

It is estimated that 100 to 140 million women around the world have undergone FGM/C, with approximately three million new cases each year [1, 4]. Recent data show decreasing acceptance of this practice even amongst countries where FGM/C is nearly universal [2].

In 2007, the WHO published a revised classification system to systematically describe the extent of FGM/C based on parts of the genitalia removed. Type I includes partial or total removal of the clitoris (clitoridectomy) while type II also includes removal of the labia minora with or without excision of the labia majora. Type III, also known as infibulation, is the most extensive form and includes narrowing of the vaginal orifice by appositioning a portion of the removed labia minora or majora. Type IV includes any other nonmedical procedures to female genitalia such as piercing, nicking, or cauterizing. Further subclassifications of FGM/C do exist and can be found in the literature [1].

Complications of FGM/C are many. Immediate complications include bleeding, infection, and pain [5, 6]. The vaginal tissue becomes more prone to tears, which increases the risk of acquiring sexually transmitted infections [7]. Women undergoing infibulation (Type III FGM/C) may be left with a small introitus, which can result in urinary tract infections and potentially prolonged, painful periods [5]. Additionally, the vagina may be scarred thus losing its elasticity, causing dyspareunia for both the patient and her partner, as well as obstetric complications during vaginal deliveries. Particularly with infibulation, women are at risk of prolonged labor and the need for cesarean section, postpartum hemorrhage, episiotomy, and prolonged maternal hospital stay. Their infants are at an increased risk of stillbirth and early neonatal death [8]. As the procedure often involves transection of the clitoris and the clitoral nerves, women are at risk of developing chronic localized pain and potentially neuroma formation [6]. Though lacking high-quality data, it is believed that the psychological consequences of this practice can be immense.

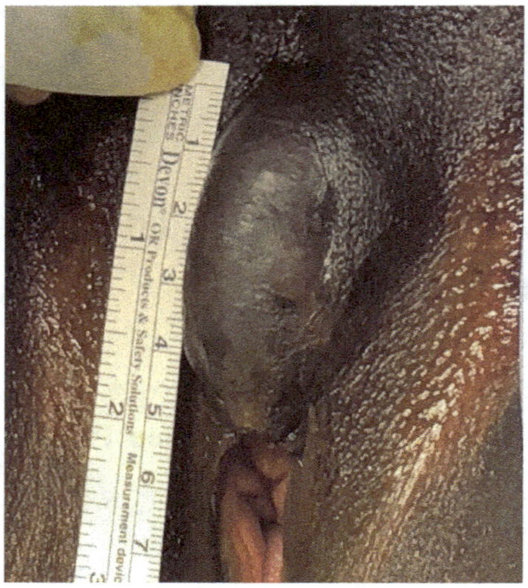

Figure 1: Preoperative view of the clitoral neuroma.

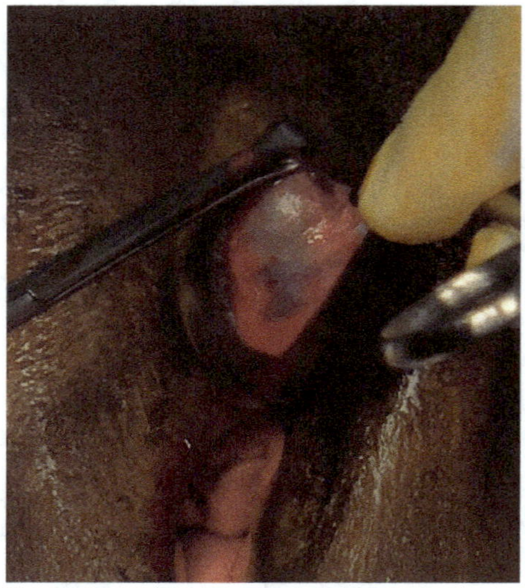

Figure 2: Cystic appearance of the neuroma.

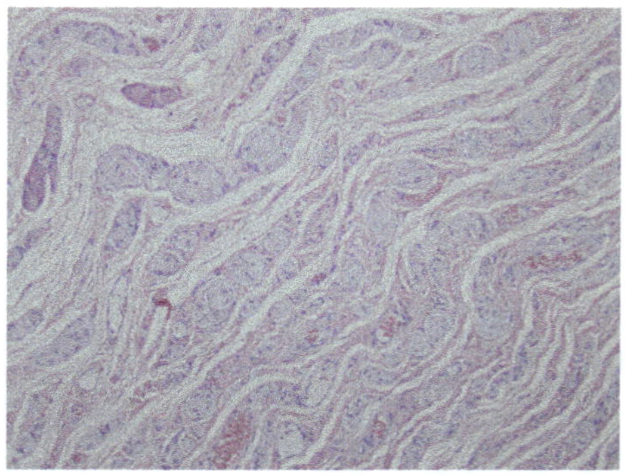

Figure 3: Microscopic view of the neuronal tissue identified within the cystic structure.

A 2015 study of Senegalese women demonstrated a 30.4% prevalence of posttraumatic stress disorder attributed to this practice [8]. Thus, the practice of FGM/C has a multitude of short and long-term consequences.

2. Case

A 39-year-old G3P2002 female of Somali origin with two prior vaginal deliveries in Somalia presented with a periclitoral swelling. This had been slowly enlarging over the previous 10 years, but the change during this pregnancy was rapid an acute. She had a history of FGM/C Type IIIb (infibulation with removal and appositioning of the labia majora) at seven years of age without reported complications. Past medical and surgical history were otherwise unremarkable. The patient had undergone prior defibulation at delivery, which was not noted to be protracted nor required operative delivery. She denied any urinary symptoms and had expectantly managed her symptoms throughout the pregnancy. Surgical management was deferred until following delivery despite the persistent periclitoral burning pain that worsened as the lesion enlarged throughout the pregnancy. The patient also noted worsening dyspareunia symptoms as the pregnancy progressed even before fetal size caused appreciable pressure. The patient delivered via cesarean section due to breech presentation and she represented during her postpartum course for surgical removal of the lesion due to persistent symptoms which negatively impacted her quality of life.

Preoperatively, physical examination demonstrated the presence of a tender 4 cm x 3 cm x 2 cm periclitoral fluctuant lesion (Figure 1). Surgically, the lesion was treated by excision and reapproximation. This was performed by infiltrating the overlying skin with Marcaine, incising vertically at midline, and then dissecting around the cyst using both blunt and sharp dissection (Figure 2). After near complete shelling of the cyst, a stalk was noted to extend across the cyst. Due to the site of attachment and origin, it was suggestive of a clitoral remnant. The neuroma stalk was noted to be firm and thick on palpation. The stalk was transected at the base where the cyst wall originated and the cyst was freed. Hemostasis was ensured. A mattress suture was used to close the defect. Excess skin was trimmed and reapproximated using a subcuticular suture for restored cosmesis.

Following excision, the cyst was opened. Gross examination of the lesion demonstrated a dark grey stalk extending throughout two ends of the cyst with a glossy green-grey viscous material and no fluid. The widest diameter of the cyst measured 3.2 cm. Pathologic analysis of the cyst wall specifically demonstrated keratinizing squamous epithelium consistent with epidermal inclusion cyst. The stalk within the cyst wall was suggestive of a traumatic neuroma demonstrating proliferation of nerve fibers within a fibrotic tissue stroma (Figure 3). No malignancy was identified.

The patient's postoperative course was uncomplicated, and she reported resolution of both discomfort and dyspareunia.

3. Discussion

Relatively few clitoral neuromas have been reported as complications of FGM/C, but it is believed that this issue may be underrecognized and under-reported [5, 6, 9]. Clitoral neuromas after FGM/C are considered a type of amputation neuroma. We believe this is what contributed to our patient's condition. These entities arise after trauma to or transection of a nerve, and they are due to disorganized proximal nerve regeneration. Histopathology of the lesion typically shows irregularly arranged nerve fascicles within a fibrous stroma [5].

Treatment options include desensitization, steroid injections, and surgical excision, the latter of which is suggested to be the most efficacious therapy for resolution of traumatic clitoral neuromas. In such cases, recurrence of the traumatic neuroma is theoretically possible, and both providers and patients should be keenly aware of this possibility. However, to date, no cases have been published regarding such a complication [5]. In similar cases of traumatic penile neuromas, standard of care for symptomatic patients is surgical excision, which often results in full recovery [10, 11]. In the setting of FGM/C, the location and presentation of the stalk within the cyst are suggestive of a clitoral neuroma; however, the differential diagnosis does include a simple inclusion cyst, malignant growth of epidermal and mesenchymal tissue, and a secondary inclusion cyst within the original cyst.

Although few similar cases of neuromas have been published, none involved expectant patients [5]. Pregnancy-associated worsening of periclitoral pain—whose origin is the remnant of the dorsal nerve of the clitoris contained within an epidermal inclusion cyst—has never reported in the literature. Furthermore, this is the first case to demonstrate the presence of a clitoral neuroma contained within an epidermal inclusion cyst.

It is important to note that clitoral neuromas after FGM/C may not always be palpable, and the patient's presenting symptoms may only be allodynia or hyperalgesia. This pain is neuropathic and thus often described as a burning, tingling, or shooting sensation [6]. Although management for this patient would have remained the same whether or not the inclusion cyst contained the neuroma, the identification of neural involvement is clinically significant as it may require further treatment at a later point. Due to the variable clinical presentation and impact that clitoral neuromas can have on a patient's life, whether pain, discomfort, or perceived disfigurement, it is crucial that providers be aware of the potential sources of pain impacting patients who have undergone FGM/C and subsequent management options.

Additional Points

Precis. Complications of female genital cutting require keen awareness of a variety of presentations and their subsequent management. *Teaching Points.* With increasingly diversified populations due to higher rates of global migration, women's healthcare providers should be aware of a variety of complications of female genital cutting. One important and likely under-reported complication is traumatic neuromas resulting in periclitoral neuropathic pain. Surgical excision has demonstrated great success and should be considered first-line management in such cases.

Authors' Contributions

D. Zoorob is project lead and contributed to manuscript writing/editing. T. Klein contributed to literature search and manuscript draft. K. Kristinsdottir contributed to literature search and initial draft. S. Seo-Patel contributed to manuscript editing.

References

[1] W. H. Organization, Ed., *Eliminating Female Genital Mutilation: An Interagency Statement*, Geneva, Switzerland, 2008.

[2] UNICEF, Ed., *Female Genital Mutilation/Cutting: A Statistical Overview and Exploration of the Dynamics of Change*, New York, NY, USA, 2013.

[3] S. Costello, "Female genital mutilation/cutting: risk management and strategies for social workers and health care professionals," *Risk Management and Healthcare Policy*, vol. 8, pp. 225–233, 2015.

[4] H. Goldberg, P. Stupp, E. Okoroh, G. Besera, D. Goodman, and I. Danel, "Female genital mutilation/cutting in the united states: updated estimates of women and girls at risk, 2012," *Public Health Reports*, vol. 131, no. 2, pp. 340–347, 2016.

[5] J. Abdulcadir, M. Pusztaszeri, R. Vilarino, J.-B. Dubuisson, and A. T. Vlastos, "Clitoral neuroma after female genital mutilation/cutting: a rare but possible event," *The Journal of Sexual Medicine*, vol. 9, no. 4, pp. 1220–1225, 2012.

[6] J. Abdulcadir, J. Tille, and P. Petignat, "Management of painful clitoral neuroma after female genital mutilation/cutting," *Reproductive Health*, vol. 14, no. 22, pp. 1–7, 2017.

[7] C. Iavazzo, T. A. Sardi, and I. D. Gkegkes, "Female genital mutilation and infections: a systematic review of the clinical evidence," *Archives of Gynecology and Obstetrics*, vol. 287, no. 6, pp. 1137–1149, 2013.

[8] D. Reisel and S. M. Creighton, "Long term health consequences of Female Genital Mutilation (FGM)," *Maturitas*, vol. 80, no. 1, pp. 48–51, 2014.

[9] H. A. Schiotz, T. Bohlin, T. A. Klingen, and T. Aaberg, "Neuroma in the clitoris after circumcision," *Journal of the Norwegian Medical Association*, vol. 6, no. 132, pp. 629-630, 2012.

[10] E. Salcedo, A. C. Soldano, L. Chen et al., "Traumatic neuromas of the penis: a clinical, histopathological and immunohistochemical study of 17 cases," *Journal of Cutaneous Pathology*, vol. 36, no. 2, pp. 229–233, 2009.

[11] H. J. Park, T. N. Kim, S. R. Baek, K. M. Lee, K. Choi, and N. C. Park, "Penile traumatic neuroma: a late complication of penile dorsal neurotomy to treat premature ejaculation," *Sexual Medicine*, vol. 4, no. 3, pp. e221–e224, 2016.

23

Efficacy of Hydroxychloroquine for Improving Pregnancy Outcomes in a Female with Systemic Lupus Erythematosus and Antiphospholipid Syndrome

Yumika Takaki, Atsushi Daimon, Misa Nunode, Tomohito Tanaka, Daisuke Fujita, and Masahide Ohmichi

Department of Obstetrics and Gynecology, Osaka Medical and Pharmaceutical University, 2-7 Daigaku-Machi, Takatsuki, Osaka 569-8686, Japan

Correspondence should be addressed to Yumika Takaki; yumika.takaki@ompu.ac.jp
and Atsushi Daimon; atsushi.daimon@ompu.ac.jp

Academic Editor: Giuseppe Gullo

The use of heparin and low-dose aspirin is the current conventional treatment for pregnant females with antiphospholipid syndrome (APS). However, there is no additional treatment recommended for cases where the standard treatment cannot prevent obstetric complications such as fetal loss and placental insufficiency. Recently, the addition of a novel antimalarial, hydroxychloroquine (HCQ), to the conventional treatment has shown the potential to prevent obstetric complications. Herein, we report a case in which the addition of HCQ improved adverse pregnancy outcomes in a pregnant female with systemic lupus erythematosus and aspirin-heparin-resistant APS.

1. Introduction

Females with antiphospholipid syndrome (APS) have an increased risk of thrombosis and pregnancy complications, such as recurrent early miscarriages and hypertensive disorders of pregnancy [1]. The use of heparin and low-dose aspirin (LDA) is the current conventional treatment for pregnant females with APS and has improved pregnancy outcomes to a live birth rate of >70% [2, 3]. Recently, an antimalarial drug, hydroxychloroquine (HCQ), was recommended, besides the conventional treatment in patients with APS and previous pregnancy failure on current therapy for APS [4]. Herein, we report a case of systemic lupus erythematosus (SLE) and aspirin-heparin-resistant APS successfully treated with HCQ in addition to the patient's existing therapy.

2. Case Presentation

A 35-year-old pregnant female (gravida 4, parity 1) with SLE without lupus nephritis and APS visited our hospital at 6 weeks of gestation (GW). The patient was diagnosed with SLE without lupus nephritis and was positive for antiphospholipid antibody (aPL), including lupus anticoagulant, anticardiolipin antibody, and antiphosphatidylserine/prothrombin antibodies at 18 years old. The patient's pregnancy history is presented in Table 1. The first pregnancy resulted in an APS diagnosis. The SLE remained in remission, and this case was diagnosed as an aspirin-heparin-resistant APS based on the patient's pregnancy history. Consequently, for the fourth pregnancy, HCQ was commenced before conception with the patient's informed consent. Immediately after a positive pregnancy test was obtained, warfarin was

Table 1: Patient's pregnancy history.

	First pregnancy	Second pregnancy	Third pregnancy
Age (y)	28	31	34
Medication during pregnancy	PSL (9 mg/day) LDA (100 mg/day)	PSL (15 mg/day) LDA (100 mg/day) UFH (10,000 units/day)	PSL (12 mg/day) LDA (100 mg/day) UFH (10,000 units/day) TAC (4 mg/day) IVIg at 9 GW (25 g/day, 5 consecutive days, total 125 g)
Complication: mother	None	HELLP syndrome	Chronic hypertension
Complication: infant	FGR, IUFD	Intact survival	IUFD
Gestational age at delivery (GW)	22	24	16
Birth weight (g)	145	498	80

PSL: prednisolone; LDA: low-dose aspirin; UFH: unfractionated heparin; TAC: tacrolimus; FGR: fetal growth restriction; IUFD: intrauterine fetal demise; HELLP: hemolysis, elevated liver enzymes, and low platelets; GW: gestational week; IVIg: intravenous immunoglobulin.

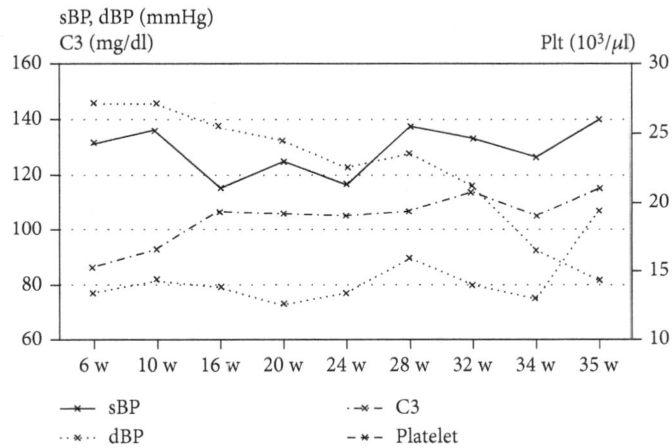

Figure 1: Changes in blood pressure and blood sampling data.

discontinued. Following that, the 6 GW embryo was confirmed, therapeutic doses of unfractionated heparin (UFH) (15,000 units/day, subcutaneously) were introduced, and intravenous immunoglobulin therapy (IVIg) (25 g/day for 5 consecutive days; total dose: 125 g) was administered without adverse effects. LDA was maintained until 34 GW, and the fetal growth was appropriate for the gestational age. However, the patient's platelet count decreased from 27.2 $\times 10^{4/}\mu$L at 6 GW to 16.5 $\times 10^{4/}\mu$L at 34 GW, and the maternal blood pressure was elevated to 133/90 mmHg (Figure 1). Contrarily, the serum C3 levels did not decrease during this pregnancy (Figure 1). The platelet count further decreased to 14.4 $\times 10^{4/}\mu$L at 35 GW (Figure 1), and we assessed that the patient's condition had worsened. Therefore, a cesarean section was performed, and a male infant weighing 2,618 g was delivered. Continuous heparin infusion was initiated 12 h after cesarean section and continued for 5 days. On postpartum day 1, LDA (100 mg/day) and warfarin (5 mg/day) were restarted. The patient and infant were discharged without complications on postpartum day 6.

3. Discussion

This case of treatment-resistant APS with SLE was treated successfully with HCQ, LDA, therapeutic doses of UFH, prednisolone (PSL), tacrolimus, and IVIg at 6 GW.

Not only autoimmune diseases, such as SLE and APS [1], but also other proinflammatory diseases, such as endometriosis [5] and polycystic ovary syndrome [6], are known to influence the reproductive outcomes. Despite receiving conventional therapy, 20–30% of females with APS continue to experience pregnancy complications. Attempts have been made to add PSL [7] or IVIg [8] to the conventional treatment; however, the best approach to improve the outcomes of these pregnancies is unknown. Recently, novel drugs, including HCQ [9] and pravastatin [10], have been considered for preventing adverse pregnancy outcomes. HCQ was recommended in addition to the conventional therapy in patients with APS and previous pregnancy failure receiving the standard treatment [4]. Thus, HCQ may benefit patients with thrombotic and obstetric APS.

Several studies have investigated the mechanism by which HCQ exerts an antithrombotic effect. In vitro, HCQ inhibited platelet aggregation and the release of arachidonic acid from aPL-induced stimulated platelets [11]. In vivo, in patients with aPL and APS, HCQ restored the destruction of the anticoagulant annexin A5 [12] and decreased soluble tissue factor [13]. The obstetric effects of HCQ have been reported in experiments with mice. In an aPL-induced fetal loss mouse model, HCQ prevented fetal death, increased placental and fetal weight, and decreased placental superoxide production, which is a marker of oxidative stress [14]. In vitro, HCQ significantly reduced the induction of endosomal nicotinamide adenine dinucleotide phosphate (NADPH), an enzyme complex involved in proinflammatory signaling pathways [15]. Clinically, HCQ is expected to prevent aPL-related adverse pregnancy outcomes, including first-trimester miscarriages and ischemic placental-mediated complications, such as preeclampsia and fetal growth restriction [9, 16].

In conclusion, HCQ may be useful in improving pregnancy outcomes in patients with previous pregnancy failure receiving the current conventional treatment for APS.

Authors' Contributions

The authors alone are responsible for the content and writing of this manuscript.

Acknowledgments

We would like to thank Editage (http://www.editage.com) for English language editing.

References

[1] K. Schreiber and B. J. Hunt, "Managing antiphospholipid syndrome in pregnancy," *Thrombosis Research*, vol. 181, Suppl 1, pp. S41–S46, 2019.

[2] G. Espinosa and R. Cervera, "Current treatment of antiphospholipid syndrome: lights and shadows," *Nature Reviews Rheumatology*, vol. 11, no. 10, pp. 586–596, 2015.

[3] M. Empson, M. Lassere, J. C. Craig, J. R. Scott, and Cochrane Pregnancy and Childbirth Group, "Prevention of recurrent miscarriage for women with antiphospholipid antibody or lupus anticoagulant," *Cochrane Database of Systematic Reviews*, vol. 2012, no. 2, article CD002859, 2012.

[4] S. Sciascia, D. W. Branch, R. A. Levy et al., "The efficacy of hydroxychloroquine in altering pregnancy outcome in women with antiphospholipid antibodies," *Thrombosis and Haemostasis*, vol. 115, no. 2, pp. 285–290, 2016.

[5] V. Šalamun, I. Verdenik, A. S. Laganà, and E. Vrtačnik-Bokal, "Should we consider integrated approach for endometriosis-associated infertility as gold standard management? Rationale and results from a large cohort analysis," *Archives of Gynecology and Obstetrics*, vol. 297, no. 3, pp. 613–621, 2018.

[6] M. N. D'Alterio, M. Sigilli, A. G. Succu et al., "Pregnancy outcomes in women with polycystic ovarian syndrome," *Minerva Obstetrics and Gynecology*, vol. 74, no. 1, pp. 45–59, 2022.

[7] K. Bramham, M. Thomas, C. Nelson-Piercy, M. Khamashta, and B. J. Hunt, "First-trimester low-dose prednisolone in refractory antiphospholipid antibody-related pregnancy loss," *Blood*, vol. 117, no. 25, pp. 6948–6951, 2011.

[8] S. Shimada, H. Yamada, T. Atsumi, T. Yamada, N. Sakuragi, and H. Minakami, "Intravenous immunoglobulin therapy for aspirin-heparinoid-resistant antiphospholipid syndrome," *Reproductive Medicine and Biology*, vol. 9, no. 4, pp. 217–221, 2010.

[9] S. Sciascia, B. J. Hunt, E. Talavera-Garcia, G. Lliso, M. A. Khamashta, and M. J. Cuadrado, "The impact of hydroxychloroquine treatment on pregnancy outcome in women with antiphospholipid antibodies," *American Journal of Obstetrics and Gynecology*, vol. 214, no. 2, pp. 273.e1–273.e8, 2016.

[10] E. Lefkou, A. Mamopoulos, T. Dagklis, C. Vosnakis, D. Rousso, and G. Girardi, "Pravastatin improves pregnancy outcomes in obstetric antiphospholipid syndrome refractory to antithrombotic therapy," *The Journal of Clinical Investigation*, vol. 126, no. 8, pp. 2933–2940, 2016.

[11] S. S. Pierangeli, M. Vega-Ostertag, and E. N. Harris, "Intracellular signaling triggered by antiphospholipid antibodies in platelets and endothelial cells: a pathway to targeted therapies," *Thrombosis Research*, vol. 114, no. 5-6, pp. 467–476, 2004.

[12] J. H. Rand, X. X. Wu, A. S. Quinn et al., "Hydroxychloroquine protects the annexin A5 anticoagulant shield from disruption by antiphospholipid antibodies: evidence for a novel effect for an old antimalarial drug," *Blood*, vol. 115, no. 11, pp. 2292–2299, 2010.

[13] K. Schreiber, K. Breen, H. Cohen et al., "HYdroxychloroquine to Improve Pregnancy Outcome in Women with AnTIphospholipid Antibodies (HYPATIA) protocol: a multinational randomized controlled trial of hydroxychloroquine versus placebo in addition to standard treatment in pregnant women with antiphospholipid syndrome or antibodies," *Seminars in Thrombosis and Hemostasis*, vol. 43, no. 6, pp. 562–571, 2017.

[14] M. L. Bertolaccini, G. Contento, R. Lennen et al., "Complement inhibition by hydroxychloroquine prevents placental and fetal brain abnormalities in antiphospholipid syndrome," *Journal of Autoimmunity*, vol. 75, pp. 30–38, 2016.

[15] N. Müller-Calleja, D. Manukyan, A. Canisius, D. Strand, and K. J. Lackner, "Hydroxychloroquine inhibits proinflammatory signalling pathways by targeting endosomal NADPH oxidase," *Annals of the Rheumatic Diseases*, vol. 76, no. 5, pp. 891–897, 2017.

[16] A. Mekinian, M. G. Lazzaroni, A. Kuzenko et al., "The efficacy of hydroxychloroquine for obstetrical outcome in antiphospholipid syndrome: data from a European multicenter retrospective study," *Autoimmunity Reviews*, vol. 14, no. 6, pp. 498–502, 2015.

24

Management of a Novel Autoimmune Disease, COPA Syndrome, in Pregnancy

Archana Ayyar,[1] **Rachel D. Seaman**,[1] **Kalpalatha Guntupalli**,[2] **and Mary C. Tolcher**[1]

[1]*Department of Obstetrics and Gynecology, Baylor College of Medicine, Houston, Texas, USA*
[2]*Department of Medicine, Pulmonary and Critical Care, Baylor College of Medicine, Houston, Texas, USA*

Correspondence should be addressed to Mary C. Tolcher; mary.tolcher@bcm.edu

Academic Editor: Daniel Martin

Background. COPA syndrome is a rare autoimmune disease, demonstrating an autosomal dominant inheritance pattern with variable penetration that occurs more frequently in females than males. This disease manifests in childhood as pulmonary hemorrhage, arthritis, and renal disease. *Case.* We present a case of obstetric management of a 20-year-old nulligravida patient with a diagnosis of COPA syndrome. Her case was further complicated by multiple antepartum admissions for hypoxemia and a complex psychosocial history of substance use. On her first antepartum admission, rheumatology recommended management with hydroxychloroquine, inhaled corticosteroids (budesonide), and bronchodilators (albuterol inhaler) as needed. On admission for induction of labor, she was again noted to have oxygen desaturations. A chronic thrombus was noted on computed tomography (CT), and a multidisciplinary team was recommended against Valsalva. Thus, she had a primary cesarean delivery. Her postpartum course was only remarkable for improved oxygenation status. *Conclusion.* Management of COPA syndrome should be performed by a multidisciplinary team including maternal-fetal medicine, rheumatology, and pulmonology specialists. Traditionally, COPA syndrome is treated with immunomodulator therapy often used to treat autoimmune syndromes. However, many of these medications are not well studied or contraindicated in pregnancy. Preconception counseling is recommended both to ensure pregnancy safe medications being prescribed and to provide information on the genetic inheritance of this disease. At time of entry to care, patients should have a baseline work-up including a radiographic imaging, complete blood count, complete metabolic panel, lactate dehydrogenase, and a 24-hour urine protein collection for baseline. Although thought to be rare, COPA syndrome has an autosomal dominance pattern of inheritance with variable penetrance that is more common in females. Thus, incidence of COPA syndrome in pregnancy will likely increase in the future. Further case studies are warranted to optimize management of patients with COPA syndrome in pregnancy.

1. Introduction

COPA syndrome, named after its affected COPα protein, is a recently identified, heritable immunodeficiency marked by dysfunctional protein transport between the Golgi complex and endoplasmic reticulum [1–3]. Under physiologic circumstances, COPα regulates the retrograde movement of proteins from the Golgi complex to the endoplasmic reticulum. One of these proteins is the stimulator of interferon gene (STING), which provides immune system equilibrium. Dysfunctional transport by mutated COPα in COPA syndrome leads to trapping of STING within the Golgi which facilitates a skewed type I interferon inflammatory response [4, 5]. This leads to the release of proinflammatory cytokines and abnormal cellular autophagy, manifesting clinically as diffuse alveolar hemorrhage (DAH), arthritis, and renal disease—often beginning before five years of age and progressing into adulthood [1–3, 6].

First identified in 2015, COPA syndrome is thought to be more common than previously believed [3]. Following an autosomal dominant inheritance pattern, the syndrome appears to have variable penetrance and affects females more commonly than males. However, to our knowledge, this is the first documented case of COPA syndrome in pregnancy.

2. Case

A 20-year-old primigravida with known COPA syndrome presented at 11 weeks gestation to establish prenatal care at our maternal-fetal medicine clinic. Her COPA disease had been diagnosed at an early age, requiring multiple admissions for pulmonary vasculitis with alveolar hemorrhage throughout her childhood. Secondary to a complex psychosocial situation and financial instability, she had been off immunosuppressive therapy for two years at the time of her entry into prenatal care. During that period, she sought symptomatic relief of episodic dyspnea through local emergency departments, with her most recent encounter occurring at 6 weeks gestation. At that visit, she presented with mild shortness of breath and was discharged with a rescue albuterol inhaler. She also endorsed long-term, regular use of cigarettes and marijuana, and smoking cessation education was provided.

On presentation to our obstetrics clinic, the patient complained of persistent shortness of breath and was found to have a peripheral oxygen saturation of 88% upon ambulation. She was directly admitted to the antepartum service for further evaluation of her hypoxemia. Chest X-ray revealed diffuse reticular opacities consistent with a history of interstitial lung disease, without any evidence of active pulmonary hemorrhage. Pulmonary function testing demonstrated a mild restrictive ventilation defect [FEV1 2.26 L (71% of predicted value), FVC 2.57 L (72%), and FEV1/FVC 88% (101%)]. Echocardiogram was normal with an ejection fraction of 60-64% and without evidence of right-sided dysfunction or pulmonary hypertension. Supplemental oxygen was not needed throughout her work-up, and her oxygen saturation remained largely within normal limits for the remainder of the admission. Following consultation with rheumatology, she was discharged home on hydroxychloroquine 300 mg daily, budesonide twice daily, and albuterol inhaler as needed, with close outpatient follow-up. She was readmitted at 21 weeks gestation for similar symptoms, thought to be due to medication nonadherence. Work-up was again unremarkable, she did not require oxygen therapy, and she was discharged to home.

At 37 2/7 weeks gestation, she was admitted for induction of labor in the setting of newly diagnosed fetal growth restriction with an estimated fetal weight at the 3rd percentile. However, upon presentation, she was again noted to be hypoxemic, with oxygen saturations ranging from 74 to 94% on room air. She required supplemental oxygenation via nasal cannula and her clinical picture was concerning for a COPA flare with possible diffuse alveolar hemorrhage (DAH). She again acknowledged nonadherence with her home medications and recent cigarette smoking at the time of admission.

An extensive work-up was commenced, and admission chest X-ray and echocardiogram remained stable from prior. Computed tomography of the chest revealed poor visualization of the superior vena cava (SVC) with extensive collateral vasculature of the left hemithorax and mediastinum, concerning for a chronic SVC thrombus with resultant collateralization and possible SVC syndrome. This was corroborated by review of outside hospital records which revealed a stable SVC thrombus for the past two years, thought to have arisen from a prior port placement. A multidisciplinary discussion was held amongst maternal-fetal medicine, cardiology, pulmonology, hematology, and radiology specialists, and ultimately, the decision was made to proceed with prednisone 30 mg daily for presumed COPA flare. Anticoagulation was deferred in the setting of suspected chronic thrombus, given the potential adverse effects of concurrent alveolar hemorrhage. The decision was also made to proceed with cesarean delivery for maternal benefit as Valsalva was felt to pose an indeterminable risk for dislodgement of the SVC thrombus and/or pulmonary decompensation.

Delivery itself was unremarkable. The patient underwent a primary low transverse cesarean delivery under neuraxial anesthesia and without cardiopulmonary complications. Her pulmonary status improved following delivery, and she was weaned off supplemental oxygen by the second postoperative day. Prophylactic anticoagulation was again deferred given remote risk for alveolar hemorrhage. The patient completed a three-day prednisone course and resumed her home medications. She was subsequently discharged on postoperative day three with close outpatient follow-up.

3. Discussion

COPA syndrome is a novel immunodeficiency due to mutations of the regulatory COPα protein and dysfunctional intracellular protein transport, resulting in interferon-mediated inflammatory response. COPA syndrome has a myriad of clinical manifestations, most commonly presenting as diffuse alveolar hemorrhage and antibody-mediated conditions (e.g., rheumatoid factor-positive arthritis, anti-neutrophil cytoplasmic antibody-positive arthritis and lung disease, isolated juvenile idiopathic arthritis, or isolated lupus-like nephropathy) [3].

Our index case was diagnosed with COPA syndrome in early childhood, and her course was complicated by discontinuity of care from diagnosis through adulthood, leading to numerous admissions for pulmonary vasculitis with alveolar hemorrhage. Her case was further complicated by numerous barriers to care leading to medication nonadherence and by marijuana and tobacco use—all of which likely exacerbated her chronic underlying pulmonary damage.

Treatment for COPA syndrome is similar to other immunodeficiency and autoimmune disorders and utilizes immunomodulators with varying safety profiles for use in pregnancy. In 2015, the Food and Drug Administration (FDA) replaced the previous pregnancy risk categories A-D and X with a new system entitled Pregnancy and Lactation Labeling Rule. This new system is aimed at providing data and clinical considerations for pregnancy, lactation, and reproduction that allow for clinical interpretation and patient-specific counseling [7]. Acute COPA exacerbations may be managed with systemic corticosteroids, cyclophosphamide, or rituximab. Maintenance therapy can include etanercept, intravenous immunoglobulin, azathioprine, hydroxychloroquine, or methotrexate [6–8]. While methotrexate is contraindicated during pregnancy, the other medications may be considered on an individual basis after appropriate discussion with specialists and patient counseling. The role of surgical management remains investigatory, although Mallea et al. report a case of a COPA patient undergoing lung transplantation with stable pulmonary function fifteen months postoperatively and without evidence of disease recurrence [9].

This case was largely managed via expert opinion, drawn from a diverse, multidisciplinary healthcare team. Although a multidisciplinary healthcare team may be involved in the care of these patients, we recommend that the obstetrical care of COPA patients be managed by maternal-fetal medicine specialists. Ideally, intensive preconception counseling should be performed in order to review patterns of transmission to offspring and to discuss potential risk of worsening maternal morbidity, particularly the risk of pulmonary decompensation. Radiographic imaging, echocardiography, and pulmonary function testing should be obtained at entry to prenatal care, serving as a baseline for comparison in event of an antepartum disease flare.

Without prior reports of COPA syndrome in pregnancy, it is difficult to discern the effects of pregnancy on COPA syndrome. However, one can infer that pregnancy increased the oxygen demands in this patient, as her previously required oxygen supplementation was weaned down postpartum. Furthermore, although there are no studies on COPA syndrome in pregnancy, there are reports of DAH secondary to systemic lupus erythematosus (SLE) [10]. Alveolar hemorrhage can cause severe hypoxemia that is unresponsive to mechanical ventilation [11]. In SLE patients, abrupt alveolar hemorrhage may develop despite concurrent immunosuppressive drugs. Treatment for active alveolar hemorrhage includes high-dose corticosteroids, possible addition of cyclophosphamide, ventilatory support, and blood resuscitation [10]. Although the patient in this index did not have acute DAH, the same treatment for DAH can be used as a model for future COPA syndrome patients with concurrent DAH.

As previously mentioned, COPA syndrome may also manifest as lupus-like nephritis, with the resultant proteinuria mimicking a common pregnancy condition, preeclampsia. Our index patient did not develop blood pressure elevation, so this conflict did not present itself. However, it is reasonable to also include preeclampsia labs (e.g., complete blood count, liver function testing, lactate dehydrogenase, creatinine, and urine protein studies) in the baseline evaluation of maternal COPA syndrome. This may aid in diagnostic clarity should the patient develop elevated blood pressures in later gestation.

Lastly, the complexities of delivery planning should not be underestimated in the setting of COPA syndrome. Mode of delivery for our index patient was determined based on multiple factors including her active COPA flare causing desaturation, chronic SVC thrombus, and possible SVC syndrome. On literature review, alveolar hemorrhage does not appear to be absolute contraindication to Valsalva; however, it is also important to note that there are no reports associating chronic SVC thrombus with COPA syndrome. Although our patient ultimately underwent a cesarean section, delivery planning for patients with COPA syndrome should be individualized without a clear contraindication to attempted vaginal delivery.

Given COPA syndrome's variable penetrance and increased expression in women, it is likely that the incidence of COPA syndrome in pregnancy will increase in the future. Further research is warranted to optimize the management of obstetrics patients with COPA syndrome.

Consent

The patient signed a waiver granting consent for this article to be published.

Authors' Contributions

AA, MCT, and KG provided care for the patient during her antepartum and intrapartum stay. AA and RS were major contributors in writing the manuscript. All authors read and approved the final manuscript.

References

[1] L. Watkin, B. Jessen, W. Wiszniewski et al., "_COPA_ mutations impair ER-Golgi transport and cause hereditary autoimmune- mediated lung disease and arthritis," *Nature Genetics*, vol. 47, no. 6, pp. 654–660, 2015.

[2] M. Frémond and N. Nathan, "COPA syndrome, 5 years after: where are we?," *Joint, Bone, Spine*, vol. 88, no. 2, article 105070, 2021.

[3] T. Vece, L. Watkin, S. Nicholas et al., "Copa syndrome: a novel autosomal dominant immune dysregulatory disease," *Journal of Clinical Immunology*, vol. 36, no. 4, pp. 377–387, 2016.

[4] Z. Deng, Z. Chong, C. Law et al., "A defect in COPI-mediated transport of STING causes immune dysregulation in COPA syndrome," *Journal of Experimental Medicine*, vol. 217, no. 11, 2020.

[5] K. Mukai, E. Ogawa, R. Uematsu et al., "Homeostatic regulation of STING by retrograde membrane traffic to the ER," *Nature Communications*, vol. 12, no. 1, p. 61, 2021.

[6] S. Krutzke, C. Rietschel, and G. Horneff, "Baricitinib in therapy of COPA syndrome in a 15-year-old girl," *European Journal of Rheumatology*, vol. 7, no. 1, pp. 78–81, 2020.

[7] S. Pernia and G. DeMaagd, "The new pregnancy and lactation labeling rule," *P T*, vol. 41, no. 11, pp. 713–715, 2016.

[8] J. Tsui, O. Estrada, Z. Deng et al., "Analysis of pulmonary features and treatment approaches in the COPA syndrome," *ERJ Open Research*, vol. 4, no. 2, pp. 00017–02018, 2018.

[9] J. Mallea, A. Kornafeld, A. Khoor, and D. Erasmus, "Lung transplantation in a patient with COPA syndrome," *Case Rep Transplant*, vol. 2020, pp. 1-2, 2020.

[10] K. Gaither, K. Halstead, and T. C. Mason, "Pulmonary alveolar hemorrhage in a pregnancy complicated by systemic lupus

erythematosus," *Journal of the National Medical Association*, vol. 97, no. 6, pp. 831–833, 2005.

[11] F. Pais, M. Fayed, and T. Evans, "The successful use of extracorporeal membrane oxygenation in systemic lupus erythematosus-induced diffuse alveolar haemorrhage," *European journal of case reports in internal medicine*, vol. 4, no. 1, article 000515, 2017.

25

Uterine Rupture with Evisceration of Intestines through the Vagina during Labour

Ubong Akpan ,[1] Chinyere Akpanika,[1] Victor Nwagbara,[2] Udeme Asibong,[3] and Saturday Etuk[1]

[1]*Department of Obstetrics and Gynaecology, University of Calabar, Calabar, Nigeria*
[2]*Department of General Surgery, University of Calabar, Calabar, Nigeria*
[3]*Department of Family Medicine, University of Calabar, Calabar, Nigeria*

Correspondence should be addressed to Ubong Akpan; ubongabasiakpan@gmail.com

Academic Editor: Kyousuke Takeuchi

Uterine rupture is a life threatening obstetric emergency and is associated with high maternal and perinatal mortality. There are some risk factors associated with uterine rupture which may include: prolonged obstructed labour, previous scarred uterus, grand-multiparity, macrosomic baby, abnormal lie, instrumental delivery, induction of labour, oxytocin stimulation and excessive uterine manipulation. Its modes of presentation have been widely reported. Here, we present a case with an unusual mode of presentation where about two-third of the small intestines protruded through the vagina following some manipulations by an unskilled birth attendant. This highlights the fact that when uterine rupture is suspected, the cord-like structure protruding per vaginum may not always be umbilical cord.

1. Background

Transvaginal bowel evisceration is rare. To date less than 100 cases have been reported in the literature. Most of the cases reported followed ruptured vaginal vault in post hysterectomized menopausal women or sexual assault [1, 2]. It may also be caused by penetrating injury involving the posterior vaginal fornix or the Pouch of Douglass or uterine perforation following unsafe abortion [3, 4].

Intestinal prolapse through the vagina has also been reported in ulcerating gynaecological malignancies [5, 6]. Cases of intra-partum visceral prolapse per vaginum, to the best of our knowledge, have not been reported in the literature. We hereby present a case which occurred as a result of excessive manipulation by an unskilled birth attendant.

2. Case Report

This was a case of a 23-year old G4 P3 A3 woman at a gestational age of 39 weeks in April, 2017 who was referred to the labour ward of the University of Calabar Teaching Hospital (UCTH), Calabar, Southern Nigeria, with a history of inability to deliver her baby after 5 days in labour prior to presentation. The patient had been managed in two different traditional birth attendant (TBA) homes. The second TBA recognized that the cause of prolonged labour was abnormal lie of the fetus and attempted to correct the lie by intrauterine manipulation through the vagina. This resulted in uterine rupture and subsequent evisceration of the intra-abdominal viscus through the vagina. The loop of the small intestine was initially mistaken for umbilical cord by the TBA who pulled several lengths of it through the vagina (Figure 1). Following the failed attempt to deliver the baby and the woman's deteriorating clinical state, the patient was subsequently rushed to UCTH.

At UCTH, the patient was resuscitated. Parenteral broad spectrum antibiotics were administered. The extruded loops of bowel were wrapped in sterile guaze soaked with warm normal saline. A general surgeon was invited to take part in the management of the patient. The patient was immediately prepared and taken to theatre for emergency laparotomy.

A midline incision was made to access the peritoneal cavity. Intra-operatively, a macerated female fetus was found in the uterine cavity. There was a left postero-lateral uterine wall

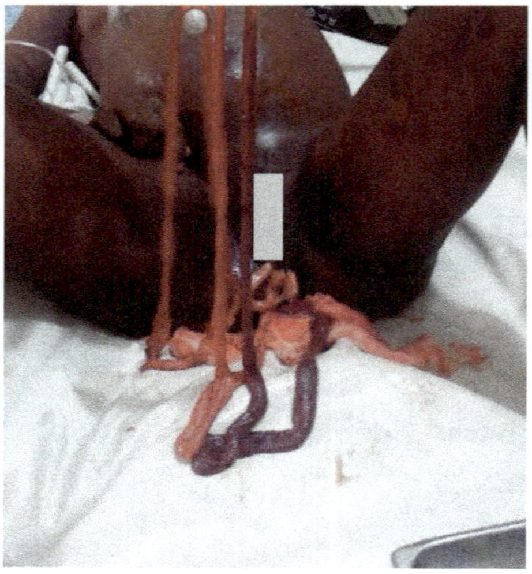

Figure 1: Extruded bowel loops through the vagina.

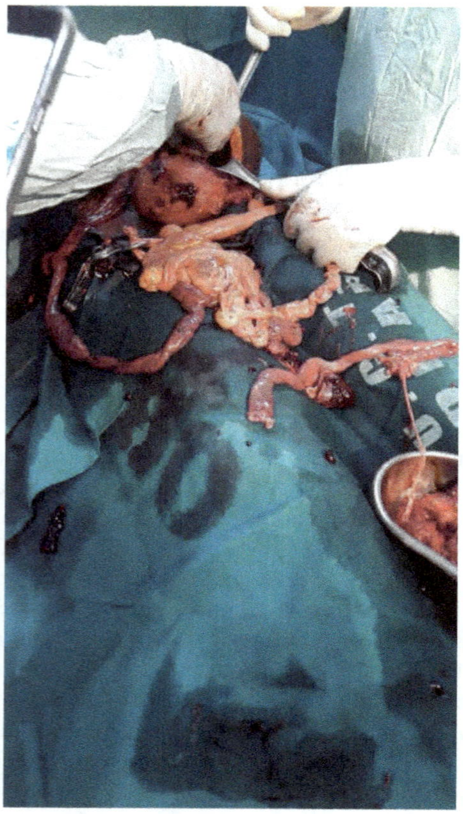

Figure 2: Ruptured uterus with devitalized intestine.

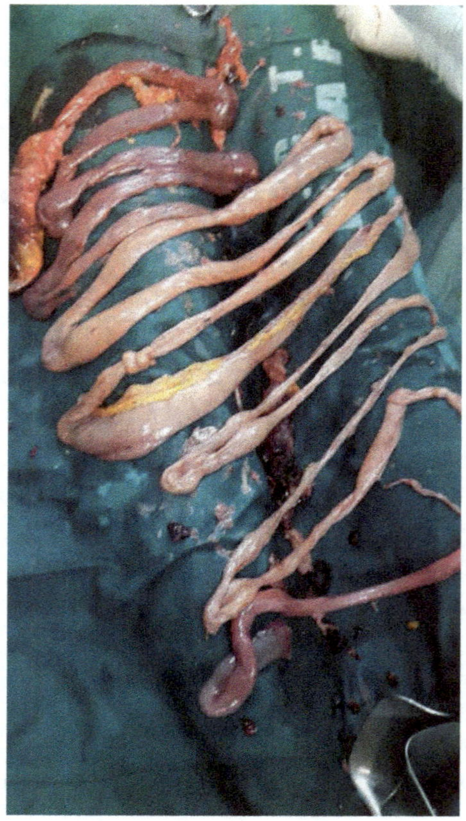

Figure 3: Resected devitalized intestine.

tear extending from the mid portion to the posterior vaginal fornix. The loops of bowel extruded through this opening. The dead fetus was extracted. About 1,200 ml of blood in the peritoneal cavity was suctioned. Total abdominal hysterectomy was performed.

The whole intestines were thoroughly examined (Figures 2 and 3); about half the length of the intestine was devitalized and therefore, resected and an end-to-end anastomosis was done. The peritoneal cavity was lavaged with warm normal saline before abdominal wall closure. Nasogastric tube was then inserted.

Post-operatively, the patient was given parenteral nutrition for 5 days. Antibiotics, analgesics and other supportive treatments were continued according to our protocols. The patient opened bowel on the eighth post-operative day. The patient was commenced on graded oral meals which the patient tolerated. Subsequent post-operative days were uneventful. The patient was later discharged home.

3. Discussion

This case highlights the grave danger of unsafe delivery especially in the hands of unskilled birth attendants. It may be difficult to assess the positive impacts of the traditional birth attendants in maternal care. In 2010, the government of the republic of Zambia discontinued the training of traditional birth attendants and banned them from conducting deliveries as they were viewed as contributing to maternal mortality [7]. A follow-up study evaluating the positive impact of such bold government decision revealed that there was remarkable improvement in maternal health which included early detection of complications and increased hospital supervised childbirths, enhanced clean and safe delivery as well as HIV/AIDS prevention [8]. Evidently, this led to a significant reduction in maternal mortality and morbidity. There may be need for gradual replacement of TBAs with skilled birth attendants in local communities in Africa.

It may be a big challenge in some African countries as many uneducated women in low-resource settings still prefer delivering under the care of TBAs as this is our index patient. This constitutes unsafe delivery and a serious challenge to safe motherhood initiative. As their activities are difficult to stop completely in our communities, training of TBAs should be gradually phased out and replaced with skilled birth attendants.

In conclusion, this case highlights that when uterine rupture occurs, any cord-like structure protruding per vaginum may not always be an umbilical cord. There is need for gradual replacement of TBAs by skilled birth attendants in our local community if we are to improve the outcome of maternal care and work towards the attainment of sustainable development goals.

References

[1] H. Kimina, Komishik Maedak, A. Tsuneda, and R. Tazawa, "Prolapse of the small intestine through a ruptured vagina caused during sexual intercourse: report of a case," *Surgery Today*, vol. 26, no. 10, pp. 846–848, 1996.

[2] P. De Laco, M. Ceccarom, C. Albonie, B. Rosit, and M. Sansorini, "Transvaginal evisceration after hystecihy: is vaginal cuff closure associated with a reduced risk?" *European Journal of Obstetrics & Gynecology and Reproductive Biology*, vol. 125, no. 1, pp. 134–138, 2008.

[3] S. Adam and O. Alomai, "Tranvaginal bowel evisceration thirteen weeks after total abdominal hysterectomy," *Journal of Obstetrics and Gynaecology*, vol. 27, no. 8, pp. 864–865, 2007.

[4] A. J. Croak, J. B. Gebhart, C. L. Klingele, G. Schroedr, R. A. Lee, and K. C. Podratz, "Characteristics of patients with vaginal rupture and evisceration," *Obstetrics & Gynecology*, vol. 103, no. 3, pp. 572–576, 2001.

[5] R. S. Parra, J. S. Ribeiro da Rocha, and O. Feres, "Spontaneous transvaginal small bowel evisceration: a case report," *Clinics*, vol. 65, no. 5, pp. 559–561, 2010.

[6] K. Yuce, P. Dursun, and M. Gültekin, "Posthysterectomy intestinal prolapse after coitus and vaginal repair," *Archives of Gynecology and Obstetrics*, vol. 272, no. 1, pp. 80–81, 2005.

[7] S. Rajeh, E. Kalu, J. Bong, and W. Wales, "Evisceration 5 years post abdominal hysterectomy," *Journal of Obstetrics and Gynaecology Research*, vol. 34, no. 3, pp. 425–427, 2008.

[8] C. Cheelo, S. Nzala, and J. M. Zulu, "Banning traditional birth attendants from conducting deliveries: experience and effects of the ban in a rural district of Kazungua in Zambia," *BMC Pregnancy and Childbirth*, vol. 16, no. 1, p. 323, 2016.

Term Delivery of a Complete Molar Pregnancy with a Coexistent Normal Pregnancy

Manisha Chhetry [1] **Aruna Pokharel** [2] **and Amar Nath Chaudhary** [2]

[1] *Department of Obstetrics and Gynecology, BP Koirala Institute of Health Science, Nepal*
[2] *Department of Obstetrics and Gynecology, Nobel Medical College and Teaching Hospital, Nepal*

Correspondence should be addressed to Manisha Chhetry; manisha.chhetry2013@gmail.com

Academic Editor: Maria Grazia Porpora

Twin pregnancy with a complete mole and a coexistent normal fetus reaching term is a rare occurrence. We report a case of a 21-yrs G2P1L0 un-booked patient at 39 weeks who was referred for the same condition diagnosed incidentally on ultrasound scan which showed a singleton pregnancy in breech presentation with a normal placenta and a heterogeneous cystic lesion seen anteriorly, suggesting a coexistent molar pregnancy. Cesarean section was done, and a healthy male baby was delivered with a grossly normal placenta and a second placenta with grape like vesicles. Histopathology confirmed the diagnosis of complete mole and normal placenta. Postoperative period was uneventful, and the patient was kept on beta hcg follow-up to monitor progression to gestational trophoblastic neoplasia, but it normalized by 12 weeks.

1. Introduction

Twin pregnancy with complete mole and a coexistent normal fetus is a rare entity with incidence quoted between 1/22,000 and 1/100,000 pregnancies [1–7]. These pregnancies rarely reach term and are usually complicated with spontaneous abortions, congenital malformations, preterm labor, early-onset preeclampsia, sudden fetal loss, and risk of progressing to persistent gestational trophoblastic neoplasia to name a few [8–14]. With the recent development of various assessment modalities, complete hydatiform mole with a coexistent live fetus continuation of pregnancy to term and delivery is becoming an acceptable option.

2. Case

A 21-yrs un-booked G2P1L0 patient at 39 weeks POG was referred from a remote hilly district for pregnancy with coexistent molar pregnancy. The patient had one previous term intrauterine fetal death delivered at home 3 yrs back, and even in this pregnancy, she only visited the local health post at term where the condition was suspected on a routine obstetric scan by the attending doctor and she was referred to our center. On examination, she was normotensive; there was no pallor or oedema. Her uterus was term size with breech presentation with reassuring fetal heart rate. Ultrasound showed a singleton pregnancy with fetal biometry corresponding to 36 weeks in breech presentation with adequate amniotic fluid and a normal placenta; additionally, a heterogeneous cystic lesion was seen anteriorly with features, suggesting a coexistent molar pregnancy (Figure 1). Her β hcg at admission was 2, 55,000 mIU, thyroid function test was normal (TSH 2 mIU/L), there was no proteinuria, and chest X-ray was normal. The counseling of patient and spouse was done, and she was taken up for cesarean section. She delivered a healthy male baby of 3.6 kg (Figure 2) with a grossly normal placenta, while the second sac had only placental tissue with grapelike vesicles (Figure 3). The intraoperative and postoperative period was uneventful, and the histopathology of placental tissue showed complete mole, while the second placenta was normal. The post-evacuation bhcg dropped to 51,000 mIU/ml. The patient was kept on two-weekly bhcg follow-up as surveillance to progression to persistent gestational trophoblastic neoplasia, but it normalized by 12 weeks.

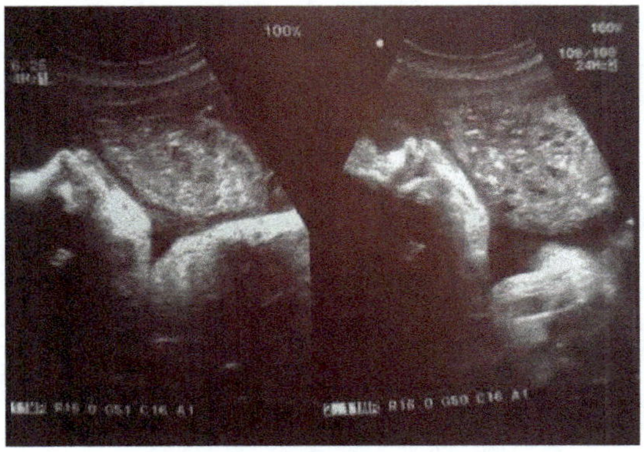

FIGURE 1: Ultrasound showing a heterogeneous cystic lesion anteriorly and a normal fetus.

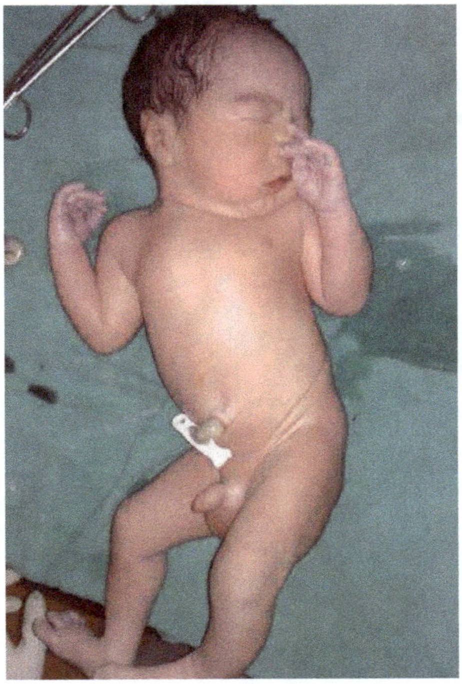

FIGURE 2: Coexistent healthy baby.

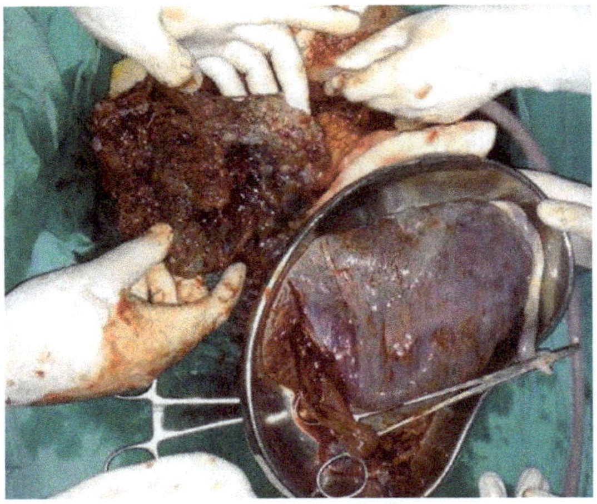

FIGURE 3: Normal placenta and second sac showing placenta with grape like vesicles and no fetal poles.

3. Discussion

Twin pregnancy with one healthy fetus and a coexistent molar pregnancy is an uncommon occurrence [1–7]. This condition is not only rare but also complex and challenging to manage as there are no clear consensuses regarding the same. Successful diagnosis requires critical interpretation of clinical symptoms, ultrasound findings, and biochemical and cytogenetic studies [8, 9]. In our patient, the condition was diagnosed in ultrasound scan in the late third trimester. Diagnosis was late as the patient did not visit any health facility for antenatal checkup. Ideally, the patient should have undergone a prenatal diagnosis by chorionic villous sampling in early pregnancy to exclude a case of partial mole and confirm uniparental disomy with cytogenetic studies [10]. This becomes important because it has been proved that complete and partial moles are two distinct pathological entities [11, 12].

All patients diagnosed with this condition have to be counseled, and pregnancy can be continued in those patients who elect to continue under proper supervision. Molar pregnancy with a coexistent live fetus is associated with severe pregnancy complications [8], so antenatal surveillance becomes all the more important, an aspect which was missed in our patient due to her late presentation. A literature review suggests that common complications include vaginal bleeding, preeclampsia, hyperemesis, hyperthyroidism, preterm birth, and fetal loss [8, 13–15]. There is more risk of persistent disease in this group of patients so they need to be followed up even after delivery [13, 15, 16].

Although there are differences in opinion regarding the management of this group of patients due to rarity of cases but it is reasonable to evaluate for metastatic disease, rule out triploidy as these fetuses are at high risk of malformation and closely monitor for possible complications like pre-eclampsia [13, 17]. Mandatory placental examination by skilled pathologist is needed in the index as well as the subsequent deliveries to rule out choriocarcinoma. The standard post-molar bhcg follow-up is to be done. Continuation of pregnancy in patients with complete mole and coexistent normal fetus is an acceptable option, provided proper surveillance is done. Proper counseling of patients and respecting patient's choice also becomes an important aspect of management.

References

[1] C. K. Anderson, R. W. Deiter, M. J. Motz, and J. A. Goldstein, "Complete hydatidiform mole with a coexistent healthy, viable fetus near term: a case report," *Journal of Reproductive Medicine*, vol. 41, no. 1, pp. 55–58, 1996.

[2] S. Vandeginste, I. B. Vergote, M. Hanssens et al., "Malignant trophoblastic disease following a twin pregnancy consisting of a complete hydatiform mole and a normal fetus and placenta. A case report," *European Journal of Gynaecological Oncology*, vol. 20, no. 2, pp. 105–107, 1999.

[3] M. Soysal, S. Kara, and E. Ekici, "Twin pregnancy with a fetus and a complete hydatidiform mole," *Archives of Gynecology and Obstetrics*, vol. 259, no. 1, pp. 41–44, 1996.

[4] D. A. Fishman, L. A. Padilla, P. Keh, L. Cohen, M. Frederiksen, and J. R. Lurain, "Management of twin pregnancies consisting

of a complete hydatidiform mole and normal fetus," *Obstetrics & Gynecology*, vol. 91, no. 4, pp. 546–550, 1998.

[5] W. Malinowski, I. Biskup, and W. Dec, "Sad fetus syndromegestational trophoblastic disease concurrent with a living fetus or fetuses," *Acta Geneticae Medicine Et Gemellologiae: Twin Research*, vol. 44, no. 3, 4, pp. 193–202, 1995.

[6] K. M. Johnston, E. K. Steele, and S. E. Magee, "Twin pregnancy with a living fetus and coexisting complete hydatidiform mole," *Ulster Medical Journal*, vol. 69, no. 2, pp. 168–170, 2000.

[7] I. Bruchim, D. Kidron, A. Amiel, M. Altaras, and M. D. Fejgin, "Complete hydatidiform mole and a coexistent viable fetus: report of two cases and review of the literature," *Gynecologic Oncology*, vol. 77, no. 1, pp. 197–202, 2000.

[8] M. Ciebiera, C. Wojtyła, G. Jakiel, and T. Roszkowski, "Molar pregnancy with a coexisting live fetus as a challenge for perinatology. A mini-review with two case reports," *Journal of Health Inequalities*, vol. 4, no. 1, pp. 39–45, 2018.

[9] V. Giorgione, P. Cavoretto, G. Cormio et al., "Prenatal diagnosis of twin pregnancies with complete hydatidiform mole and coexistent normal fetus: a series of 13 cases," *Gynecologic and Obstetric Investigation*, vol. 82, no. 4, pp. 404–409, 2017.

[10] A. Vimercati, A. C. Gennaro, I. Cobuzzi et al., "Two cases of complete hydatidiform mole and coexistent live fetus," *Journal of Prenatal Medicine*, vol. 7, no. 1, pp. 1–4, 2013.

[11] A. E. Szulman and U. Surti, "The syndromes of hydatidiform mole. I. Cytogenetic and morphologic correlations," *American Journal of Obstetrics and Gynecology*, vol. 131, no. 6, pp. 665–671, 1978.

[12] M. A. Steller, D. R. Genest, M. R. Bernstein, J. M. Lage, D. P. Goldstein, and R. S. Berkowitz, "Natural history of twin pregnancy with complete hydatidiform mole and coexisting fetus," *Obstetrics and Gynecology*, vol. 83, no. 1, pp. 35–42, 1994.

[13] M. A. Steller, D. R. Genest, M. R. Bernstein, J. M. Lage, D. P. Goldstein, and R. S. Berkowitz, "Clinical features of multiple conception with partial or complete molar pregnancy and coexisting fetuses," *Journal of Reproductive Medicine*, vol. 39, no. 3, pp. 147–154, 1994.

[14] L. Wee and E. Jauniaux, "Prenatal diagnosis and management of twin pregnancies complicated by a co-existing molar pregnancy," *Prenatal Diagnosis*, vol. 25, no. 9, pp. 772–776, 2005.

[15] "Forum: twin gestation comprising mole in concert with normal fetus: Test, treat, abort or let them go to term," *Trophoblastic Disorders Update*, vol. 3, p. 3, 1999.

[16] RCOG, *The Management of Gestational Trophoblastic Disease*, College of obstetricians and Gynecologists, London, 1999.

[17] Committee on practice bulletins-Gynecology, American College of Obstetricians and gynecologists, "Diagnosis and treatment of gestational trophoblastic disease: ACOG Practice Bulletin No. 53," *Obstetrics & Gynecology*, vol. 103, no. 6, p. 1365, 2004.

27

Systemic Thrombolysis for Treatment of Postpartum Saddle Embolism Complicated by Postpartum Hemorrhage: A Case Report and Brief Literature Review

Kathy Mostajeran, Hillary Boswell, and Ziad Haidar

Gulf Coast Educational Consortium/HCA Houston Healthcare West, 12141 Richmond Ave. Houston, TX 77082, USA

Correspondence should be addressed to Kathy Mostajeran; kathy.mostajeran@hcahealthcare.com

Academic Editor: Maria Grazia Porpora

Venous thromboembolic events (VTE), specifically pulmonary embolisms, account for a significant portion of maternal morbidity and mortality. Due to the procoagulant physiological changes that occur, pregnancy and the postpartum period are known risk factors for thromboembolic events. The risk is greatest during the first-week postpartum and remains elevated for up to six weeks as compared to the general population. Treatment guidelines regarding the use of thrombolytics for massive pulmonary embolism occurring in pregnancy and the postpartum are not well established. In nonpregnant populations, thrombolytic agents are well known to decrease the mortality in the setting of a massive pulmonary embolism. However, in the absence of management guidelines, thrombolysis in pregnancy remains guided by case reports and case series. We present a case of a massive pulmonary embolism (PE) causing hemodynamic instability during the postpartum period treated with tissue plasminogen activator (tPA). The case was complicated by delayed postpartum hemorrhage successfully managed with the uterotonic methylergometrine. The patient was started on oral anticoagulation and continued for six months without recurrent VTE. Our case demonstrates a rare occurrence of a saddle embolism after a vaginal delivery within the first postpartum week which was successfully managed with the use of systemic thrombolysis and minimal intervention to manage the iatrogenic delayed postpartum hemorrhage. To the authors' knowledge, no other similar case report exists. This case highlights the need to develop guidelines for the use of thrombolysis in mothers who present with massive pulmonary embolus and a noninvasive means to manage adverse bleeding events in the puerperium.

1. Introduction

According to the Center of Disease Control Pregnancy Mortality Surveillance System, pulmonary embolism accounted for approximately 9.4% ($n = 281$) of the maternal deaths between 2011 and 2015 in the United States [1]. The rate of venous thromboembolism (VTE) is approximately 1.72 per 1,000 deliveries with 1.1 deaths per 100,000 [2]. While pulmonary embolism is a rare occurrence in pregnancy and the puerperium, it can have devastating consequences when not recognized early and treated aggressively.

Pregnancy and the postpartum period exemplify Virchow's triad of initiating factors for venous thrombosis, namely, hypercoagulability, increased venous stasis, and vascular damage. Pomp et al. published data findings of thromboembolic events that occurred during pregnancy and the postpartum period in the MEGA study [3]. Researchers discovered an increased relative risk of thromboembolic events during the first 6-week postpartum, with the highest risk for occurrence during the second postpartum week [3]. When compared to the third trimester, the risk of pulmonary embolism was greater during the postpartum period [3].

Pregnancy and the postpartum period are considered a relative contraindication for the use of thrombolytics, due to the lack of controlled studies and the fear of life-threatening hemorrhage [4]. Relative contraindications to the use of thrombolytics include recent surgery and active bleeding, common scenarios in the postpartum state [4].

Published research is limited to case studies and systematic reviews of published case studies which highlight the beneficial effects of thrombolysis in treatment of pulmonary embolism in pregnancy. Fewer case studies exist to evaluate the use of thrombolytic treatment in the postpartum period. Systematic reviews of case studies have revealed that in the setting of massive pulmonary embolism in the postpartum period, the maternal survival rate is 86.4%; however, the bleeding risk is approximately 58.3% [5].

We present a case of a 30-year-old female who was diagnosed with a saddle pulmonary embolism and acute hemodynamic decompensation six days after a normal spontaneous vaginal delivery. She was treated successfully with systemic thrombolysis with recovery of right ventricular function. The case was complicated by a delayed postpartum hemorrhage managed with only uterotonics. The patient was successfully transitioned to Rivaroxaban and treated for six-month duration without recurrence of VTE.

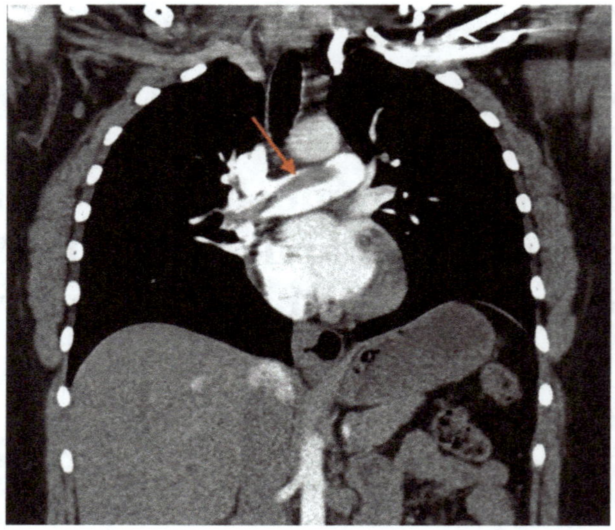

FIGURE 1: Computed tomography angiography coronal view demonstrated a large saddle embolism as shown by the red arrow.

2. Case Report

A 30-year gravida 2 para 2002 female presented to an outside facility's emergency department with a chief complaint of syncopal episodes on postpartum day number 6 after a normal spontaneous vaginal delivery and a right mediolateral episiotomy. Her past medical history was significant for pregestational type 2 diabetes mellitus, reportedly well controlled with metformin, with a BMI of 40 kg/m^2. She reported that she had been active at home with no history of recent prolonged travel or bed rest during the postpartum period. The patient's obstetrical history was previously uncomplicated. However, delayed placenta delivery and a right mediolateral episiotomy during her most recent vaginal delivery were reported. She had no personal or family history of thromboembolic events. She had one syncopal episode the night prior to her presentation followed by a second one the next morning while washing her face. After the second episode, she sought treatment at the closest emergency department and reported having had two additional syncopal episodes, one of which occurred in the emergency department. Shortly after arrival, the patient became hypoxic and hypotensive, with blood pressure measuring 88/50 and 88% oxygen saturation. She developed shortness of breath, and a stat computed tomography angiography of the chest demonstrated a saddle pulmonary embolus as seen in Figures 1 and 2. The decision was made to begin the infusion protocol of 100 mg tissue plasminogen activator (tPA) over the course of two hours prior to transfer to our hospital for a higher level of care in the intensive care unit.

The patient reported that prior to receiving the tPA infusion, her lochia was minimal but had increased since the tPA infusion. At the outlying facility, the patient's hemoglobin was 12.7 g/dL upon presentation. Upon arrival at our hospital, the patient's initial hemoglobin and hematocrit were 10.7 g/dL and 33.5%, respectively. The patient complained of shortness of breath; however, she remained hemodynamically stable and maintained an oxygen saturation of 100% while receiving 2 L of oxygen via nasal cannula. Her shortness of breath improved shortly after admission to the intensive care unit. The tPA infusion was completed at our hospital. An activated partial thromboplastin time (aPTT) at baseline was 42 seconds, and the patient was started on intravenous unfractionated heparin at a rate of 18 units/kilograms/hour without a bolus. The choice of unfractionated heparin was made due to its shorter half-life and ability to be reversed with protamine in an event of life-threatening uncontrollable hemorrhage requiring surgical intervention. The aPTT was trended based on hospital protocol to ensure therapeutic range. Inspection of the mediolateral episiotomy did not reveal any oozing, and the source of bleeding was suspected to be from the uterus. Upon discovering that the lochia had been increasing, the patient was started on 60 mg of megestrol acetate twice daily on day one with minimal improvement. The decision to start megestrol acetate was made due to the presumed subinvolution of the placenta site and limited evidence of the efficacy of megestrol acetate in treatment of subinvolution in animal models [6]. However, given the massive blood loss and the diagnosis of delayed postpartum hemorrhage, this strategy was quickly abandoned.

On hospital day 2, the patient continued to complain of progressively increasing vaginal bleeding and passage of clots. She was then started on 40 mg of oxytocin intravenously to encourage uterine contractions. Later in the evening, she reported some minimal improvement in vaginal bleeding. Over the course of 24 hours 12 peripads were soaked with blood and clots. By the end of day 2, the patient's hemoglobin and hematocrit were 9.1 g/dL and 28.1%, respectively. The oxytocin was continued for 24 hours, and bleeding was reassessed the following day. An echocardiogram was performed and demonstrated only mildly reduced right ventricular systolic function with no other abnormalities.

On hospital day 3, the patient continued to have excessive lochia and complained of uterine cramping. On day 3, her hemoglobin and hematocrit were 7.4 g/dL and 22.8%, respectively. Subsequently, the patient was given an intramuscular dose of 0.2 mg of methylergometrine, which was deemed to be safe in the setting of greater than 24 hours since tPA

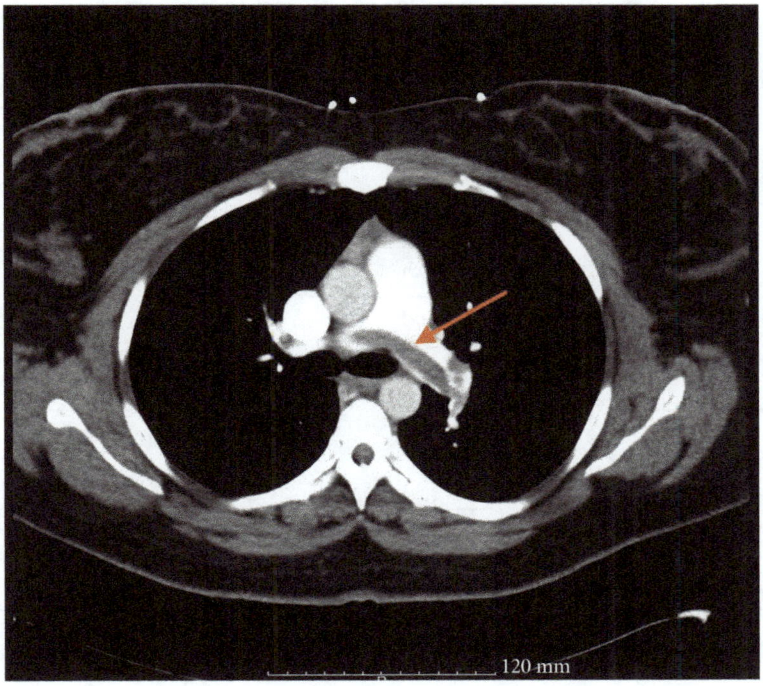

Figure 2: Computed tomography of the chest, transverse view, demonstrated a large saddle embolus as indicated by the red arrow.

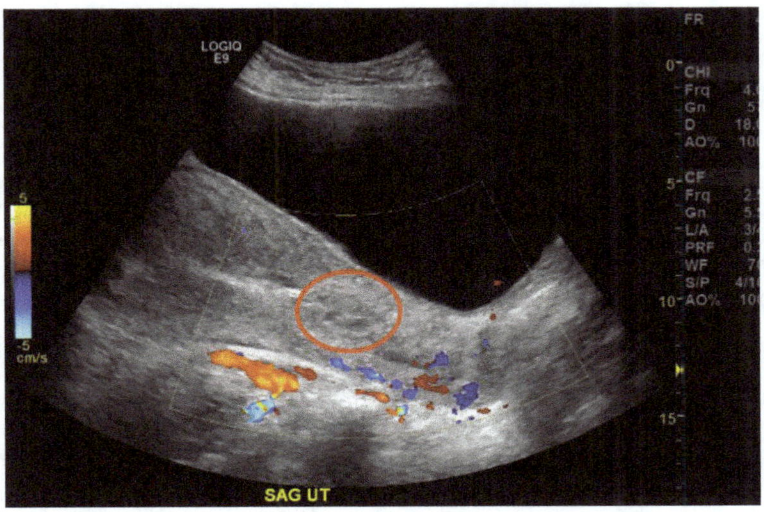

Figure 3: Transvaginal ultrasound of the uterus. Sagittal view of the uterus demonstrated complex echogenic area in the lower uterine segment without Doppler flow, consistent with a blood clot (encircled in red) measuring approximately 2.9 cm in diameter.

infusion. A transvaginal ultrasound was performed and revealed a complex echogenic focus without Doppler flow in the lower uterine segment consistent with a blood clot as seen in Figure 3.

On hospital day 4, she reported great improvement in her lochia overnight. However, by this point, her hemoglobin had dropped to 6.4 g/dL and her hematocrit was 19.5%. Subsequently, two units of packed red blood cells were transfused. Repeat hemoglobin was collected eight hours later and noted to be 8.4 g/dL. At this point, the patient's lochia had returned to minimal.

While the patient had been titrated to therapeutic levels of anticoagulation with unfractionated heparin, a discussion regarding the patient's lack of desire to breastfeed, and the difficulty she would encounter with the monitoring required with warfarin treatment, unfractionated heparin was discontinued, and Rivaroxaban was started. The regimen was 15 mg twice per day for 21 days then 20 mg once per day for a treatment duration of 6 months. She was advised to be aware of adverse events including black tarry stools, heavy menstrual bleeding, bleeding gums, back pain, or bowel or bladder dysfunction. She was advised that bruising and bleeding from cuts would be more pronounced.

The patient was discharged home on hospital day five and was followed up as outpatient intermittently for monitoring of ongoing treatment. The patient had a thrombophilia panel 6

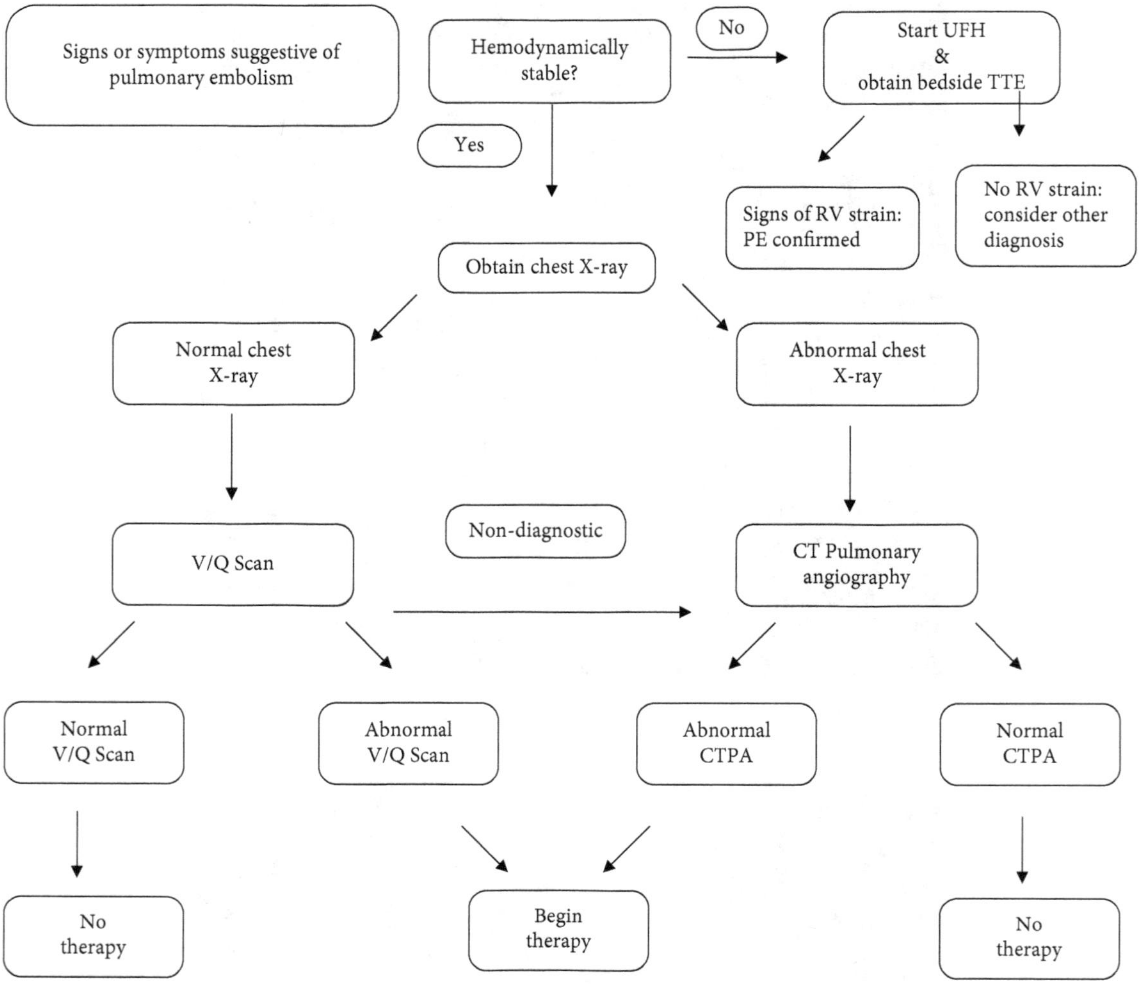

FIGURE 4: Algorithm for diagnosing pulmonary embolism in pregnancy and the postpartum period in a hemodynamically stable and unstable patient. V/Q: ventilation-perfusion; CTPA: computed tomographic pulmonary angiography; TTE: transthoracic echocardiogram; UFH: unfractionated heparin; RV: right ventricle.

weeks after her last dose of Rivaroxaban. The thrombophilia panel testing was normal.

3. Discussion

Pregnancy and the postpartum period are known risk factors for thromboembolic events. Factors which confer an additional risk in this population include cesarean delivery, obesity, smoking, thrombophilia, lupus, heart disease, diabetes, sickle cell disease, postpartum infection, postpartum hemorrhage, and blood transfusion [7]. However, approximately 25% of venous thromboembolic events in pregnancy are recurrent and personal history of a previous VTE confers the highest risk [7]. Researchers found that VTE was 38% higher in women aged 35 and older and 64% higher in black women [2]. Of the VTE events that occurred in pregnancy and the postpartum period, approximately 80% were deep vein thrombosis while the other 20% were pulmonary emboli [2]. Our patient denied any personal or family history of previous venous thromboembolism, and this was her first episode of pulmonary embolism. Her risk factors included obesity and pregestational diabetes in addition to being six-day postpartum. While she reported a delayed delivery of her placenta, she did not require any blood transfusion or experience postpartum hemorrhage or infection.

Diagnosis of VTE in pregnancy and the postpartum period can be difficult due to nonspecific signs and symptoms. Specifically, the presenting symptoms of a pulmonary embolism in the postpartum period include syncope, tachycardia, chest pain, and hypotension. Oxygen desaturation is rare as a presenting sign and often associated with a large saddle embolism. Recommendations are that any woman presenting in pregnancy or the postpartum period with symptoms suggestive of pulmonary embolism should receive the appropriate imaging if hemodynamically stable [8–10]. First, a chest X-ray should be obtained. If results of the X-ray are normal, then a ventilation perfusion (V/Q) scan should be obtained next [8–10]. If chest X-ray is found to be abnormal, follow-up imaging should be a computed tomography pulmonary angiography [8–10]. Figure 4 demonstrates the basic algorithm for diagnosing pulmonary embolism in pregnancy and the postpartum period in a hemodynamically stable and unstable patient. In cases of unstable hemodynamic status, the patient should be started on therapeutic anticoagulation therapy prior to diagnostic modalities [8–10]. A bedside echocardiogram may also aid in quick diagnosis by demonstrating changes associated with right-sided heart strain (dilated right atrium/right ventricle) if computed tomography pulmonary angiography is not immediately available [8, 9]. In the present case, the patient became hemodynamically unstable, and the decision was quickly made to obtain a computed tomography angiography of the chest, which demonstrated a large saddle embolism as seen in Figures 1 and 2.

The treatment of pulmonary embolism (PE) in a non-pregnant population is based on risk stratification. The most important determinant of outcomes is hemodynamic instability. In an American Heart Association scientific statement, massive PE was defined as an acute pulmonary embolism with sustained hypotension not due to a cause other than PE, pulselessness, or persistent and profound bradycardia [11]. Patients with high risk or massive PE have been demonstrated to profoundly benefit from thrombolytic therapy in the absence of contraindications. A meta-analysis of randomized control trials, in which thrombolysis was compared with heparin in the treatment of pulmonary embolisms, found that, when used in the setting of major pulmonary embolism causing hemodynamic instability, there was a decreased rate of mortality as compared to the use of heparin alone [12]. The researchers concluded that there was benefit to the use of thrombolysis to treat hemodynamically unstable patients in the acute setting of massive pulmonary embolism with approximately a 12% bleeding risk [12]. Currently, the administration of thrombolytic therapy to individuals presenting with massive pulmonary embolisms is considered standard of care and a life-saving intervention.

While thrombolysis for the treatment of pulmonary embolism in the nonpregnant population has been demonstrated to decrease mortality, pregnancy is considered a relative contraindication [4]. Although recent surgery and bleeding are also considered relative contraindications, no mention of the postpartum period is made in the guidelines set by the American College of Chest Physicians on the use of antithrombotic therapy in VTE disease [4]. This is likely due to the lack of controlled studies and the fear of life-threatening hemorrhage in pregnancy and particularly the postpartum period. Published research is limited to multiple case studies which highlight the beneficial effects of thrombolysis in the treatment of pulmonary embolism in pregnancy. Fewer case studies exist to evaluate the use of thrombolytic treatment in the postpartum period.

A systematic review of case reports analyzed the outcomes of thrombolytics used for treatment of massive pulmonary embolism in pregnancy and the early postpartum period (limited to 48 hours after delivery) and found that there were favorable maternal outcomes [13]. However, the same study also found that there was a substantial bleeding risk that mostly pertained to the postpartum period [13]. Another systematic review of case reports analyzed the outcomes of massive and submassive pulmonary embolisms that occurred in pregnancy and up to six-week postpartum treated with thrombolysis [5]. Researchers found that in the postpartum period, when thrombolysis was used, the maternal survival rate was 86.4% but the hemorrhage rate was 58.3% when treatment occurred after delivery [5]. When stratified by the thrombolytic agent utilized, the same authors discovered that tPA had a hemorrhage risk of 5% while the hemorrhage risk after administering streptokinase was 50% when administered in the postpartum period [5]. Urokinase was also used, but less frequently [8, 13]. The most common postpartum hemorrhages were intra-abdominal bleeding in women who underwent cesarean delivery and vaginal hemorrhage in those who underwent vaginal delivery [5]. This is in contrast to a nonpregnant population with massive pulmonary embolism who receives thrombolysis, where the survival rate is estimated to be 50% to 70% and the risk of hemorrhage is approximately 12% [4, 12]. The difference in survival rate most likely reflects the younger population and better cardiovascular reserve of the pregnant and postpartum population. On the other hand, bleeding risk is significantly higher in the postpartum patient. This is due in part to recent surgery in patients after cesarean delivery, who demonstrated higher rates of intra-abdominal bleeding after administration of systemic thrombolytics [5]. Vaginal bleeding significant enough to be considered a massive postpartum hemorrhage after a vaginal delivery in the setting of systemic thrombolytics for treatment of massive pulmonary embolism can be explained by the necessity of deposition of fibrin over the placenta site as well as clots within the supplying vessels to aid in postpartum uterine involution [5].

Only case reports and case series analyzing the use of thrombolytic therapy for treatment of life-threatening embolism during pregnancy and the postpartum period exist. After reviewing the literature by searching PubMed using the words "postpartum," "pulmonary embolism," and "thrombolysis," only nineteen cases could be found, derived from systematic reviews, which reported pulmonary embolism in the postpartum period treated with only thrombolytic agents in addition to therapeutic heparin [5, 8, 13, 14]. Most of these cases were either directly after delivery or prior to hospital discharge within the first two-day postpartum. Interestingly, very few case reports of pulmonary embolism utilizing thrombolytic treatment in postpartum women during the period of highest risk, as previously discussed, have been published [5, 8, 13, 14]. Only six cases have been reported of massive pulmonary embolism treated with only systemic thrombolysis after a vaginal delivery [5, 8, 13, 14]. Of those, only 2 cases occurred greater than or equal to 1-week postpartum after a vaginal delivery [5]. To the authors' knowledge, this is the only case of massive saddle pulmonary embolism occurring within the first-week postpartum after the patient was discharged home following a routine uncomplicated vaginal delivery, successfully treated exclusively with systemic thrombolysis. Furthermore, this case represents the successful use of systemic thrombolysis for the treatment and management of subsequent delayed postpartum hemorrhage with uterotonics in the setting of massive maternal pulmonary embolism.

4. Conclusion

This case highlights the maternal benefits of using systemic thrombolysis in the acute setting of hemodynamic decompensation secondary to a massive pulmonary embolism in the postpartum period. Given the contribution of VTE to the incidence of maternal mortality, more studies need to explore the potential beneficial effects that thrombolysis may have on decreasing maternal mortality and morbidity during pregnancy and the postpartum period. Clinicians should be aware of the potential use of thrombolysis in life-threatening cases of VTE; however, more research is needed to validate its usefulness during pregnancy and the postpartum period.

Disclosure

The views expressed in this publication represent those of the authors and do not necessarily represent the official views of HCA or any of its affiliated entities.

Acknowledgments

This research was supported in part by HCA Healthcare and/or an HCA Healthcare-affiliated entity.

References

[1] E. E. Petersen, N. L. Davis, D. Goodman et al., "Vital signs: pregnancy-related deaths, United States, 2011–2015, and strategies for prevention, 13 states, 2013–2017," *Morbidity and Mortality Weekly Report*, vol. 68, no. 18, pp. 423–429, 2019.

[2] A. H. James, M. G. Jamison, L. R. Brancazio, and E. R. Myers, "Venous thromboembolism during pregnancy and the postpartum period: incidence, risk factors, and mortality," *American Journal of Obstetrics and Gynecology*, vol. 194, no. 5, pp. 1311–1315, 2006.

[3] E. R. Pomp, A. M. Lenselink, F. R. Rosendaal, and C. J. M. Doggen, "Pregnancy, the postpartum period and prothrombotic defects: risk of venous thrombosis in the MEGA study," *Journal of Thrombosis and Haemostasis*, vol. 6, no. 4, pp. 632–637, 2008.

[4] C. Kearon, E. A. Akl, A. J. Comerota et al., "Antithrombotic therapy for VTE disease: antithrombotic therapy and prevention of thrombosis, 9th ed: American College of Chest Physicians Evidence-Based Clinical Practice Guidelines," *Chest*, vol. 141, no. 2, pp. e419S–e496S, 2012.

[5] G. Martillotti, F. Boehlen, H. Robert-Ebadi, N. Jastrow, M. Righini, and M. Blondon, "Treatment options for severe pulmonary embolism during pregnancy and the postpartum period: a systematic review," *Journal of Thrombosis and Haemostasis*, vol. 15, no. 10, pp. 1942–1950, 2017.

[6] D. Kumar, A. Kumar, P. Kumar, C. L. Yadava, and S. PrakashYadav, "Sub-involution of placental sites (SIPS): an overview," *JournalofEntomologyandZoologyStudies*, vol. 6, no. 6, pp. 65–67, 2018.

[7] A. H. James, "Venous thromboembolism in pregnancy," *Arteriosclerosis, Thrombosis, and Vascular Biology*, vol. 29, no. 3, pp. 326–331, 2009.

[8] D. Rodriguez, C. Jerjes-Sanchez, S. Fonseca et al., "Thrombolysis in massive and submassive pulmonary embolism during pregnancy and the puerperium: a systematic review," *Journal of Thrombosis and Thrombolysis*, vol. 50, no. 4, pp. 929–941, 2020.

[9] C. McLintock, T. Brighton, S. Chunilal et al., "Recommendations for the diagnosis and treatment of deep venous thrombosis and pulmonary embolism in pregnancy and the postpartum period," *Australian and New Zealand Journal of Obstetrics and Gynaecology*, vol. 52, no. 1, pp. 14–22, 2012.

[10] M. R. Toglia and J. G. Weg, "Venous thromboembolism during pregnancy," *New England Journal of Medicine*, vol. 335, no. 2, pp. 108–114, 1996.

[11] M. R. Jaff, M. S. McMurtry, S. L. Archer et al., "Management of massive and submassive pulmonary embolism, iliofemoral deep vein thrombosis, and chronic thromboembolic pulmonary hypertension: a scientific statement from the American Heart Association," *Circulation*, vol. 123, no. 16, pp. 1788–1830, 2011.

[12] S. Wan, D. J. Quinlan, G. Agnelli, and J. W. Eikelboom, "Thrombolysis compared with heparin for the initial treatment of pulmonary embolism: a meta-analysis of the randomized controlled trials," *Circulation*, vol. 110, no. 6, pp. 744–749, 2004.

[13] M. Akazawa and M. Nishida, "Thrombolysis with intravenous recombinant tissue plasminogen activator during early postpartum period: a review of the literature," *Acta Obstetricia et Gynecologica Scandinavica*, vol. 96, no. 5, pp. 529–535, 2017.

[14] E. Jackson, K. M. Curtis, and M. E. Gaffield, "Risk of venous thromboembolism during the postpartum period: a systematic review," *Obstetrics & Gynecology*, vol. 117, no. 3, pp. 691–703, 2011.

28

Unexplained First Trimester Intrahepatic Cholestasis of Pregnancy: A Case Report and Literature Review

Anastasia A. Salame, Mohammad J. Jaffal, Marco A. Mouanness, Amal R. Nasser Eddin, and Labib M. Ghulmiyyah

American University of Beirut Medical Center, Beirut PO Box: 11-0236, Lebanon

Correspondence should be addressed to Labib M. Ghulmiyyah; lg08@aub.edu.lb

Academic Editor: Maria Grazia Porpora

Intrahepatic cholestasis of pregnancy (ICP) is a condition that usually affects the 3rd trimester-pregnant women and is associated with adverse pregnancy outcomes. We present a 31-year-old G2P1 patient with symptoms of ICP as early as 10 weeks of gestation (WG). Her pruritis was initially attributed to eczema. Due to the intensity of her discomfort and failure of topical treatment, ICP was suspected, total bile acid salt levels were taken and ursodeoxycholic acid was subsequently started at 18 WG. The patient was followed closely during her pregnancy to adjust the dose of the medication accordingly. Induction of labor was performed at 37 WG without complications. This case demonstrated the importance of clinical suspicion in the setting of such symptomatology in order not to miss or delay treatment of threatening conditions such as ICP.

1. Introduction

Intrahepatic cholestasis of pregnancy (ICP) is a suspected endocrino-metabolic disease that affects pregnant women usually during the third trimester of pregnancy when the sex steroids reach their highest levels. While its maternal repercussions are somehow limited to minor symptoms of pruritis and related discomfort, pregnancy outcomes might be severely affected. Preterm labor and delivery, fetal hypoxia, and intra-uterine fetal demise (IUFD) are well known complications of ICP that has driven guidelines to recommend induction of labor during the early third trimester period [1]. The overall estimated rate of adverse pregnancy events ranges between 19.2% and 64.1% [2]. The exact pathophysiology of ICP leading to the accumulation of bile acid, the increasing serum liver enzymes, and the unfavorable pregnancy outcomes, remains unknown [2, 3].

Suggested risk factors for ICP include elevated estrogen levels, genetic causes, ethnicity, anticardiolipin antibodies, hepatitis C infection, multiple pregnancies, pregnancies resulting from assisted reproductive technologies as well as a personal history ICP [2, 4–6].

The diagnosis of ICP is made by the documentation of elevated bile acid serum levels (≥10 micro-mol/L). Depending on the serum bile acid levels, ICP can be classified as either mild (10 and 40 micro-mol/L, with the usual symptom of itching) or severe (>40 micro-mol/L, or concomitant gestational hypertension, IUFD and/or recurrent ICP) [7, 8].

ICP is considered as a disease of the third and/or late second trimester; however, recent evidence suggests that in rare situations ICP can be diagnosed as early as the first trimester. Numerous studies have suggested a link between the gestational age at which ICP was diagnosed and the pregnancy outcomes (increased risks of preterm delivery, small for gestational age, and stillbirth with earlier onset types of ICP) [9, 10]. We present a case of severe ICP in a spontaneous first trimester pregnancy with a successful outcome.

2. Case Report

A 31-year-old G2P1A0L1 presented to our clinic for follow up at 20 weeks of gestation with the diagnosis of ICP. The patient reported that her symptoms started as early as 10 weeks of gestation of her spontaneously conceived pregnancy. Initially the patient used topical steroids in an attempt to relieve her symptoms to no avail. She later sought medical attention from several dermatologists who prescribed creams for eczema and

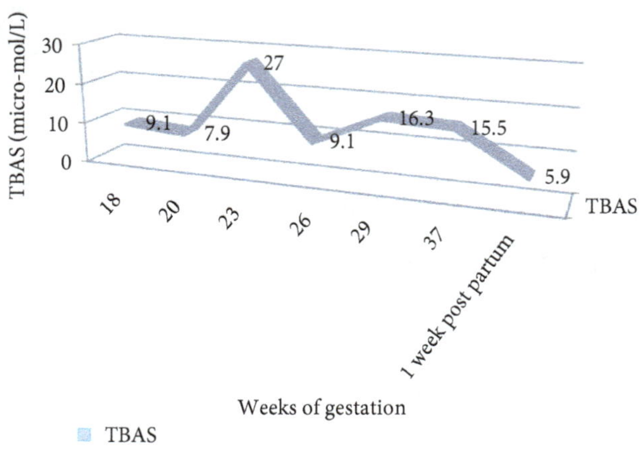

FIGURE 1: TBAS values in micro-mol/L as a function of weeks of gestation.

dermatitis that included lotions, antihistamines and oral steroids reaching 40 mg daily also to no avail. Despite two weeks of treatment the pruritis increased in severity and at this point ICP was suspected for which total bile acid salts TBAS as well as liver function tests were ordered. The patient discontinued her previous medications and was started prophylactically on ursodeoxycholic acid (UDCA) at a dose of 250 mg TID. At 18 weeks of gestation the results of her laboratory tests showed an increase in TBAS of 9.1. At this point the patient was referred to a maternal fetal medicine specialist at our center.

At our clinic, the patient was followed every 3 weeks with out-patient clinic visits until 33 weeks of gestation and then weekly afterwards. Nonstress tests were performed twice weekly as of 28 WG and follow up growth scans at 2-3 week intervals. The estimated fetal weight was within 50th percentile range at all times. The levels of TBAS were measured every 3 weeks. Her UDCA doses were modified depending on her serum bile salt values. The patients' TBAS values are presented in Figure 1.

By the end of her pregnancy she was receiving 2000 mg daily of UDCA with mild tolerable symptoms. Her liver function tests were within the normal limits at all times during pregnancy. SGOT values ranged between 13 and 20 U/L, SGPT values ranged between 8 and 14 U/L, while bilirubin was less than 0.1 mg/dl.

The patient was induced at 37+1 weeks of gestation using misoprostol and then followed by oxytocin for labor augmentation. The patient progressed smoothly to full dilation within 12 hours of induction. She delivered a live born male of weight 3340 grams and Apagr score of 8 and 9 at 1 and 5 minutes respectively. The patient and her child were discharged home on the day 1 post vaginal delivery in a stable condition. Follow up TBAS 1-week post-partum revealed a value of 5.9 micro-mol/L, with complete resolution of symptoms. The patient provided an informed consent with which we were given permission to access her medical chart.

3. Discussion

The prevalence of ICP during pregnancy varies geographically from 0.1 to 15.6% [11]. The potential poor pregnancy outcomes push obstetricians towards a closer follow up of affected pregnancies. One of the challenges that primary care physicians face is the ability to make a timely diagnosis of such a threatening condition, especially when symptoms appear early on during pregnancy. The cut-off gestational age for differentiation between early and late onset is set at 34 weeks of gestation [5]. It is believed that elevated levels of estrogen as well as progesterone might play an inducing factor in the onset of ICP [12, 13]. Add to that, genetic predisposition might lead to malfunction in the bile acid transmembrane hepatocyte transporters, causing accumulation of bile acid. In fact, in the setting of hyperestrogenism (i.e. pregnancy or oral contraceptive pill intake), this malfunction becomes evident and the patient develops the typical symptomatology [14]. Most of the data documented that early onset first trimester ICP cases are concomitant with supra-physiological estrogen levels during the first trimester. Such elevated sex steroid levels are usually noted in multiple gestations or pregnancies complicated by ovarian hyperstimulation syndrome. Add to that, pregnancies conceived via ovarian stimulation cycles with subsequent embryo transfer are at a higher risk of developing early onset ICP [15]. However, our patient conceived spontaneously and already had a noncomplicated pregnancy before which only strengthens the fact that the cause-effect relationship leading to ICP is weak and still needs to be fully clarified. Table 1 shows the published cases of first trimester ICP along with the identified risk factors and the pregnancy outcomes.

J. Lin et al. showed that adverse pregnancy outcomes were higher in patients diagnosed to have early onset ICP compared to the late-onset ICP group, the analysis revealed significantly higher rates of fetal distress, intrauterine growth restriction, preterm birth, and low birth weight in the early-onset ICP group [5]. The overall preterm delivery rate was 34.15% in comparison to the worldwide numbers that range between 19 and 60% [5, 9, 16]. This is due in part to the induction of labor at earlier gestational ages to avoid fetal adverse events. Add to that, elevated bile acid concentrations alter cell membrane permeability and stimulate prostaglandin release, thus leading to increased uterine reactivity as well as increased sensitivity to oxytocin which might cause preterm labor [17]. On another level, it has been postulated that bile acid salts deposit in the placenta and lead to edema, strictures, and acceleration of placental cell apoptosis with subsequent alteration of the placental function [9]. Also, elevated maternal and amniotic fluid levels of bile acids can lead to umbilical vessels spasms with resultant reduction in the trans-placental nutrient exchange and fetal oxygenation. It has been postulated as well that, elevated fetal levels of acids might cause end organ damage resulting in fetal hypoxia and death [18]. Finally, recent studies have showed that fetal cardiomyocytes harbor receptors for bile acids known as the nuclear BA receptor farnesoid-X receptor (FXR) that have been found to be involved in cardiac injury and cardiomyocyte apoptosis [19]. Elevated levels of bile acids might therefore be potentially cardio-toxic with resultant life threatening arrhythmias, cardiac dysfunction, and intrauterine fetal death (relative risk of 2.58 in comparison with non-ICP pregnancies) [20]. In the setting of early onset ICP, the duration of fetal and placental exposure to abnormally elevated bile acid salt levels is significantly prolonged and thus

TABLE 1: Characteristics of all cases of first trimester ICP documented in the literature.

Article title	Number of cases	Predisposing factor	Ethnicity	Gestational age at diagnosis/onset of symptoms	Bile acid level at the time of diagnosis (micro-mol/L)	Pregnancy Outcome
Kirkinen et al. 1995	1	(i) Triploid fetus (ii)Elevated alpha Fetoprotein	Not available	Not available	Not available	Not specified
Brites et al. 1998	1	Not specified	Not available	11 weeks of gestation	198 at 20 weeks of gestation	IOL at 36 weeks of gestation. Baby had intestinal stenosis
Zamah et al. 2008	2	(i) IVF treatment	Asian	8 weeks of gestation	137.2	IOL at term due to oligohydramnios
		(ii) Moderate OHSS	East Indian	6 weeks of gestation	308	Spontaneous miscarriage at 9 weeks of gestation
Steele et al. 2012	1	(i) First pregnancy No obvious risk factors	British	11 weeks of gestation	205 at 16 weeks of gestation	Emergency cesarean for nonreassuring fetal heart at 32^{+2} weeks of gestation
Johnston et al. 2014	1	(i) Recurrent ICP (ii) Heterozygous mutation of ABCB4 gene	Not available	8 weeks of gestation	217	PPROM at 30^{+5} weeks of gestation c/s for malpresentation
Hubschmann et al. 2016	1	(i) Recurrent ICP	Guatemalan	7^{+5} weeks of gestation	243.6 at 13^{+5} weeks of gestation	Elective cesarean section at 31^{+6} weeks of gestation
Mutlu et al. 2017	2	(i) IVF treatment	Turkish	6 weeks of gestation	166.8	Blighted ovum
		(ii) Moderate OHSS	Turkish	5 weeks of gestation	122	PPROM at 36 WG with delivery of twins via cesarean section
Our case	1	(i) No known risk factors	Lebanese	10 weeks of gestation	9.1 at 18 weeks of gestation	IOL at 37 weeks of gestation

the cytotoxic effects are more likely to take place. This mandates a closer follow up of patients diagnosed to have ICP at an early stage of pregnancy as well as timed intervention to interrupt pregnancy [9, 18].

Until today, many studies have been performed to assess the effectiveness and safety profile of the widely used Ursodeoxycholic acid (UDCA). It has been suggested that it not only improves the severity of the symptoms related to ICP, but also decreases the level of bile acid salts and potentially improves the pregnancy outcome especially in the setting of early onset ICP [21, 22]. The exact mechanism by which UDCA improves the outcome of ICP patients is unknown so far. It is believed that UDCA normalizes hepatic metabolism, improves transplacental bile acid transport, and/or prevents the oxidative stress and cellular death [23]. Furthermore, UDCA is believed to be cardio-protective and thus an enhancer of the fetal cardiac function. This is vital in the setting of the suspicion that elevated bile acid salts can cause cardiac arrest of the fetus [24]. In Lebanon, clear and independent guidelines are absent, thus the guidelines of the American college of obstetrics and Gynecology (ACOG) as well as the Society for Maternal-Fetal Medicine (SMFM) are adapted in our daily practice. However, given that this particular patient did not improve on the recommended doses of UDCA, the decision was taken to treat her with the highest level recommended in the literature which is equivalent to 2000 mg/day [8]. Other newer approaches to ICP medical treatment such as Resveratrol, a Silent Information Regulator 1 (SIRT1) is thought to activate SIRT1 with resultant reduction in the levels of pro-inflammatory cytokines and bile acids [25]. The use of Resveratrol in the context of ICP however is still limited pending more conclusive data.

The ideal time of delivery is determined based on the severity of maternal symptoms, onset of ICP, and maternal discomfort as well as assessment of fetal well-being [5]. Mild ICP patients can be managed till 38 WG, while severe cases of ICP should be delivered at maximum of 37 WG. Recent investigations have showed that ICP patients are more prone to serious conditions such as preeclampsia, gestational diabetes, as well as nonpregnancy related hepatobiliary disease such portal hypertension and liver failure [26–28].

4. Conclusion

First trimester ICP is a rare condition that physicians need to be aware of particularly in the setting of typical symptomatology. So far, close follow-up, fetal monitoring, and UDCA are the mainstay of treatment to avoid poor neonatal outcomes. Further studies are needed to better understand the pathophysiology and find the ultimate treatment for ICP.

Acknowledgment

This work was carried out at the American University of Beirut Medical Center (AUBMC), Beirut-Lebanon.

References

[1] Šimják, Patrik, A. Pařízek et al., "Fetal complications due to intrahepatic cholestasis of pregnancy," *Journal of Perinatal Medicine*, vol. 43, no. 2, pp. 133–139, 2015.

[2] A. Floreani and M. T. Gervasi, "New insights on intrahepatic cholestasis of pregnancy," *Clinics in Liver Disease*, vol. 20, no. 1, pp. 177–189, 2016.

[3] P. H. Dixon and C. Williamson, "The pathophysiology of intrahepatic cholestasis of pregnancy," *Clinics and Research in Hepatology and Gastroenterology*, vol. 40, no. 2, pp. 141–153, 2016.

[4] Z. Jie, D. Yiling, and Y. Ling, "Association of assisted reproductive technology with adverse pregnancy outcomes," *Iranian Journal of Reproductive Medicine*, vol. 13, no. 3, p. 169, 2015.

[5] J. Lin, W. Gu, and Y. Hou, "Diagnosis and prognosis of early-onset intrahepatic cholestasis of pregnancy: a prospective study," *The Journal of Maternal-Fetal & Neonatal Medicine*, vol. 7, pp. 1–7, 2017.

[6] M. F. Mutlu, K. Aslan, I. Guler et al., "Two cases of first onset intrahepatic cholestasis of pregnancy associated with moderate ovarian hyperstimulation syndrome after IVF treatment and review of the literature," *Journal of Obstetrics and Gynaecology*, vol. 37, no. 5, pp. 547–549, 2017.

[7] J. Ribalta, H. Reyes, M. C. Gonzalez et al., "S-Adenosyl-L-methionine in the treatment of patients with intrahepatic cholestasis of pregnancy: a randomized, double-blind, placebo-controlled study with negative results," *Hepatology*, vol. 13, no. 6, pp. 1084–1089, 1991.

[8] A. Glantz, H. U. Marschall, and L. Å. Mattsson, "Intrahepatic cholestasis of pregnancy: relationships between bile acid levels and fetal complication rates," *Hepatology*, vol. 40, no. 2, pp. 467–474, 2004.

[9] T. T. Chao and J. S. Sheffield, "Primary dermatologic findings with early-onset intrahepatic cholestasis of pregnancy," *Obstetrics & Gynecology*, vol. 117, no. 2, pp. 456–458, 2011.

[10] R. Madazli, M. A. Yuksel, M. Oncul, A. Tuten, O. Guralp, and B. Aydin, "Pregnancy outcomes and prognostic factors in patients with intrahepatic cholestasis of pregnancy," *Journal of Obstetrics and Gynaecology*, vol. 35, no. 4, pp. 358–361, 2015.

[11] S. Ozkan, Y. Ceylan, O. V. Ozkan, and S. Yildirim, "Review of a challenging clinical issue: intrahepatic cholestasis of pregnancy," *World Journal of Gastroenterology: WJG*, vol. 21, no. 23, pp. 7134–7141, 2015.

[12] H. Reyes and J. Sjövall, "Bile acids and progesterone metabolites intrahepatic cholestasis of pregnancy," *Annals of Medicine*, vol. 32, no. 2, pp. 94–106, 2000.

[13] S. Abu-Hayyeh, G. Papacleovoulou, A. Lövgren-Sandblom et al., "Intrahepatic cholestasis of pregnancy levels of sulfated progesterone metabolites inhibit farnesoid X receptor resulting in a cholestatic phenotype," *Hepatology*, vol. 57, no. 2, pp. 716–726, 2013.

[14] A. G. Hubschmann, K. M. Orzechowski, and V. Berghella, "Severe first trimester recurrent intrahepatic cholestasis of pregnancy: a case report and literature review," *American Journal of Perinatology Reports*, vol. 06, no. 01, pp. e38–e41, 2016.

[15] C. Feng, W. J. Li, R. H. He, X. W. Sun, G. Wang, and L. Q. Wang, "Impacts of different methods of conception on the perinatal outcome of intrahepatic cholestasis of pregnancy in twin pregnancies," *Scientific Reports*, vol. 8, no. 1, p. 3985, 2018.

[16] R. Smolarczyk, M. Grymowicz, J. Sienko, and K. Czajkowski, "Successful perinatal outcome in an early onset intrahepatic cholestasis of pregnancy with extremely high serum hepatic function tests," *Gynecological Endocrinology*, vol. 25, no. 7, pp. 475–476, 2009.

[17] A. M. Germain, S. Kato, J. A. Carvajal, G. J. Valenzuela, G. L. Valdes, and J. C. Glasinovic, "Bile acids increase response and expression of human myometrial oxytocin receptor," *American Journal of Obstetrics and Gynecology*, vol. 189, no. 2, pp. 577–582, 2003.

[18] N. Favre, N. Bourdel, V. Sapin, A. Abergel, and D. Gallot, "Importance of bile acids for intra-hepatic cholestasis of pregnancy," *Gynecologie, Obstetrique & Fertilite*, vol. 38, no. 4, pp. 293–295, 2010.

[19] J. Pu, A. Yuan, P. Shan et al., "Cardiomyocyte-expressed farnesoid-X-receptor is a novel apoptosis mediator and contributes to myocardial ischaemia/reperfusion injury," *European Heart Journal*, vol. 34, no. 24, pp. 1834–1845, 2012.

[20] O. Kirbas, E. H. Biberoglu, A. Kirbas et al., "Evaluation of ventricular repolarization in pregnant women with intrahepatic cholestasis," *International Journal of Cardiology*, vol. 15, no. 189, pp. 25–29, 2015.

[21] Y. Bacq, L. Sentilhes, H. B. Reyes et al., "Efficacy of ursodeoxycholic acid in treating intrahepatic cholestasis of pregnancy: a meta-analysis," *Gastroenterology*, vol. 143, no. 6, pp. 1492–501, 2012.

[22] X. Kong, Y. Kong, F. Zhang, T. Wang, and J. Yan, "Evaluating the effectiveness and safety of ursodeoxycholic acid in treatment of intrahepatic cholestasis of pregnancy: a meta-analysis (a prisma-compliant study)," *Medicine*, vol. 95, no. 40, p. e4949, 2016.

[23] T. Kagawa, R. Orii, S. Hirose et al., "Ursodeoxycholic acid stabilizes the bile salt export pump in the apical membrane in MDCK II cells," *Journal of Gastroenterology*, vol. 49, no. 5, pp. 890–899, 2014.

[24] M. Rodríguez, A. Sprohnle, J. Muñoz, C. Cadena, R. Corvalán, and A. Sepúlveda-Martínez, "Treatment of intrahepatic cholestasis of pregnancy with ursodeoxycholic acid associated with improvement of fetal first-degree atrioventricular block," *Ultrasound in Obstetrics & Gynecology*, vol. 52, no. 6, pp. 801–802, 2018.

[25] E. Liao, Z. Li, and Y. Shao, "Resveratrol regulating SIRT1-NF-κB signal pathway in intrahepatic cholestasis of pregnancy," *Hepatology Research*, vol. 48, no. 12, pp. 1031–1044, 2018.

[26] C. Labbe, C. Delesalle, C. Creveuil, and M. Dreyfus, "Early and later intrahepatic cholestasis of pregnancy (ICP): study of adverse pregnancy outcomes," *Gynecologie, Obstetrique, Fertilite & Senologie*, vol. 46, no. 4, pp. 388–394, 2018.

[27] M. Martineau, C. Raker, R. Powrie, and C. Williamson, "Intrahepatic cholestasis of pregnancy is associated with an increased risk of gestational diabetes," *European Journal of Obstetrics & Gynecology and Reproductive Biology*, vol. 176, pp. 80–85, 2014.

[28] E. Wikström Shemer, H. U. Marschall, J. F. Ludvigsson, and O. Stephansson, "Intrahepatic cholestasis of pregnancy and associated adverse pregnancy and fetal outcomes: a 12-year population-based cohort study," *BJOG: An International Journal of Obstetrics & Gynaecology*, vol. 120, no. 6, pp. 717–723, 2013.

Benign Recurrent Intrahepatic Cholestasis in Pregnancy: Fetal Death at 36 Weeks of Gestation

Mariam Ayyash[1] **Nicolina Smith,**[1] **Madhurima Keerthy,**[1] **Ashina Singh,**[2] **and Majid Shaman**[3]

[1]*Department of Obstetrics and Gynecology, Henry Ford Health System, Detroit, Michigan, USA*
[2]*Department of Gastroenterology and Hepatology, Henry Ford Health System, Detroit, Michigan, USA*
[3]*Division of Maternal and Fetal Medicine, Department of Obstetrics and Gynecology, Henry Ford Health System, Detroit, Michigan, USA*

Correspondence should be addressed to Mariam Ayyash; mayyash1@hfhs.org

Academic Editor: Daniel Martin

Introduction. Benign recurrent intrahepatic cholestasis is a rare hepatologic disorder characterized by recurrent, self-limited episodes of severe pruritus, jaundice, and elevated bile acids. While there are guidelines for the management of intrahepatic cholestasis of pregnancy, the literature regarding benign recurrent intrahepatic cholestasis and pregnancy is limited. *Case.* A 29-year-old G1P0 woman, with history of liver toxicity, had elevated total serum bile acid levels and liver enzymes documented at 8 weeks of gestation and throughout her pregnancy. She had a reactive nonstress test just 3 days prior to her induction. Fetal demise was noted when she presented at 36 weeks for her induction. *Conclusion.* We recommend that women with elevated total serum bile acid early in pregnancy due to a separate entity relative to intrahepatic cholestasis of pregnancy be managed in a more individualized approach.

1. Introduction

Benign recurrent intrahepatic cholestasis (BRIC) was first described in 1959 [1]. It can present any time in life, from infancy to late adulthood, and is characterized by recurrent self-limited episodes of severe pruritus and jaundice that can last from several weeks to months [2]. BRIC does not lead to progressive liver dysfunction and cirrhosis, but the symptoms associated with each attack may be associated with significant morbidity [2]. The pathophysiology of BRIC is poorly understood, and treatment remains empiric, primarily aimed at symptom relief [3]. The literature addressing BRIC during pregnancy is limited, and many patients with an abnormal liver profile and total serum bile acids (TSBA) are managed as having intrahepatic cholestasis of pregnancy (ICP).

ICP is generally characterized by pruritus and an elevation in liver enzymes and/or TSBA concentrations, and importantly, it typically develops in the second or third trimester [4, 5]. The etiology of ICP is not fully understood; it is associated with adverse fetal outcomes such as increased risk of preterm delivery, intrapartum fetal heart rate abnormalities, meconium-stained fluid, neonatal respiratory distress syndrome, and fetal death [5, 6]. The severity of ICP ranges from mild itching during pregnancy to fetal death [7]. Given the risk of fetal death within the context of ICP, the Society for Maternal-Fetal Medicine recommends induction of labor for women with ICP in the late preterm/early term period, specifically between 36 weeks and 39 weeks if TSBA is under 100 μmol/L and at 36 weeks if TSBA is more than or equal to 100 μmol/L [8]. Because such recommendations are specifically for ICP, there are no particular guidelines for labor induction within the setting of BRIC or other cholestatic liver disorders, when bile acid levels may be elevated within the first trimester.

We present the case of a patient with presumed BRIC for whom we followed the guidelines for women with ICP for

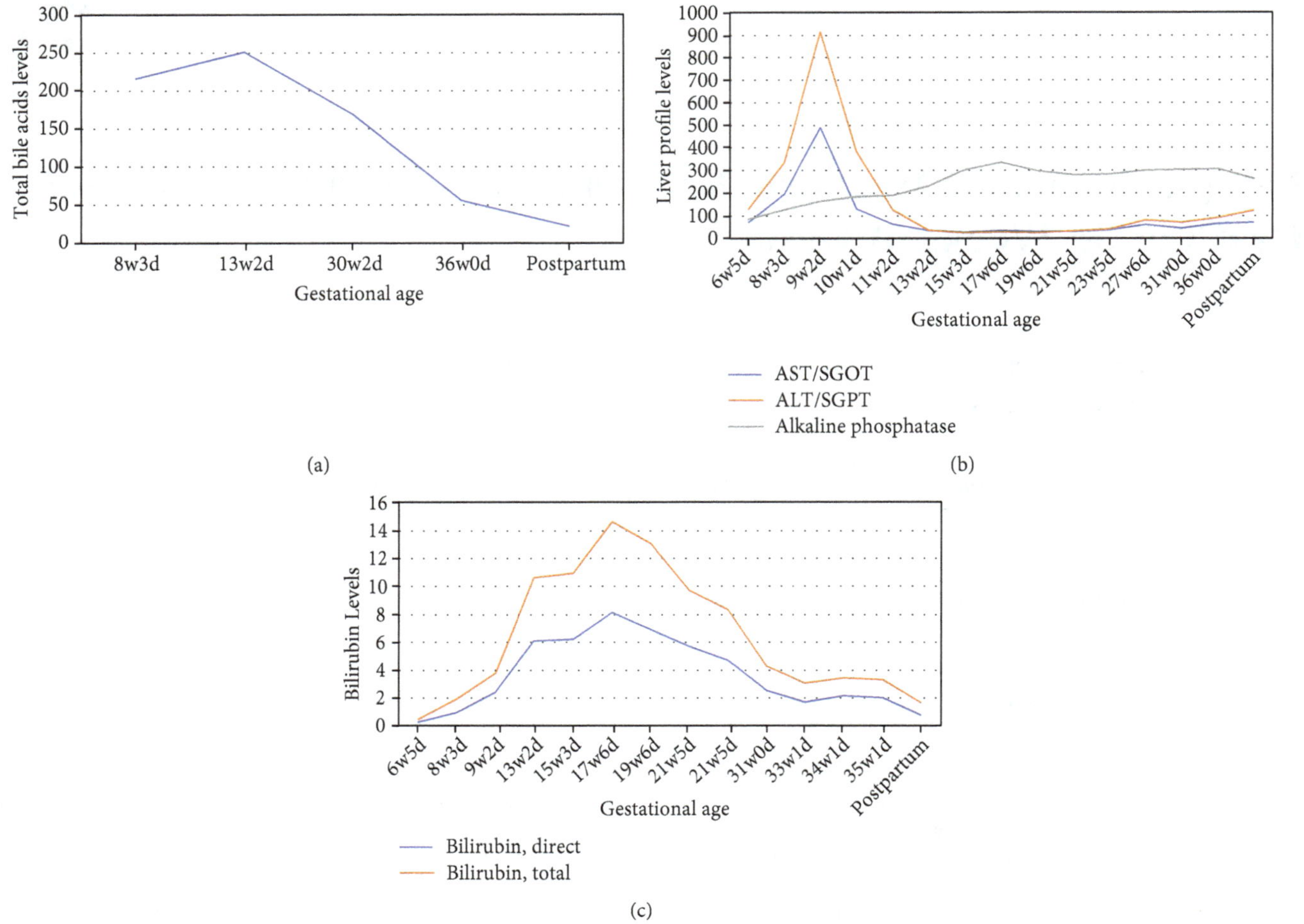

FIGURE 1: (a) Trend in bile acid levels. (b) Trend in liver profile values. (c) Trend in bilirubin levels (note: "postpartum" refers to 12 days following delivery).

delivery with induction at 36 weeks. However, upon presenting at her 36-week gestation mark for induction of labor, the patient had fetal death.

2. Case Presentation

A 29-year-old gravida 1 woman presented at 6 weeks and 2 days of gestational age for prenatal care. She had a history of liver toxicity that occurred in 2009 and again in 2014, which was thought to be related to drug-induced liver injury caused by oral contraceptive pills. At the time of her liver toxicity episodes, she had had an extensive infectious and autoimmune workup, which included testing for acute and chronic hepatitis A, hepatitis E, hepatitis B, hepatitis C, Epstein-Barr virus, cytomegalovirus, and human herpesvirus, all of which were negative. A liver biopsy was taken in 2014 which was consistent with possible drug-induced cholestasis. At the beginning of her pregnancy, she started having symptoms of pruritus, dark urine, and pale stool. She was followed by the hospital's monthly maternal critical care conference meetings from the beginning of her pregnancy because of her cholestasis diagnosis, elevated liver enzymes, and initial elevated TSBA levels of 215 μmol/L at 8 weeks and 3 days of gestation.

She was being followed by hepatology experts and was initially started on ursodeoxycholic acid (UDCA) 300 mg 3 times a day, which was subsequently increased to 600 mg 2 times a day in her first trimester. She reported mild improvement in her symptoms after she was started on ursodiol. Her liver enzymes, which had been in a mixed hepatocellular and cholestatic pattern, improved after starting the UDCA. An underlying genetic cause within the differential diagnosis was suspected as the culprit of her clinical presentation, especially because of the patient's previous recurrent cholestatic episodes before her pregnancy. The follow-up plan during her pregnancy included liver profile and bile acid monitoring every 2 to 4 weeks (Figures 1(a) and 1(b)), weekly bilirubin checks (Figure 1(c)), serial growth ultrasounds every 4 weeks, nonstress tests twice weekly starting at 32 weeks of gestation, and ultimately delivery via induction of labor at 36 to 37 weeks and pending maternal and fetal status. Her growth ultrasounds were within normal limits with the last growth done at 32 weeks of gestation. Because of her increasing TSBA levels, the patient's UDCA dose was increased to 600 mg 3 times daily (15 mg/kg/day) (Figure 1). The plan was then to schedule induction of labor at 36 weeks with administration of 2 doses of betamethasone before her scheduled induction. When she presented for her betamethasone, she had a reactive nonstress test and received her first dose of betamethasone followed by a second dose the next day.

She arrived at 36 weeks and 0 days for induction of labor. She reported having contractions and leakage of yellow-brown fluid, with decreased fetal movement. The patient's cervix was 4 cm dilated with no evidence of prelabor preterm rupture of the membrane. No fetal heart tones were noted, and fetal death was confirmed upon evaluation by 2 health-care providers. The patient was induced at that time with oxytocin and vaginally delivered a male newborn a few hours after the start of her induction. The newborn had normal anatomy. The patient had fetal death laboratory workup that included assessment of Kleihauer-Betke fetal hemoglobin, complete blood count, thyroid-stimulating hormone, and lactate dehydrogenase levels, in which all were within the reference range, as well as testing for the presence of toxoplasmosis, parvovirus, and antiphospholipid syndrome, all of which were negative. Her liver enzymes remained elevated (Figure 1(b)). A karyotype was performed on the newborn and showed a normal male karyotype. The patient underwent genetic testing after delivery, and her result showed a heterozygous variant of *ABCB11*, which is one of several recessive alleles associated with BRIC.

3. Discussion

Our patient had a unique presentation of cholestasis during pregnancy, which was later confirmed as BRIC. Her TSBA levels had remained above 200 μmol/L after the first trimester and went under 100 μmol/L only when she presented with the fetal death at the time of her scheduled labor induction. At that time, though, the value remained above 40 μmol/L, a cutoff value that traditionally defines severe ICP and is associated with increased incidence of adverse fetal outcomes [5]. The mechanism by which elevated TBSA levels lead to adverse pregnancy outcomes, including fetal death, has not been well established. While there is an increased rate of fetal death with higher-than-normal TSBA levels, the literature suggests that the risk of fetal demise is significantly higher for women with TSBA levels specifically 100 μmol/L or higher [9, 10]. It is also worth noting that the impact of the timing of TSBA elevation on pregnancy outcomes, particularly when it occurs in the first trimester, has not been well explored in the literature, probably because there is a paucity of knowledge on the natural history of BRIC and ICP when bile acids are elevated early in pregnancy. In patients who have particularly severe TSBA elevation early in pregnancy, individualized plans need to be made for monitoring the fetus, and consideration should be given to the timing of induction possibly before 36 weeks and should be based on specific TSBA values.

The literature has cited 3 case reports describing pregnancy outcomes of women with the ICP onset in the first trimester due to elevation in bile acids then [11–13]. While these cases were labeled as first trimester ICP, they could very well have been BRIC, given the recurrence of cholestasis episodes outside of pregnancy and the early onset of TBSA elevation in the first trimester. In fact, it is thought that BRIC among most women is underdiagnosed because the two most common features of BRIC, pruritus and jaundice, are misattributed to either pregnancy or to the use of oral contraceptive pills [14].

Our patient was treated per the ICP guidelines, with appropriate monitoring and a plan for labor induction at 36 weeks of gestation, but ultimately had fetal death. Our patient's presentation of cholestasis was unique, as her TSBA levels were over 200 μmol/L in her first trimester and then gradually decreased to the 100 s μmol/L range throughout the remainder of her pregnancy. At the time of labor induction, her TSBA level was at 56 μmol/L, well under 100 μmol/L; however, it is still within the relatively severe range during pregnancy, and no literature has evaluated the impact on pregnancy outcomes of such TSBA elevations in the first trimester. The current Society for Maternal-Fetal Medicine guidelines recommend induction at 36 weeks of gestation for women with ICP and TSBA greater than or equal to 100 μmol/L [8]. The American College of Obstetricians and Gynecologists has also suggested that delivery before 36 weeks of gestation may be indicated depending on laboratory and clinical circumstances; however, clear-cut timeframes or criteria were not defined [15]. Often, TSBA levels are not assessed in cases of cholestasis at all because of lengthy lab resulting times, which can take anywhere between 2 and 6 days. While TSBA enzymatic test processing can be done within less than two hours, due to the low number of samples requested to be processed, technicians often wait to add more samples to cover the processing cost. This often results in the few days of delays in reporting results. Designing individual tests or evaluating TSBAs on a routine basis can help resolve such processing concern. In fact, due to its association with adverse pregnancy outcomes, we suggest that TSBA be routinely ordered for women with a history of liver/biliary disease in the first trimester as elevated TSBA results can influence management plans throughout pregnancies. In situations where a patient's TSBA levels are known and an alternative diagnosis to ICP is suspected because of TSBA elevation in the first trimester (particularly with levels over 100 μmol/L), it is important to take these circumstances into account when considering the induction timeframe for pregnant women with ICP in the setting of likely a coexisting cholestatic disease. Little is known about the natural history of women with cholestatic disorders that are separate from ICP, and because reliable research on how these women fare during pregnancy is lacking, an individualized approach to care should be taken. Additionally, it is recommended that in cases where abnormally high TSBA levels occur within a setting of pruritus and elevated transaminase levels early in pregnancy, patients should be sent for genetic testing. In fact, this is recommended in the newly outlined practice guidelines on reproductive health in liver disease from the American Association for the Study of Liver Diseases [16].

We presented the case of a woman with presumed BRIC who was treated per the current ICP guidelines and yet had fetal death at 36 weeks of gestation, on the day of her planned labor induction. We recommend that women in early pregnancy who have elevated TSBA levels that may be the result of a cholestatic condition other than ICP should not be restricted to the current treatment and delivery guidelines that are specific for ICP. Regardless of whether they have BRIC or another cholestatic liver disorder, these women should be cared for with a more individualized approach: better established guidelines regarding the standardization and frequency of bile acid testing, antepartum testing, and patient education are needed, and more attention should be given to patients with a history of fetal death and cholestasis, with considerations such as antepartum admission with regular nonstress testing monitoring close to the timing of delivery, with induction earlier than the recommended 36 weeks. Lastly, we hope that a national registry can be established to improve the study of cholestatic disorders that are distinct from ICP to better guide treatment plans for these patients.

Acknowledgments

The authors thank Karla D. Passalacqua, PhD, at Henry Ford Hospital for her editorial assistance and Stephanie Stebens, MLIS, at Sladen Library, Henry Ford Hospital, for her input in reviewing this manuscript.

References

[1] W. H. J. Summerskill and J. M. Walshe, "Benign recurrent intrahepatic " Obstructive " Jaundice," *Lancet*, vol. 2, no. 7105, pp. 686–690, 1959.

[2] V. A. Luketic and M. L. Shiffman, "Benign recurrent intrahepatic cholestasis," *Clinics in Liver Disease*, vol. 3, no. 3, pp. 509–528, 1999.

[3] N. Tygstrup and B. Jensen, "Intermittent intrahepatic cholestasis of unknown etiology in five young males from the Faroe Islands," *Acta Medica Scandinavica*, vol. 185, p. 523, 1969.

[4] N. Roncaglia, A. Arreghini, A. Locatelli, P. Bellini, C. Andreotti, and A. Ghidini, "Obstetric cholestasis: outcome with active management," *European Journal of Obstetrics, Gynecology, and Reproductive Biology*, vol. 100, no. 2, pp. 167–170, 2002.

[5] A. Glantz, H.-U. Marschall, and L.-A. Mattsson, "Intrahepatic cholestasis of pregnancy: relationships between bile acid levels and fetal complication rates," *Hepatology*, vol. 40, no. 2, pp. 467–474, 2004.

[6] B. A. Mullally and W. F. Hansen, "Intrahepatic cholestasis of pregnancy: review of the literature," *Obstetrical & Gynecological Survey*, vol. 57, no. 1, pp. 47–52, 2002.

[7] C. A. Riely and Y. Bacq, "Intrahepatic cholestasis of pregnancy," *Clinics in Liver Disease*, vol. 8, no. 1, pp. 167–176, 2004.

[8] R. H. Lee, M. Greenberg, T. D. Metz, and C. M. Pettker, "Society for Maternal-Fetal Medicine Consult Series 53: Intrahepatic cholestasis of pregnancy: Replaces Consult 13, April 2011," *American Journal of Obstetrics and Gynecology*, vol. 224, no. 2, pp. B2–B9, 2021.

[9] C. Ovadia, P. T. Seed, A. Sklavounos et al., "Association of adverse perinatal outcomes of intrahepatic cholestasis of pregnancy with biochemical markers: results of aggregate and individual patient data meta-analyses," *Lancet*, vol. 393, no. 10174, pp. 899–909, 2019.

[10] D. di Mascio, J. Quist-Nelson, M. Riegel et al., "Perinatal death by bile acid levels in intrahepatic cholestasis of pregnancy: a systematic review," *The Journal of Maternal-Fetal & Neonatal Medicine*, vol. 19, pp. 1–9, 2019.

[11] V. Keitel, C. Vogt, D. Haussinger, and R. Kubitz, "Combined mutations of canalicular transporter proteins cause severe intrahepatic cholestasis of pregnancy," *Gastroenterology*, vol. 131, no. 2, pp. 624–629, 2006.

[12] A. G. Hubschmann, K. M. Orzechowski, and V. Berghella, "Severe first trimester recurrent intrahepatic cholestasis of pregnancy: a case report and literature review," *AJP Reports*, vol. 6, no. 1, pp. e38–e41, 2016.

[13] M. Stulic, D. Culafic, I. Boricic et al., "Intrahepatic cholestasis of pregnancy: a case study of the rare onset in the first trimester," *Medicina (Kaunas, Lithuania)*, vol. 55, no. 8, p. 454, 2019.

[14] R. Brenard, A. P. Geubel, and J. P. Benhamou, "Benign recurrent intrahepatic cholestasis," *Journal of Clinical Gastroenterology*, vol. 11, no. 5, pp. 546–551, 1989.

[15] "ACOG Committee Opinion No. 764: Medically indicated late-preterm and early-term deliveries," *Obstetrics and Gynecology*, vol. 133, no. 2, pp. e151–e155, 2019.

[16] M. Sarkar, C. W. Brady, J. Fleckenstein et al., "Reproductive health and liver disease: practice guidance by the American Association for the Study of Liver Diseases," *Hepatology*, vol. 73, no. 1, pp. 318–365, 2021.

30

Silicone Plate for the Prevention of Postoperative Adhesions in Patients with Asherman Syndrome

Maho Miyagi, Keiko Mekaru, Sugiko Oishi, Chiaki Urasoe, Kozue Akamine, and Yoichi Aoki

Department of Obstetrics and Gynaecology, Graduate School of Medicine, University of the Ryukyus, 207 Uehara, Nishihara, Okinawa 903-0215, Japan

Correspondence should be addressed to Keiko Mekaru; f041252@eve.u-ryukyu.ac.jp

Academic Editor: Julio Rosa e Silva

Purpose. Re-adhesion rates following hysteroscopic adhesiolysis have remained high. Accordingly, we present a case involving temporary placement of an intrauterine silicone plate to prevent re-adhesions following hysteroscopic adhesiolysis in a 36-year-old woman with Asherman syndrome. *Methods.* After hysteroscopic adhesiolysis, a silicone plate molded to the uterine cavity's shape was inserted into the uterine cavity and left in place for 1 month. *Results.* The patient had a history of endometrial curettage for endometrial polyps. After the procedure, she developed amenorrhea and experienced infertility for 5 years despite four cycles of *in vitro* fertilization and embryo transfer. Following admission to our hospital, hysteroscopic examination showed a wide area of intrauterine adhesions for which hysteroscopic adhesiolysis and silicone plate insertion were performed. The silicone plate was removed after 1 month. No intrauterine adhesions were observed during the subsequent hysteroscopic examination. After a thawed embryo transfer, the patient became pregnant and delivered a healthy baby. *Conclusions.* A silicon plate may be considered a useful tool for preventing re-adhesion following hysteroscopic adhesiolysis without serious complications.

1. Introduction

Intrauterine adhesions, such as those observed in patients with Asherman syndrome, can lead to embryo implantation disorders, causing infertility and recurrent miscarriages. This is believed to be due to endometrial damage, often caused by endometrial curettage. Specifically, each procedure carries a 16% risk of intrauterine adhesion that increases with the number of procedures performed [1]. Severe intrauterine adhesions could lead to uterine amenorrhea. Therefore, patients who plan to bear children should undergo hysteroscopic adhesiolysis. However, this procedure carries a high re-adhesion rate, reaching 62.5% in severe cases [2]. Even without severe adhesions, the re-adhesion rate following adhesiolysis is 27.2% in patients with Asherman syndrome [3]. Although an intrauterine device (IUD) is traditionally placed to prevent postoperative adhesions, its effects remain insufficient. In the field of otorhinolaryngology, medical silicone plates are being used to prevent adhesions during tympanoplasty. Here, we present a case involving temporary intrauterine placement of a silicone plate to prevent re-adhesions with successful outcomes, accompanied by a literature review.

2. Case Summary

Our patient was a 36-year-old G0P0 female with an unremarkable medical history except for a 5-year history of infertility. The patient sought infertility treatment from a previous physician when she was 31 years old and subsequently underwent endometrial curettage for endometrial polyps. After the procedure, she developed amenorrhea with small menstrual blood loss despite Kaufmann therapy. The patient then underwent four cycles of *in vitro* fertilization and embryo transfer. Though biochemical pregnancy was confirmed once, the patient was referred to our department for further examination and treatment.

A hysteroscopic examination performed at our department confirmed a wide area of intrauterine adhesions

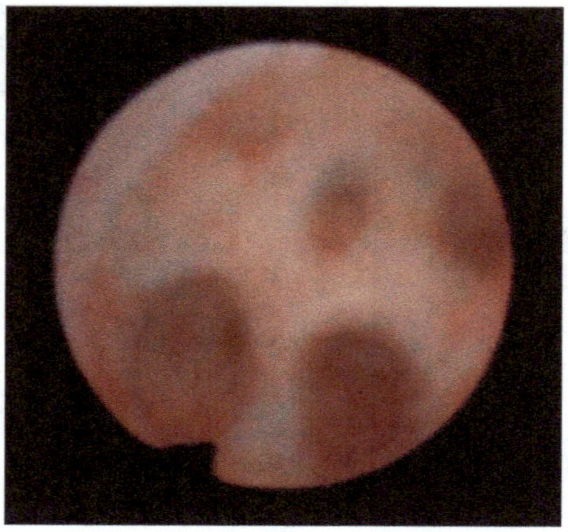

FIGURE 1: Hysteroscopic examination.

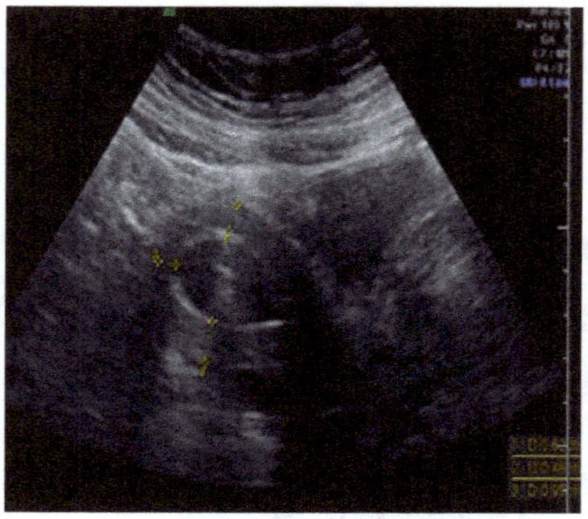

FIGURE 2: Transabdominal ultrasound was used to measure the balloon size.

(Figure 1), which led to a diagnosis of Asherman syndrome. In the present case, Asherman syndrome severity was evaluated using the European Society of Gynecological Endoscopy classification of intrauterine adhesions based on hysteroscopic findings. Due to their honeycomb-like appearance, the intrauterine adhesions were classified as stage III multiple dense adhesions (moderate).

2.1. Honeycomb-Like Adhesions and Fibrosis can be Observed in the Uterine Cavity. Hysteroscopic adhesiolysis was subsequently performed under general anesthesia. Initially, a 14-F urinary catheter with a balloon was inserted into the uterine cavity, after which 5 mL of saline was slowly injected into the balloon. Following blunt adhesiolysis with the balloon, partially tough, cord-like tissues were resected using an electric scalpel. Thereafter, a urinary catheter was inserted into the uterine cavity and an additional 5 mL of saline was injected. The balloon's transverse and longitudinal diameters were measured using ultrasound with the information obtained used to mold the silicone plate (Figure 2). The transverse diameter of the balloon was 3 cm, while the longitudinal diameter from the fundus to the internal ostium in the sagittal section was 3.6 cm. The silicone plate had the following characteristics: 200 × 150 mm silicone sheet with a thickness of 0.5 mm (Koken Co., Ltd. Bunkyo ward, Tokyo, Japan). The plate was molded into an inverted triangle, resembling the previously measured uterine cavity's shape (Figure 3). A nylon thread was sewn to the tail of the silicone plate to facilitate traction and removal. Finally, the silicon plate was inserted using transabdominal ultrasound and placenta forceps to match the uterine cavity's shape. The position of the inserted silicone plate was confirmed through hysteroscopy and ultrasound (Figure 4). The patient received one preoperative intravenous administration of antibiotics (1 g viccillin/administration), followed by continuous administration of the same antibiotics until postoperative day 1 (1 g viccillin/8 h) to prevent infection. The patient had an uneventful postoperative course and was discharged on postoperative day 2. She began hormone replacement therapy (HRT) 1 week post-surgery. No signs of infection were observed, and the silicone plate was removed

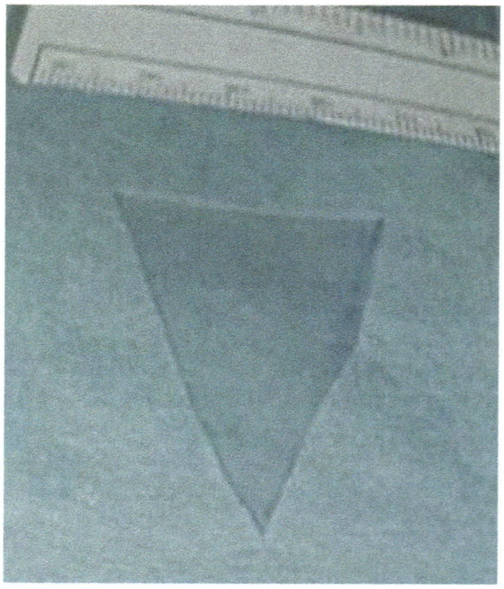

FIGURE 3: The silicone plate (200 × 150 mm silicone sheet with a thickness of 0.5 mm; Koken Co., Ltd. Bunkyo ward, Tokyo, Japan) was molded into an inverted triangle, comparable to the shape of the uterine cavity.

after 1 month. The patient continued to receive two cycles of HRT. No intrauterine adhesions were found during the subsequent hysteroscopic examination (Figure 5).

In vitro fertilization began 9 weeks post-surgery. After a short protocol which was used for ovarian stimulation, five oocytes were retrieved under local anesthesia. Four embryos were obtained through insemination, and four day 2 early cleavage-stage embryos were frozen. Subsequently, one thawed 4-cell embryo was transferred under HRT, and the patient became pregnant.

Labor was induced with oxytocin at 41 weeks and 0 days of gestation. Due to weak uterine contractions and arrested labor, an emergency cesarean section was performed at 41 weeks and 2 days of gestation.

The infant was a male weighing 3070 g with an Apgar score of 8 at both 1 and 5 min. Umbilical cord blood gas analysis showed a pH of 7.184. No intrauterine adhesions or placenta

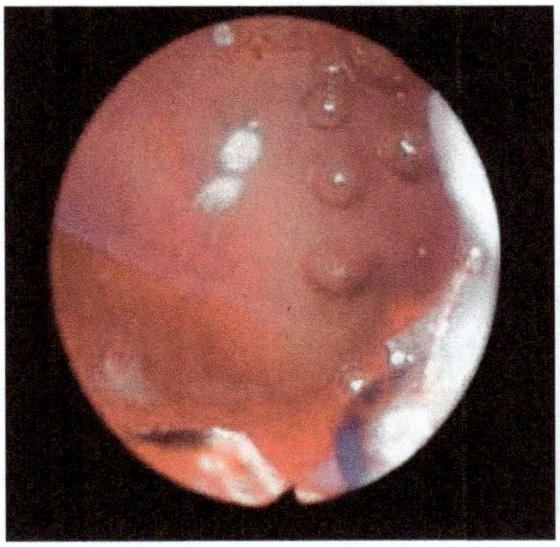

(a)

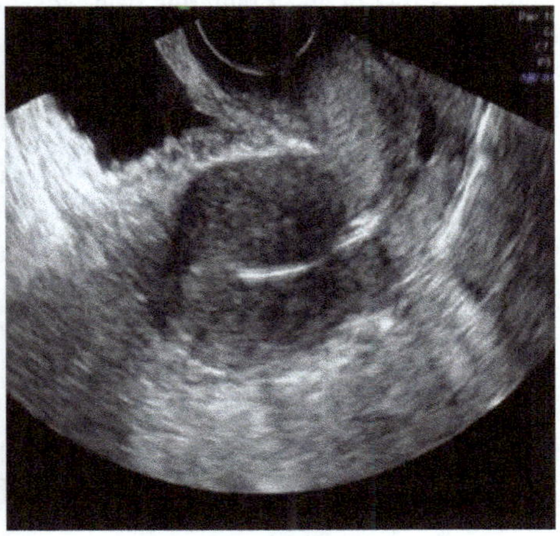

(b)

FIGURE 4: Hysteroscopic (a) and transabdominal ultrasound (b) findings for the intrauterine placement of the silicone plate.

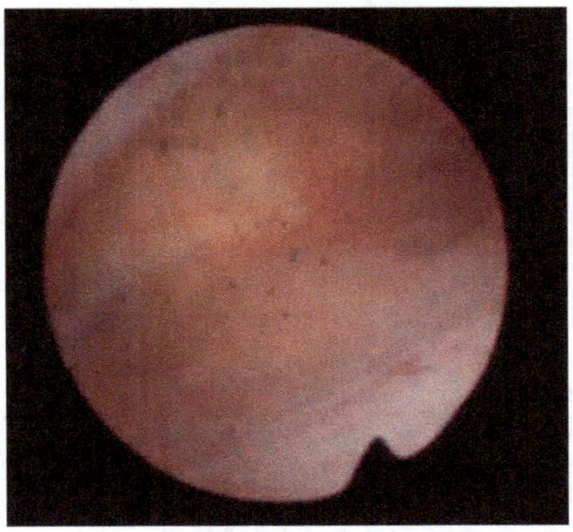

FIGURE 5: Hysteroscopic findings following silicone plate removal.

accreta were observed intraoperatively. The patient had a good postoperative course and was discharged on postoperative day 7.

The patient provided written informed consent before surgery. This study was conducted according to the principles stated in the 1964 Declaration of Helsinki, and all subsequent revisions, and was approved by the Institutional Review Board of our university (approval number: 941).

3. Discussion

Asherman syndrome, which refers to the presence of partial or complete adhesions in the uterine cavity, is caused by damage to the endometrium following endometrial curettage, endometritis, transcervical resection of uterine myoma, enucleatic myomectomy reaching the endometrium intraoperatively, or a cesarean section. Considering that such adhesions can be responsible for uterine amenorrhea, infertility, and recurrent miscarriages, women with this condition who wish to bear children require appropriate treatment. Although hysteroscopic adhesiolysis of the uterine cavity has been generally performed, postoperative re-adhesion rates have remained at 27.2–62.5% [2, 3].

An earlier report had addressed this issue by temporarily inserting a medical silicone plate into the uterus to prevent adhesions [4], indicating its utility. In the field of otorhinolaryngology, medical silicone plates are also being used *in vivo* to prevent adhesions during tympanoplasty. Although our institution had previously practiced the insertion of IUDs to prevent postoperative adhesions, re-adhesions were still observed in a subset of cases. Hysteroscopic findings indicated that re-adhesion occurred on the lateral margins or fundus of the uterus, which are not in contact with the IUD. Accordingly, an IUD may have too small an area to cover the entire uterine cavity, unlike a silicone plate.

Table 1 summarizes recent prospective randomized studies investigating the role of an IUD, Foley catheter, and uterine balloon in preventing postoperative re-adhesion. Some studies have suggested that several anti-adhesion therapies may offer a potential benefit for decreasing postoperative re-adhesion in women undergoing operative hysteroscopy.

However, no strategies have been strongly recommended to decrease the recurrence rate of intrauterine adhesions [9].

One study involving Foley catheter insertion in 25 patients achieved a pregnancy rate of 33.9%, as well as a menstrual resumption rate of 81%. However, due to uterine perforation in two cases [10], this technique's safety and efficacy remains uncertain. While no uterine perforation had been in the present case, the main concern with silicone plate placement is infection. Although silicone can be placed *in vivo*, leaving it in place for 1 month increases the patient's susceptibility to endometritis or pelvic peritonitis due to increased risk of infection. To address this issue, prophylactic antibiotic administration should be considered. In the present case, prophylactic antibiotics had been administered preoperatively and 1 day postoperatively. Unlike in previous reports, our patient did not receive long-term antibiotic administration. Nonetheless, no serious complications, including infection and uterine perforation, had been observed.

During pregnancy following treatment for Asherman syndrome, incidences of premature delivery, intrauterine growth retardation, and placenta accreta had been reported [11, 12]. A 2010 review by Deans et al. found that premature delivery

Table 1: Studies investigating the role of an intrauterine devicefoley catheter, and uterine balloon in preventing intrauterine adhesion formation after hysteroscopic surgery.

	Study design	Devices	Recurrence rate	*p*
Gan et al. (2017) [5]	Prospective randomized	Foley catheter + freeze-dried amnion graft	28% (11/40)	0.24
		Foley catheter only	40%(16/40)	
Wang et al. (2016) [6]	Prospective randomized	Amniotic scaffold balloon	21% (6/29)	0.25
		Foley catheter only	36% (10/28)	
Xiao et al. (2015) [7]	Prospective randomized	Auto-crosslinked hyaluronic acid gel + foley catheter	13% (7/55)	0.0006
		Foley catheter only	38% (21/56)	
Lin et al. (2015) [8]	Prospective randomized	Heart-shaped balloon	30% (25/82)	NS
		Intrauterine device	35% (28/80)	

occurred in nearly half of the 696 cases previously treated for adhesiolysis. Additionally, the authors reported 17 cases of placental malposition, such as placenta accreta and placenta previa, and two cases of uterine rupture [11]. Due to the risk for such serious complications, pregnancy and delivery must be managed carefully, and patients must have sufficient understanding of the aforementioned risks. For severe Asherman syndrome cases, pregnancy and delivery must be managed carefully, with detailed informed consent from the patients. The present case experienced a normal pregnancy except for a short period of vaginal bleeding wherein the patient was hospitalized due to a threatened miscarriage. Finally, a healthy infant was delivered with no intrauterine adhesions or placental malposition.

4. Conclusion

A silicon plate may be considered a useful tool for preventing re-adhesion following hysteroscopic adhesiolysis without serious complications.

Authors' Contributions

(i) Protocol/Project development: Maho Miyagi, Keiko Mekaru. (ii) Data collection: Sugiko Oishi, Chiaki Urasoe. (iii) Data analysis: Kozue Akamine, and Yoichi Aoki. (iv) Manuscript writing: Maho Miyagi, Keiko Mekaru.

References

[1] S. Friedler, E. J. Margalioth, I. Kafka, and H. Yaffe, "Incidence of post-abortion intrauterine adhesions evaluated by hysteroscopy-a prospective study," *Human Reproduction*, vol. 8, no. 3, pp. 442–444, 1993.

[2] D. Yu, Y. M. Wong, Y. Cheong, E. Xia, and T. C. Li, "Asherman syndrome-one century later," *Fertility and Sterility*, vol. 89, no. 4, pp. 759–779, 2008.

[3] M. M. Hanstede, E. Van Der Meij, L. Goedemans, and M. H. Emanuel, "Results of centralized asherman surgery, 2003–2013," *Fertility and Sterility*, vol. 104, no. 6, pp. 1561–1568, 2015.

[4] H. Henmi, A. Azumaguchi, M. Saito, T. Kita, T. Akashi, and K. Nagasawa, "A method preventing intrauterine adhesion after hysteroscopic surgery," *Journal of Fertilization Implantation*, vol. 27, no. 1, pp. 268–271, 2010.

[5] L. Gan, H. Duan, F. Q. Sun, Q. Xu, Y. Q. Tang, and S. Wang, "Efficacy of freeze-dried amnion graft following hysteroscopic adhesiolysis of severe intrauterine adhesions," *International Journal of Gynaecology & Obstetrics*, vol. 137, no. 2, pp. 116–122, 2017.

[6] X. Wang and H. Duan, "Clinical evaluation of amniontic products after transcervical resection of intensive degree of intrauterine adhesions," *Chinese Journal of Obstetrics and Gynecology*, vol. 51, no. 1, pp. 27–30, 2016.

[7] S. Xiao, Y. Wan, F. Zou et al., "Prevention of intrauterine adhesion with auto-crosslinked hyaluronic acid gel: a prospective, randomized, controlled clinical study," *Chinese Journal of Obstetrics and Gynecology*, vol. 50, no. 1, pp. 32–36, 2015.

[8] X. N. Lin, F. Zhou, M. L. Wei et al., "Randomized, controlled trial comparing the efficacy of intrauterine balloon and intrauterine contraceptive device in the prevention of adhesion reformation after hysteroscopic adhesiolysis," *Fertility and Sterility*, vol. 104, no. 1, pp. 2352–2340, 2015.

[9] J. Bosteels, S. Weyers, T. M. D'Hooghe et al., "Anti-adhesion therapy following operative hysteroscopy for treatment of female subfertility," *Cochrane Database of Systematic Reviews*, vol. 27, no. 11, 2017.

[10] M. I. Amer and K. H. Abd-El-Maeboud, "Amnion graft following hysteroscopic lysis of intrauterine adhesions," *Journal of Obstetrics Gynaecology Research*, vol. 32, no. 6, pp. 559–566, 2006.

[11] R. Deans and J. Abbott, "Review of intrauterine adhesions," *Journal of Minimally Invasive Gynecology*, vol. 17, no. 5, pp. 555–569, 2010.

[12] L. Engelbrechtsen, J. Langhoff-Roos, J. J. Kjer, and O. Istre, "Placenta accreta: adherent placenta due to asherman syndrome," *Clinical Case Reports*, vol. 3, no. 3, pp. 175–178, 2015.

31

A Case of Bilateral Anesthesia Mumps after Cesarean Section under Spinal Anesthesia: A Rare Case and Literature Review

Narges Montazeri,[1] Mohammad Hassan Darabi,[1] Kamran Hessami,[2] Ramin Shekouhi,[3] Maryam Sohooli,[3] Tahereh Shamsi,[4] Fateme Bagheri,[4] and Mohammad Amin Shahrbaf[5]

[1]*Maternal-Fetal Medicine Research Center, Shiraz University of Medical Sciences, Shiraz, Iran*
[2]*Department of Obstetrics and Gynecology, Baylor College of Medicine, Houston, TX, USA*
[3]*Colorectal Research Center, Department of Surgery, Shiraz University of Medical Sciences, Shiraz, Iran*
[4]*School of Medicine, Shiraz University of Medical Sciences, Shiraz, Iran*
[5]*Faculty of Medicine, Shahid Beheshti University of Medical Sciences, Tehran, Iran*

Correspondence should be addressed to Tahereh Shamsi; t_shamsi@sums.ac.ir

Academic Editor: Daniel Martin

A 30-year-old pregnant female presented to the emergency department with labor pain in her 39th week of pregnancy. Cesarean section under spinal anesthesia was the chosen route of delivery for this patient due to previous cesarean section in her first pregnancy. The delivery itself was uneventful but seven hours after the surgery, bilateral swelling of parotid glands were noted. Rehydration therapy and a single dose of hydrocortisone (100 mg IV route) were administered, and swellings were completely resolved on postoperative day 2. This is one of the rare cases of anesthesia mumps after spinal anesthesia, and we think rehydration therapy and the single dose corticosteroid may prove useful in these cases.

1. Introduction

Acute temporary swelling of the salivary glands, especially parotid glands, termed as “anesthesia mumps” usually occurs during or after surgery and is one of the rare complications of general anesthesia. [1] While majority of reported cases are surgery related, it should be noted that this disease is not exclusive to operation and recovery rooms as it may arise from bedridden Intensive Care Unit patients, too [2]. It often presents as a painless unilateral parotid enlargement that subsides within few days without further sequelae [3]. Scarcely, respiratory distress occurs which requires immediate intervention aiming at securing airway. [4, 5]

In this study, we report a rare case of bilateral postoperative sialadenitis in a young female who underwent caesarian section (C/S) after the spinal anesthesia. To the best of our knowledge, this is one of the few cases of anesthesia mumps occurring after spinal anesthesia. Another unique aspect of this case is the fact that symptoms resolved rather quickly, with the left side enlargement disappearing in ten hours and the right side resolving in less than 24 hours.

2. Case Presentation

2.1. Present Illness. A 30-year-old female, Gravid 2 Para 1 Live 1, was scheduled for cesarean section (C/S) at gestational age of 39 weeks and 5 days due to a history of previous cesarean section. The patient was a known case of epilepsy which was controlled by Lamotrigine during pregnancy. Her prior obstetrical history included a C/S for delivery of a term newborn due to severe preeclampsia, while the current pregnancy had been uncomplicated. Pelvic examination revealed a 2 centimeters cervical dilation as the fetus presentation was vertex with a longitudinal lie. Membranes were intact, and there were no signs of leakage. All other physical examination findings and routine laboratory tests were found to be normal. The ultrasound studies of the current gestation were normal throughout pregnancy.

2.2. Operative Data. After consulting with neurology service 1600 mg of sodium valproate was administered for the patient before performing routine anesthesia monitoring and supportive O_2 therapy. Induction of spinal anesthesia was performed by injection of 8 milliliters of Marcaine 0.5% and 10 micrograms of fentanyl, through a 12.5 cm, 27-gauge spinal needle in sitting position at the lumbar level of L_3-L_4 interspace. After confirmation of the anesthesia, C/S was performed by a Pfannenstiel incision. The surgical procedure was uneventful, and five minutes after the incision, a healthy male newborn with 2750 grams of weight and 1- and 5-minute Apgar score of 10 was born. After delivery, 4 mg of intravenous (IV) ondansetron was administrated for its antiemetic effect.

2.3. Follow-Up. The vital signs of patient were normal after the operation, and recovery was uneventful. The patient was transferred to obstetric ward and got out of bed three hours after the surgery. Seven hours after operation, the patient complained from "bilateral facial swelling" (Figure 1).

Physical examination showed bilateral enlargement of parotid regions expanding down to the mandibular angle (Figure 2). There was no pain, redness, or any other sign and symptoms of inflammation. Vital signs including respiratory rate were well within normal values and patient did not complain from dyspnea. Intraoral examination showed patency of Steensen's duct, and no purulent discharge could be seen or elicited by massaging parotid glands. Routine laboratory data including Complete Blood Count were normal with a leucocyte count of 8400/microliter (Table 1). After consultation with Ear Nose Throat (ENT) service, a diagnosis of acute postoperative sialadenitis or anesthesia mumps was established. The patient was hydrated by 1000 cc of normal saline and received one dose of 100 mg IV hydrocortisone afterwards with no antibiotic therapy. The patient was observed every 2 hours, and there was no development of purulent discharge and the left sided swelling healed completely by 10 hours and in postoperative day (POD) 2 the right sided swelling also diminished, although a rise in leucocyte count was observed. On POD 3, patient's general condition, respiration, and the ability to swallow were all normal and she was discharged without any complications.

POD 1: postoperative day 1; POD 2: postoperative day 2.

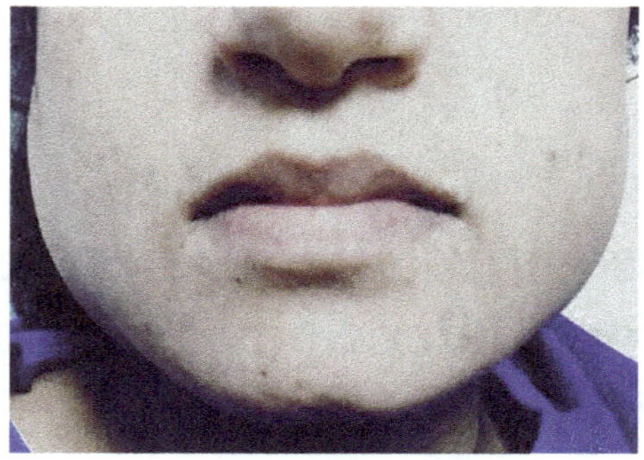

FIGURE 1: Front face view of the patient at 7 hours after surgery.

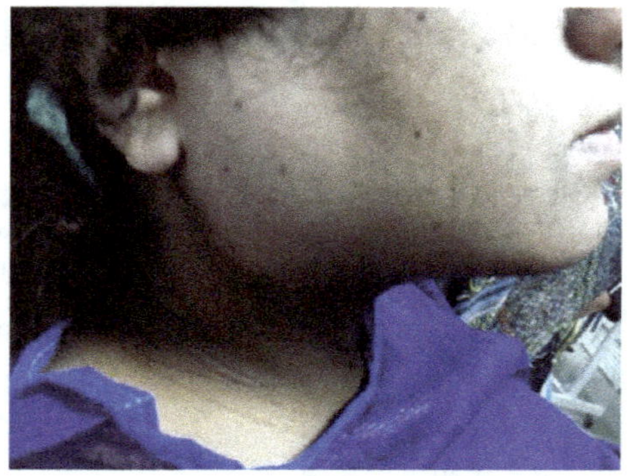

FIGURE 2: Lateral face view of the patient at 7 hours after surgery.

TABLE 1: Laboratory findings of the patient.

Variable	POD 1	POD 2
White cell count (per μL)	8400	11900
Lymphocyte count (%)	21.90	20
Neutrophil count (%)	71.8	73
Platelet count (per μL)	230000	180000
Hemoglobin (gr/dL)	10.7	9.3
Red blood cell count $\times 10^6$ (per μL)	4.93	4
Hematocrit (%)	35.2	27.4
Mean cell volume (FL)	71.4	68.5
Mean corpuscular hemoglobin (Pg)	21.7	23.25
Mean corpuscular hemoglobin concentration (gr/dL)	30.4	33.94
Prothrombin time, control (sec)	12.5	
Prothrombin time, patient (sec)	11.9	
International normalized ratio	1	
Partial thromboplastin time, control (sec)	33	
Partial thromboplastin time, patient (sec)	32	
Blood sugar (mg/dL)	82	
Blood urea nitrogen (mg/dL)	6	
Creatinine (mg/dL)	0.7	
Sodium (mMOL/L)	137	
Potassium (mMOL/L)	3.6	
Blood group & rhesus	A+ positive	

3. Discussion and Literature Review

Acute postoperative sialadenitis was first described by Munde in 1878 after an oophorectomy surgery [6]. It is a noninfectious process with an unknown etiology. However, some etiologies have been proposed throughout the years as more reports surfaced about this benign self-limiting

TABLE 2: Published cases of anesthesia mumps following spinal anesthesia in the English literature.

Case	Year	Age	Sex	Symptoms	Surgical procedure	Type of anesthesia	Anesthetic medication	Respiratory distress	Treatment	Complications
1 (11)	2009	89	F	Bilateral painless submandibular gland enlargement	Right partial hip arthroplasty	Combined spinal–epidural anesthesia	15 mg of 0.5% heavy bupivacaine	No	Supportive	Full recovery (5 days)
2 (10)	2013	37	F	Painless bilateral parotid swelling	Breast surgery and abdominoplasty	Thoracic block between T2 and T3 intervertebral spaces, and lumbar epidural block between L1 and L2	13 mL of 0.5% bupivacaine and 50 lg of fentanyl	No	Supportive (IV fluid hydration)	Full recovery (12 hours)
3 (10)	2013	45	F	Painless bilateral parotid swelling	Subglandular breast implantation, and body contouring(liposuction)	Thoracic block between T4 and T5 intervertebral spaces, and lumbar epidural block between L1 and L2	10 mL of 0.5% Marcaine and 100 lg of fentanyl	No	Supportive (IV fluid hydration)	Full recovery (36 hours)
4 (10)	2013	30	F	Painless bilateral parotid swelling	Subglandular breast implantation, and liposuction	Thoracic block between T5 and T6 intervertebral spaces, and lumbar epidural block between L1 and L2	10 mL of 1% lidocaine and 100 lg of fentanyl	No	Dexamethasone injection, and IV fluid hydration	Full recovery (48 hours)
5 (12)	2017	38	F	Mild respiratory distress, and bilateral enlarged parotid gland	Elective cesarean section	Spinal anesthesia	Not mentioned	Yes	Antihistamines, and anti-inflammatory agents, supportive therapy	Full recovery (10 hours)
6 (13)	2021	31	F	Painless swelling in both parotid glands	Elective cesarean section	Spinal anesthesia between L3-L4 intervertebral spaces	12 mg bupivacaine, 100 mcg morphine, and 10 mcg fentanyl	No	Intravenous injection of 45.5 mg pheniramine maleate, 20 mg tenoxicam, IV fluid hydration	Full recovery (9 hours)
7[our case]	2021	30	F	Painless bilateral parotid swelling	Elective cesarean section	Spinal anesthesia between L3-L4 intervertebral spaces	8 mL of Marcaine 0.5%, and 10 micrograms of fentanyl	No	Intravenous injection of 100 mg IV hydrocortisone, IV fluid hydration	Full recovery (24 hours)

enlargement of parotid glands. These included factors such as dehydration, hyperflexion of neck during surgery, Stensen duct obstruction, prolonged general anesthesia, venous congestion of head and neck, overreactive parasympathetic tone, and adverse drug reactions like succinylcholine-induced profuse saliva production [1, 4, 7, 8]. Anesthesia mumps clearly have a tendency to present as a unilateral swelling after general anesthesia [1]. This can be explained by the potentially significant role of patient positioning in prolonged surgeries under general anesthesia, as these cases usually develop a unilateral enlargement possibly due to an obstruction of Stensen duct. This was the case in a 3-year-old patient reported by Mutaf and Büyükgüral [9]

Our case developed anesthesia mumps after spinal anesthesia. All of the previous cases of spinal anesthesia were females that developed bilateral swellings just like our case did. [10–13] Our patient had no obvious predisposing factor and review of medications proved fruitless, but we can assume that dehydration has played a role in the development of anesthesia mumps [13] since pregnant women with labor pain tend to forget sufficient water intake. For a comparison between our case and previous cases of anesthesia mumps after spinal anesthesia refer to Table 2.

Postoperative sialadenitis is generally considered a self-limited benign disease that will be healed within hours to days in the affected individuals [9]. However, some therapies including rehydration and administrating anti-inflammatory medications such as nonsteroidal anti-inflammatory drugs (NSAIDs) or corticosteroids can be helpful for the treatment of this complication [14]. Our patient was hydrated and received a single dose of hydrocortisone, and the results were more promising than what we originally thought, as the patient healed completely in less than 24 hours. We can assume rehydration therapy as a proper first step in management of this disorder. Nevertheless, the definite therapy for anesthesia mumps remains to be found. Protective measures including hydration before surgery, optimal positioning of the patient in operation room, and choosing the best method of anesthesia can be effective for preventing this complication.

All in all, acute unilateral or bilateral swelling of the parotid gland after anesthesia, particularly of spinal type, is a very rare occurrence. Physicians should be familiar with the transient and benign nature of this anesthesia-related complication which can present itself even after local anesthesia. They should be also prepared for very rare urgent cases that require immediate intervention for securing the airway. According to our case and the review of literature, we can conclude that rehydration therapy with crystalloids such as normal saline is the best first step in management of this disease, although more studies on this matter are required.

Consent

Written informed consent was obtained from the patient.

References

[1] E. C. E. Cem and P. Uzgur, "Case report: postoperative parotitis and review of the literature," *Journal of Emergency Medicine Case Reports*, vol. 11, no. 3, pp. 88-89, 2020.

[2] T. Ghatak, M. Gurjar, S. Samanta, and A. Baronia, "A case of "anesthesia mumps" from ICU," *Saudi Journal of Anaesthesia*, vol. 7, no. 2, pp. 222-223, 2013.

[3] İ. Katı, Z. Kurdoğlu, U. Göktaş, O. Ç. Aytekin, and S. Avcu, "Anesthesia mumps after the cesarean section in pregnant woman," *European Journal of General Medicine*, vol. 8, no. 4, pp. 342–344, 2011.

[4] T. Hamaguchi, N. Suzuki, and I. Kondo, "A case of anesthesia mumps that required postoperative re-intubation," *JA Clinical Reports*, vol. 4, no. 1, pp. 1–4, 2018.

[5] F. Cavaliere, G. Conti, M. G. Annetta, A. Greco, A. Cina, and R. Proietti, "Massive facial edema and airway obstruction secondary to acute postoperative sialadenitis or" anesthesia mumps": a case report," *Journal of Medical Case Reports*, vol. 3, no. 1, pp. 1–4, 2009.

[6] A. W. Schwartz, K. D. Devine, and O. H. Beahrs, "Acute postoperative parotitis ("surgical mumps")," *Plastic and Reconstructive Surgery*, vol. 25, no. 1, pp. 51–58, 1960.

[7] K. I. Avgerinos, N. Degermetzoglou, S. Theofanidou, G. Kritikou, and I. Bountouris, "Acute parotitis after lower limb amputation: a case report of a rare complication," *Case Reports in Otolaryngology*, vol. 2018, Article ID 3714214, 2018.

[8] D. Jain, I. Bala, and D. Dwivedi, "Anaesthesia mumps in a child: a rare entity," *Indian Journal of Anesthesia*, vol. 58, no. 4, pp. 500-501, 2014.

[9] M. Mutaf and B. Büyükgüral, "An unusual postoperative complication: anesthesia mumps," *European Journal of Plastic Surgery*, vol. 29, no. 7, pp. 335–338, 2007.

[10] M. J. F. Rosique, R. G. Rosique, I. R. Costa, B. R. Lara, J. L. F. Figueiredo, and D. G. B. Ribeiro, "Parotitis after epidural anesthesia in plastic surgery: report of three cases," *Aesthetic Plastic Surgery*, vol. 37, no. 4, pp. 838–842, 2013.

[11] A. Pirat, A. Camkiran, S. Balci, P. Zeyneloglu, and Z. Kayhan, "Bilateral submandibular salivary gland swelling following regional anesthesia for hip replacement," *Acta Anaesthesiologica Scandinavica*, vol. 53, no. 2, p. 272, 2009.

[12] C. Moisei, R. M. Sima, and L. Pleş, "Acute parotiditis after cesarean section; case report," *Journal of Clinical and Investigative Surgery*, vol. 2, no. 2, pp. 110–113, 2017.

[13] B. Günaydın, S. Bağcaz, G. İnan, E. Tekin, and D. Karcaaltıncaba, "Postoperative acute parotitis after cesarean delivery under spinal anaesthesia," *Turkish Journal of Anaesthesiology and Reanimation*, vol. 49, no. 2, pp. 159–162, 2021.

[14] A. Asghar, K. Karam, and S. Rashid, "A case of anesthesia mumps after sacral laminectomy under general anesthesia," *Saudi Journal of Anaesthesia*, vol. 9, no. 3, pp. 332-333, 2015.

32

Rudimentary Horn Pregnancy Diagnosed after Laparotomy

Kurabachew Mengistu,[1] Tufa Bobe,[2] Gashaw Tilahun,[2] Kibru Kifle,[3] and Dereje Geleta[4]

[1]*Department of Anesthesiology, College of Medicine and Health Sciences, Hawassa University, Hawassa, Ethiopia*
[2]*Department of Obstetrics and Gynaecology, College of Medicine and Health Sciences, Madda Wallabu University, Robe, Ethiopia*
[3]*Department of Obstetrics and Gynaecology, College of Medicine and Health Sciences, Hawassa University, Hawassa, Ethiopia*
[4]*School of Public and Environmental Health, College of Medicine and Health Sciences, Hawassa University, Hawassa, Ethiopia*

Correspondence should be addressed to Kurabachew Mengistu; kurabachewmengistu@rocketmail.com

Academic Editor: Edi Vaisbuch

Müllerian abnormalities are present in 0.17% of fertile women and 3.5% of infertile women, and a unicornuate uterus is observed in 0.4% of women. The uterus is normally formed during embryogenesis by the fusion of the two Müllerian ducts. If one of the ducts does not develop, only one Müllerian duct contributes to the uterine development. We report a case of Gravida II, abortion I referred from a primary hospital with a referral paper and sonography stating she had IUFD. She had regular antenatal care follow-up at the primary hospital and had 8 months of amenorrhea. Our ultrasound assessment confirmed the intrauterine fetal demise, but the rudimentary horn pregnancy was missed. Repeated attempts at the induction of labor were tried but unsuccessful. The diagnosis was confirmed at laparotomy. She underwent cesarean section with right intact rudimentary horn removal. A nonviable male fetus with birth weight of 1.2 kg was delivered. Women with this abnormality are asymptomatic and unaware of having a unicornuate uterus. Abdominal pain is the most common presenting symptom with the rudimentary horn, but communicating horn pregnancy is generally asymptomatic in early pregnancy. Early awareness of this rare clinical condition is so crucial especially in developing countries where the availability of new technologies is scarce to explore uterine abnormalities. The patient had uneventful postoperative recovery and was discharged after 3 postoperative days.

1. Introduction

Congenital malformations of the female genital tract are defined as deviations from normal anatomy resulting from embryological maldevelopment of the Müllerian or paramesonephric ducts. They represent a rather common benign condition with a prevalence of 4–7% [1].

The incidence of pregnancy occurring in a rudimentary horn of the unicornuate uterus is very rare ranging from 1 in 75,000 to 150,000 pregnancies [2].

As most of the rudimentary horns are asymptomatic, only 8% of rudimentary horn pregnancies are diagnosed before the symptoms appear [3].

Expert ultrasonography can reveal some Müllerian anomalies, but confirmation requires magnetic resonance imaging [4].

Cases with rudimentary horn pregnancy usually result in the rupture of the horn in the second or third trimester, typically between the 10th and 20th week of gestation, although a rupture has been reported at 34 weeks [5].

This is a case demonstrating a communicating rudimentary horn connected to a unicornuate uterus, where the diagnosis was revealed after surgery.

2. Case Presentation

A 22-year-old Gravida II, abortion I came to our institution on referral from a primary hospital with a referral paper and sonography showing that she had IUFD. She had a spontaneous abortion for which dilation and curettage (D&C) was performed at the primary hospital 16 months back. She had no remarkable medical and surgical histories. She had regular antenatal care follow-up at the primary hospital and had 8 months of amenorrhea.

Upon admission, the patient was clinically asymptomatic and stable, showing no uterine contractions and no cervical

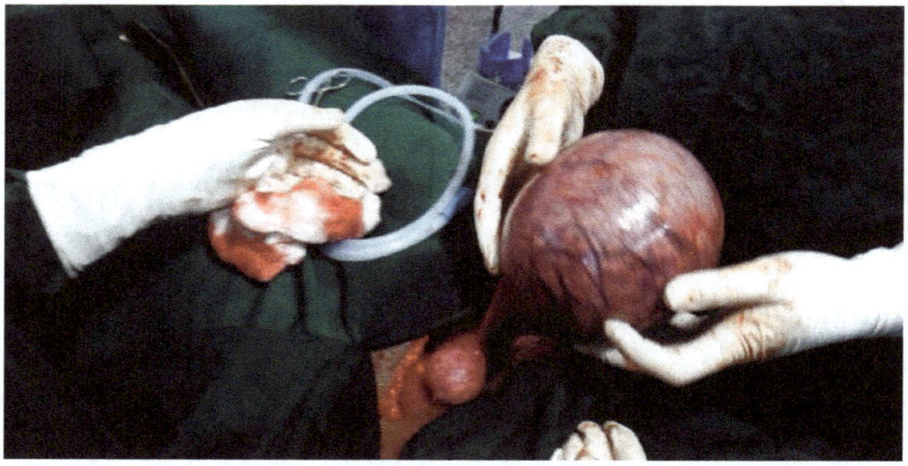

Figure 1: Intraoperative finding of intact rudimentary horn pregnancy.

dilatation. On abdominal examination, the uterus was enlarged equivalent in size to 30 weeks of pregnancy.

On examination, her BP was 120/75 mm of Hg, pulse 85/minute, temperature 36.5°C, and respiratory rate 22/minute. FHS was absent

Obstetric ultrasonography revealed a singleton, intrauterine fetal demise with a gestational age of 32 weeks, estimated fetal weight of 1.3 kg, and negative fetal heartbeat. The placenta was fundal and anteriorly. The cervix was closed, uneffaced, and posterior. All laboratory investigations were normal.

Initially, she was administered 50 mcg of vaginal misoprostol at 6-hour intervals, without response after the 6th dose. Then, she was given an infusion of normal saline 0.9% with 5 IU of oxytocin, followed by increasing concentrations of the same infusion. Just then, there was no cervical dilation, despite the onset of contractions.

Cervical effacement with no dilatation was seen. Finally, a Foley catheter was used. All attempts were unsuccessful. The patient was counselled and underwent a cesarean section horizontally under spinal anaesthesia.

The intraoperative finding was intact rudimentary horn pregnancy. Clamps were applied over the fibrous band on the medial side and the fallopian tube and ovarian and round ligaments on the lateral side; the accessory horn was excised with the dead fetus; and right salpingo-oophorectomy was performed (Figures 1 and 2).

On releasing the forceps applied to the fibrous band and probing, a canal was detected between the rudimentary horn and the uterine cavity at the level of the isthmus. The round ligament, ovarian ligament, and tube were connected to the right cornua of the uterus.

The patient was advised to follow up. The patient had uneventful postoperative recovery and was discharged after 3 postoperative days.

3. Discussion

A unicornuate uterus with a rudimentary horn is a congenital uterine anomaly which results from the developmental arrest of the two Müllerian ducts with the simultaneous incomplete fusion of the opposite side [6].

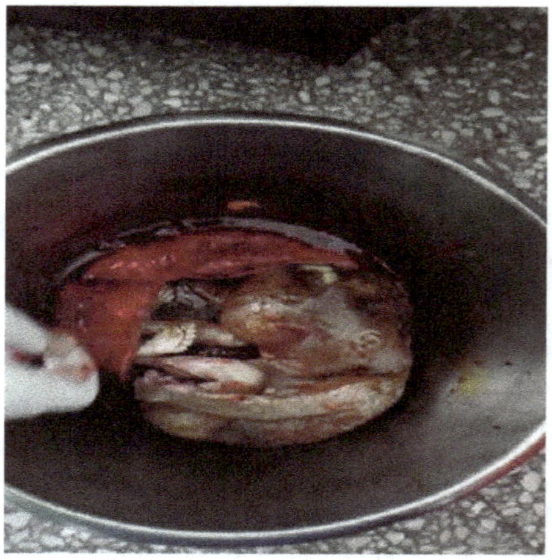

Figure 2: Excised rudimentary horn with the dead fetus.

The unicornuate uterus with rudimentary horn may have a cavity that is either in communication with (type A1a) or sealed off from (type A1b) the primary uterine cavity, or it may have failed to canalize entirely and is without a cavity (type A2, [7]).

When a rudimentary horn is present, it is the noncavitary type in 33% of cases, the cavitary but noncommunicating type in 22% of cases, and the cavitary and communicating type in 10% of cases [8].

Most cases of rudimentary horn pregnancy (RHP) provide a diagnostic challenge and are diagnosed after rupture, which leads to emergency surgery, blood transfusions, and increased morbidity [8].

Diagnosis is challenging in this malformation due to a limited field of sonographic view compared to other diagnostic imaging modalities and lateral deviation of the rudimentary horn [9].

Sonographic sensitivity is only 26%, and as the pregnancy advances, the specificity goes down [10].

The common misdiagnosis on ultrasound includes a bicornuate uterus with pregnancy in one horn, uterus didelphys, abdominal pregnancy, or even normal intrauterine pregnancy with an adnexal mass undergoing torsion [11].

It is shown that 62% of the rudimentary horn is preferentially placed on the right, which was revealed in our case report because the left Müller's canal progresses more caudally than the right [9].

Our patient had no renal abnormalities despite approximately 38% of patients having coexisting renal abnormalities. Unilateral renal agenesis is most commonly found; this is always ipsilateral with the rudimentary horn [12].

The literature presently supports prompt excision of the horn, pregnancy, and ipsilateral once a rudimentary horn pregnancy has been diagnosed [13].

4. Conclusion

Early awareness of this rare clinical condition is so crucial especially in developing countries where the availability of new technologies is scarce to explore uterine abnormalities. A high index of suspicion should be made if there is no response to repeated failed attempts at the induction of labor.

References

[1] G. F. Grimbizis, S. Gordts, A. di Spiezio Sardo et al., "The ESHRE/ESGE consensus on the classification of female genital tract congenital anomalies," *Human Reproduction*, vol. 28, no. 8, pp. 2032–2044, 2013.

[2] M. G. Tesemma, "Pregnancy in noncommunicating rudimentary horn of unicornuate uterus: a case report and review of the literature," *Case Reports in Obstetrics and Gynecology*, vol. 2019, Article ID 1489751, 3 pages, 2019.

[3] V. Malhotra, M. Chauhan, S. Nanda, N. Attri, and S. Mann, "Suspect rudimentary horn pregnancy in failed induction," *Journal of Gynecologic Surgery*, vol. 31, no. 2, pp. 95–97, 2015.

[4] F. Y. Fouelifack, J. T. Fouogue, J. O. Messi, D. T. Kamga, J. H. Fouedjio, and Z. Sando, "Spontaneous second-trimester ruptured pregnancy of rudimentary horn: a case report in Yaounde, Cameroon," *Pan African Medical Journal*, vol. 18, pp. 2–4, 2014.

[5] Q. Ambusaidi and C. Jha, "Pregnancy in the rudimentary uterine horn case report of an unusual presentation," *Sultan Qaboos University Medical Journal*, vol. 14, no. 1, pp. 134–138, 2014.

[6] M. Lallar, R. Nandal, and D. Sharma, "Unruptured rudimentary horn pregnancy presenting with acute haemoperitoneum with combined intrauterine pregnancy: a case report," *Iranian Journal of Reproductive Medicine*, vol. 13, no. 1, pp. 49–52, 2015.

[7] D. Reichman, M. R. Laufer, and B. K. Robinson, "Pregnancy outcomes in unicornuate uteri: a review," *Fertility and Sterility*, vol. 91, no. 5, pp. 1886–1894, 2009.

[8] X. Li, P. Peng, X. Liu et al., "The pregnancy outcomes of patients with rudimentary uterine horn: a 30-year experience," *PLoS One*, vol. 14, no. 1, article e0210788, 2019.

[9] M. Bruand, T. Thubert, N. Winer, P. Gueudry, and V. Dochez, "Rupture of non-communicating rudimentary horn of uterus at 12 weeks' gestation," *Cureus*, vol. 12, no. 3, 2020.

[10] S. Goyal, A. Mahajan, and S. Goyal, "Rudimentary horn of uterus : a diagnostic challenge in pregnancy," *International Journal of Biomedical and Advance Research*, vol. 8, no. 9, pp. 366–368, 2017.

[11] S. Siwatch, R. Mehra, D. K. Pandher, and A. Huria, "Rudimentary horn pregnancy: a 10-year experience and review of literature," *Archives of Gynecology and Obstetrics*, vol. 287, no. 4, pp. 687–695, 2013.

[12] G. Angu, A. Pradhan, and S. Kamble, "A case of pregnancy in the rudimentary horn of unicornuate uterus," *International Journal of Reproduction, Contraception, Obstetrics and Gynecology*, vol. 5, no. 10, article 3646, 2016.

[13] L. E. Fitzmaurice, R. M. Ehsanipoor, and M. Porto, "Rudimentary horn pregnancy with herniation into the main uterine cavity," *American Journal of Obstetrics and Gynecology*, vol. 202, no. 3, pp. e5–e6, 2010.

Streptococcus constellatus Peritonitis and Subsequent Septic Shock following Intrauterine Device Removal

Joan Tymon-Rosario,[1] Jessica M. Atrio,[1,2] Hyun Ah Yoon,[3] David Erlichman,[4] and Veronica Lerner[1,5]

[1]*Department of Obstetrics & Gynecology and Women's Health, Albert Einstein College of Medicine, Montefiore Medical Center, Bronx, NY, USA*
[2]*Division of Family Planning, Department of Obstetrics & Gynecology and Women's Health, Bronx, NY, USA*
[3]*Department of Pathology, Albert Einstein College of Medicine, Montefiore Medical Center, Bronx, NY, USA*
[4]*Department of Radiology, Albert Einstein College of Medicine, Montefiore Medical Center, Bronx, NY, USA*
[5]*Division of Minimally Invasive Surgery, Department of Obstetrics & Gynecology and Women's Health, Bronx, NY, USA*

Correspondence should be addressed to Joan Tymon-Rosario; jtr2577@gmail.com

Academic Editor: Giovanni Monni

Background. Previous reports have described cases of abscess formation by *Streptococcus constellatus* involving the oral cavity, gastrointestinal tract, and septic thrombophlebitis of the right ovarian vein with subsequent bacteremia and septic shock. Ascending infection from the genital tract to the fallopian tubes resulting in peritonitis from *Streptococcus constellatus* is a rare clinical circumstance where there is minimal information in the literature to guide its diagnosis, management, and expected prognosis. *Case.* A 36-year-old G3P0111 developed a tubo-ovarian abscess two weeks after intrauterine device (IUD) removal and then rapidly decompensated with septic shock from peritonitis due to *Streptococcus constellatus* infection. The patient was also newly diagnosed with diabetes and in diabetic ketoacidosis (DKA) on presentation. She received broad-spectrum antibiotic coverage and required two exploratory surgical procedures to obtain source control. Two Interventional Radiology- (IR-) guided drainage procedures were subsequently performed to drain remaining fluid collections. Her recovery involved a prolonged ICU stay. On hospital day seventy-three, after receiving approximately 8 weeks of antibiotics and the above noted procedures the patient was discharged to a subacute rehabilitation facility. *Conclusion. Streptococcus constellatus* is a highly pathogenic organism once a systemic septic infection has become established that can cause an ascending genital tract infection resulting in tubo-ovarian abscess formation, peritonitis, and septic shock.

1. Introduction

Pelvic inflammatory disease (PID) comprises a spectrum of inflammatory disorders of the upper female genital tract as well as the surrounding organs. This includes any combination of endometritis, salpingitis, oophoritis, peritonitis, perihepatitis, and/or tubo-ovarian abscess [1]. Recent studies have demonstrated that the proportion of PID cases that are attributable to *Neisseria gonorrhoeae or Chlamydia trachomatis* are declining, as <50% of women who are diagnosed with PID are found to be positive for either of these organisms [1–4]. The various microorganisms that comprise the vaginal flora such as the anaerobes, enteric Gram-negative rods, *Gardnerella vaginalis, Haemophilus influenza, Mycoplasma hominis, Ureaplasma urealyticum, Mycoplasma genitalium,* and *Streptococcus agalactiae* have been associated with PID [5, 6].

Streptococcus constellatus collectively with *Streptococcus anginosus* and *Streptococcus intermedius* constitute the *Streptococcus anginosus* (formerly *Streptococcus milleri*) group [7]. *Streptococcus constellatus* is a commensal organism of the human oral cavity, urogenital region, and intestinal tract.

The distinguishing feature of this organism is its ability to form abscesses. In rare cases these abscesses can spread hematogenously and result in bacteremia with metastatic abscesses in other organs, subsequent septic emboli, septic thrombophlebitis, and septic shock as a rare complication. Previous reports in the literature have described such cases of abscess formation involving the oral cavity, upper gastrointestinal tract, and even septic thrombophlebitis of the right ovarian vein that have resulted in bacteremia and septic shock [7, 8].

Ascending infection from the genital tract to the fallopian tubes resulting in peritonitis in previously healthy women after intrauterine device (IUD) placement has been described in the literature; however, there is general consensus that this incidence is very low with PID occurring in 0.1-0.5 percent of patients after IUD placement [9, 10]. The causative pathogenic species that have been associated with serious infections with IUD use include *Staphylococcus, Streptococcus,* and *Actinomyces* species [9, 11–17]. We report a unique clinical circumstance in which *Streptococcus constellatus* caused an aggressive ascending genital infection with an unusual clinical course after IUD removal.

2. Case Description/Summary

A 36-year-old G3P0111 with a past medical history significant for seizure disorder and morbid obesity (Body Mass Index 33 kg/m^2) presented with a chief complaint of progressively worsening abdominopelvic pain, nausea, and vomiting for one day. Two weeks prior she presented to an outside facility for right-sided abdominopelvic pain and dyspareunia at which time her intrauterine device was found to be malpositioned with the IUD was low lying and predominantly in the cervix but otherwise there was no evidence of pelvic pathology on transvaginal ultrasound imaging. She subsequently had the intrauterine device removed by an outside gynecologist prior to her presentation to our facility. On presentation to the emergency room, she was found to be tachycardic but normotensive and afebrile. Her laboratory values were significant for white blood cell count of 18.4-cells/mm^3 and a glucose level of 443 mg/dL. Computed tomography (CT) scan of the abdomen and pelvis demonstrated a right-sided tubo-ovarian abscess that was 8 cm in diameter with foci of internal air and extensive surrounding inflammatory changes (Figure 1).

The patient had not received primary care for a prolonged period of time. She was subsequently found to be in diabetic ketoacidosis with newly diagnosed type 2 diabetes mellitus and a hemoglobin A1c level of 14% requiring aggressive intravenous fluid hydration and insulin. She also had a low grade temperature so one set of blood cultures were obtained and she was initiated on empiric antibiotics with intravenous gentamicin and clindamycin pending complete work-up. Interventional radiology (IR) was consulted for possible drainage of the tubo-ovarian abscess but the location of the abscess was not amenable for a safe percutaneous approach secondary to bowel loops and major arteries being in close proximity to the abscess. While she initially had mild improvement of her abdominal pain with downtrending fever curve and leukocytosis, her clinical course was complicated by oliguria and acute renal insufficiency which was thought to be due to administration of gentamicin in the setting of intravascular volume depletion. In light of the patient's deteriorating renal function and reported IgE-mediated allergy to penicillin, the antibiotic regimen was changed to oral levofloxacin and metronidazole.

On hospital day three, the patient was noted to be somnolent with decreased mentation and labored breathing. Her capillary blood glucose level was 74 mg/dL and she had fevers up to 102.9°F with the initial blood culture detecting growth of *Streptococcus constellatus*. Critical care medicine and infectious diseases consultations were obtained for impending septic shock and the antimicrobial regimen was empirically broadened to vancomycin, meropenem, and micafungin. She subsequently underwent endotracheal intubation for airway protection and was initiated on vasopressor support and transferred to the intensive care unit (ICU). Consent for surgical source control was obtained from the health care proxy, who endorsed that the patient desires to preserve her fertility.

On hospital day four, the patient underwent laparoscopic lysis of adhesions, drainage, and debridement of a presumed right tubo-ovarian complex, partial right salpingectomy, and abdominal washout. Upon entry into the abdominal cavity there were copious purulent fluid and diffuse inflammatory changes throughout the abdomen and pelvis. Secondary to inflammation and friability of the tissue, the superior and medial portion of the right tubo-ovarian complex was resected with sufficient distance from the sidewall and the remaining small portion of the wall was left in situ. Of note, mostly blood clot was noted in the cavity of the complex, which was consistent with hemorrhagic cyst; however, extreme inflammation and friability of the complex made it difficult to clearly identify structures but no frank pus was noted within the adnexal structures. The uterus did not appear to be involved with any of these inflammatory processes. Postoperatively, the patient still had persistent high-grade fevers and continued to remain intubated on vasopressor support. On postoperative day two, a discussion was held with her health care proxy about her lack of clinical improvement and agreement for reoperation with possible hysterectomy. She was brought back to the operating room where she underwent an exploratory laparotomy, abdominal washout, lysis of adhesions, partial omentectomy, right salpingo-oophorectomy, right ureterolysis, and cholecystectomy in an attempt for further source control. During the procedure, multiple pockets of pus in the middle and upper abdomen between loops of bowel and omentum were noted and drained, with extensive fibrinous exudate noted to be overlying the small bowel, large bowel, and pelvis. Right salpingo-oophorectomy was performed to assure that no potential source for infection was being left behind but no frank pockets of pus were noted at this time which were similar to her initial intraoperative findings. The gallbladder was noted to be gangrenous consistent with acalculous gangrenous cholecystitis, which prompted cholecystectomy

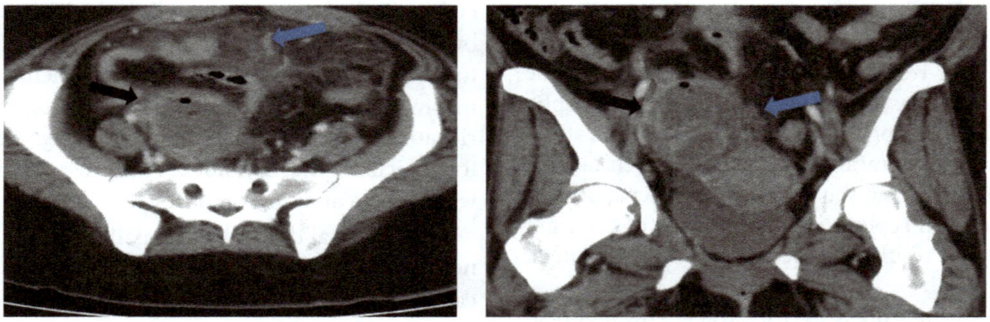

(a) (b)

Figure 1: Patient's computed tomography (CT) scan of the abdomen and pelvis before surgery. Figure 1(a) Transverse view. Figure 1(b) Coronal view. Black arrow demonstrates right adnexal peripherally enhancing mass with extensive surrounding inflamatory changes and foci of air compatible with tubo-ovarian absess (TOA). Blue arrow demonstrates extensive inflitration of teh mesentery with inflamatory changes as well as fluid concerning for TOA rupture and seeding of the mesentary.

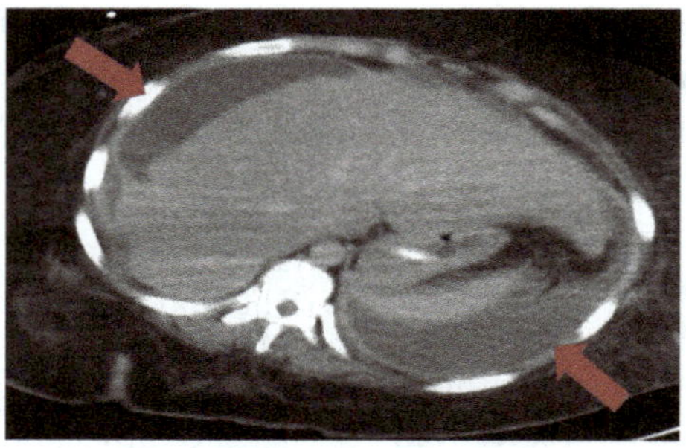

Figure 2: Patient's computed tomography (CT) scan of the abdomen and pelvis after her two surgeries looking for collections that remained. Red arrows demonstrate complex perihepatic and perisplenic ascites with peritoneal enhancement concerning for postoperative purulent collections. The collections were subsequently drained percutaneously and found to represent abscesses.

to be performed. Drains were placed and the fascia was closed, but the incision was left open to heal via secondary intention.

After undergoing the above procedures, the patient remained intubated on vasopressor support with high-grade fevers and persistent leukocytosis. She slowly was weaned off of vasopressor support, had an improvement in her ventilator settings, and became more responsive. Overall, her postoperative course was complicated by anemia necessitating blood transfusions and a left-sided lower extremity deep venous thrombosis with a right subsegmental pulmonary embolus requiring therapeutic anticoagulation. Transthoracic echocardiography did not reveal any valvular vegetations. The patient also developed a sacral decubitus ulcer as a result of her physical deconditioning. In addition, a wound vacuum was also placed over her abdominal incision secondary to poor wound healing. A peritoneal fluid culture from her initial procedure had detectable growth of *Streptococcus constellatus* that was susceptible to penicillin and ceftriaxone identical to the organism from the initial blood culture. The final pathology from her initial procedure demonstrated a hemorrhagic cyst with necrotic tissue and blood clot. The final pathology from her second procedure demonstrated right ovarian tissue with a hemorrhagic corpus luteum, fallopian tube, and fibroadipose tissue showing acute suppurative and chronic inflammation. It also demonstrated the gallbladder had acute suppurative and chronic inflammation, predominantly seen in the serosal surface. Another CT scan of the abdomen and pelvis was performed demonstrating bilateral upper quadrant fluid collections (Figure 2). Successful IR-guided drainage of the upper abdominal fluid collections was performed with drain placement. She was maintained on broad-spectrum antibiotics coverage with vancomycin and meropenem for approximately 2 weeks given persistent high grade fevers with high pressor requirements and a high concern for an uncontrolled source. As repeated blood cultures and repeated abdominal drainage cultures did not detect any bacteria so the regimen was deescalated to ceftriaxone and metronidazole.

It was also discussed that given the patients poor respiratory status with ventilation settings of both high fraction of inspired oxygen (Fi02) and positive end-expiratory pressure (PEEP) requirements that if further surgical intervention was indicated it would likely require use of extracorporeal membrane oxygenation (ECMO). Further surgery would also put her at high risk of a surgical complication such as enterotomy. Moreover, additional surgical intervention was deferred as the likely source of infection at this time was abdominal and successful IR-guided drainage with peritoneal fluid cultures demonstrated no growth of any organisms.

On postoperative day 16 after her second procedure, the patient remained ventilator dependent and thus underwent tracheostomy placement with concurrent abdominal wound debridement and replacement of the wound vacuum. Vaginal cultures were also obtained at the time of this procedure and demonstrated *Candida albicans* for which the patient received antifungal treatment. She then subsequently had a percutaneous endoscopic gastrostomy (PEG) tube placed but it failed so she remained on nasogastric tube feeds. Despite continued treatment with broad-spectrum IV antibiotics, the patient still had persistent fevers and thus the decision was made to perform another CT chest, abdomen, and pelvis to evaluate for any further intra-abdominal collections or alternative source of infection. Imaging demonstrated a significant decrease in size of the prior collections and concern for pneumonia. The patient's antibiotic regimen was adjusted per the infectious disease consultation recommendations. The intraperitoneal drains were removed as they had minimal output and could pose as a potential nidus for infection. The patient still remained intermittently febrile and thus on postoperative day 30 from her exploratory laparotomy she obtained another CT chest, abdomen, and pelvis which demonstrated an interval decrease in small bilateral pleural effusions and bibasilar atelectasis/consolidation but with upper abdominal collections again present. IR-guided drainage was again successfully performed after which the patient defervesced. The patient was afebrile after postoperative day 36 from her second procedure, without a leukocytosis and she was able to converse coherently with a tracheostomy collar in situ. Her upper abdominal drain was removed and she completed additional two weeks of ceftriaxone and metronidazole from time of last abdominal drainage. In total, she had received antibiotic coverage for approximately 8 weeks during her complicated clinical course. On hospital day seventy-three, the patient was discharged in stable condition to a subacute rehabilitation facility.

3. Discussion

This case presents a rare clinical scenario wherein a patient developed a tubo-ovarian abscess two weeks after intrauterine device (IUD) removal and then rapidly decompensated with resulting peritonitis and septic shock from the organism *Streptococcus constellatus* with a prolonged hospitalization due to metastatic spread of the infection. The spectrum of inflammatory disorders of the upper female genital tract typically results from the infection of various microorganisms that comprise the vaginal flora. Although *Streptococcus constellatus* is a commensal of the human oral cavity, urogenital and intestinal tract, there have been rare case reports of its abscess-forming capabilities that led to bacteremia, septic shock, and potentially death. Haidar et al. presented a case of *Streptococcus constellatus* bacteremia associated with septic thrombophlebitis to the right ovarian vein extending into the inferior vena cava [7]. Our case adds new insight on the management and treatment of severe life-threatening complications resulting from the abscess formation by *Streptococcus constellatus* in the female genital tract with resulting peritonitis and septic shock [7, 8].

Ascending infection from the genital tract to the fallopian tubes resulting in peritonitis in previously healthy women after intrauterine device placement (IUD) has been described in the literature [9]. The causative pathogenic organism described in these case reports is *Streptococcus pneumoniae. Streptococcus constellatus* although well known for its abscess-forming capability potentially resulting in septic shock has not yet been described as a causative organism from ascending genital infection resulting in tubo-ovarian abscess formation with septic shock. Therefore, the severe pathologic potential of *Streptococcus* organisms and their role in pelvic inflammatory disease is an area of research that warrants further investigation. Additionally, although one cannot make an exact causal relationship between the patient's IUD removal and subsequent infection, ascending genital infection after IUD removal rather than only after placement is also an area of investigation, which should be further explored.

The care of this patient exemplifies the importance of a multidisciplinary team approach in the management of a medically complex patient with an unusual disease process. Given the patient's tenuous clinical course, a multidisciplinary team conference was held to discuss her treatment plan. During the conference, it was postulated that *Streptococcus constellatus*, a commensal of the human genitourinary and gastrointestinal tract, may have had spread due to mucosal injury in the setting of the intrauterine device malposition and/or removal that was complicated by hematogenous spread to the fallopian tube, intraperitoneal cavity, and the gastrointestinal tract causing likely polymicrobial abscesses. In addition, new diagnosis of diabetes mellitus complicated by diabetic ketoacidosis likely contributed to dysfunctional host defense against this pathogen allowing aggressive spread. This theory was consistent with the fact that the final pathology was more consistent with serositis and there was no purulent material noted along the pelvic organs on the second case after the partial tubo-ovarian abscess. Additionally, *Streptococcus constellatus* is known to create extensive local abscesses and to cause septic emboli with a high morbidity and mortality rate [7, 8].

We acknowledge that a shortcoming to our findings is that this is a single case report of a personalized treatment plan, which limits the application of our findings to other patients. However, this case highlights the morbidity and potential mortality that can result from a pelvic infection with *Streptococcus constellatus* causing peritonitis and septic shock. Therefore, care for those patients with such a pelvic infection caused by *Streptococcus constellatus* likely will require not only medical management with broad-spectrum antibiotics as the abscesses are often polymicrobial with other anaerobic organisms and gram negative pathogens but also early surgical intervention(s) for complete source control. The various treatment options and the management of the possible complications of *Streptococcus constellatus* infection require further assessment in order to improve future patient care.

Additional Points

(1) *Streptococcus constellatus* can cause rapidly progressing and life-threatening ascending genital tract infections that

can cause abscess formation, peritonitis, and septic shock. (2) Rapid clinical deterioration in a patient diagnosed with a tubo-ovarian abscess must prompt one to consider infection with unconventional microorganisms such as *Streptococcus constellatus*. (3) Peritonitis and septic shock may complicate the medical management of a tubo-ovarian abscess caused by *Streptococcus constellatus* necessitating early surgical intervention.

Authors' Contributions

Dr. Tymon-Rosario and Dr. Lerner conceived the presented ideas. Dr. Tymon-Rosario abstracted the data from the medical records and wrote the manuscript in consultation with Dr. Lerner, Dr. Atrio, and Dr. Yoon. Input from all of the authors was used for the final editions to the manuscript.

References

[1] CDC, *2015 Sexually Transmitted Diseases Treatment Guidelines*, US Department of Health and Human Services, Atlanta, GA, USA, 2015.

[2] H. C. Wiesenfeld, S. L. Hillier, L. Meyn et al., "Mycoplasma genitalium—is it a pathogen in acute pelvic inflammatory disease (PID)?" in *Proceedings of the STI & AIDS World Congress 2013 (Joint Meeting of the 20th ISSTDR and 14th IUSTI Meeting)*, Vienna, Austria, 2013.

[3] R. B. Ness, D. E. Soper, R. L. Holley et al., "Effectiveness of inpatient and outpatient treatment strategies for women with pelvic inflammatory disease: results from the Pelvic Inflammatory Disease Evaluation and Clinical Health (PEACH) randomized trial," *American Journal of Obstetrics & Gynecology*, vol. 186, pp. 929–937, 2002.

[4] A. M. Burnett, C. P. Anderson, and M. D. Zwank, "Laboratory-confirmed gonorrhea and/or chlamydia rates in clinically diagnosed pelvic inflammatory disease and cervicitis," *The American Journal of Emergency Medicine*, vol. 30, no. 7, pp. 1114–1117, 2012.

[5] R. B. Ness, K. E. Kip, S. L. Hillier et al., "A cluster analysis of bacterial vaginosis-associated microflora and pelvic inflammatory disease," *American Journal of Epidemiology*, vol. 162, no. 6, pp. 585–590, 2005.

[6] C. L. Haggerty, P. A. Totten, S. G. Astete, and R. B. Ness, "Mycoplasma genitalium among women with nongonococcal, nonchlamydial pelvic inflammatory disease," *Infectious Diseases in Obstetrics and Gynecology*, vol. 2006, Article ID 30184, 2006.

[7] A. Haidar, A. Haddad, A. Naqvi, N. U. Onyesoh, R. Malik, and M. Williams, "*Streptococcus constellatus* causing septic thrombophlebitis of the right ovarian vein with extension into the inferior vena cava," *Case Reports in Infectious Diseases*, vol. 2015, Article ID 495898, 5 pages, 2015.

[8] K. W. P. Ng and A. Mukhopadhyay, "Streptococcus constellatus bacteremia causing septic shock following tooth extraction: a case report," *Cases Journal*, vol. 2, no. 5, article 6493, 2009.

[9] J. A. Goldman, A. Yeshaya, D. Peleg, A. Dekel, and D. Dicker, "Severe pneumococcal peritonitis complicating IUD: case report and review of the literature," *Obstetrical & Gynecological Survey*, vol. 41, no. 11, pp. 672–674, 1986.

[10] T. M. M. Farley, M. J. Rosenberg, P. J. Rowe, J.-H. Chen, and O. Meirik, "Intaruterine devices and pelvic inflammatory disease: An international perspective," *The Lancet*, vol. 339, no. 8796, pp. 785–788, 1992.

[11] C. D. Klug, C. R. Keay, and A. A. Ginde, "Fatal toxic shock syndrome from an intrauterine device," *Annals of Emergency Medicine*, vol. 54, no. 5, pp. 701–703, 2009.

[12] C. M. Herzer, "Toxic shock syndrome: broadening the differential diagnosis," *The Journal of the American Board of Family Practice / American*, vol. 14, pp. 131–136, 2001.

[13] E. E. Cho and D. Fernando, "Fatal streptococcal toxic shock syndrome from an intrauterine device," *The Journal of Emergency Medicine*, vol. 44, no. 4, pp. 777–780, 2013.

[14] C. Westhoff, "IUDs and colonization or infection with Actinomyces," *Contraception*, vol. 75, no. 6, pp. S48–S50, 2007.

[15] F. Sergeant and L. Marpeau, "Actinomycosis abdominopelvic: tumor syndrome associated with a bacterium," *Journal of Chiropractic Medicine*, vol. 141, pp. 150–156, 2004.

[16] P. Michel, "Pelvic actinomycosis revealed by pelvic inflammatory disease," *Annals of Surgery*, vol. 129, pp. 96–99, 2004.

[17] S. R. Henderson, "Pelvic actinomycosis associated with an intrauterine device," *Obstetrics & Gynecology*, vol. 41, pp. 726–732, 1973.

34

Uterine Trauma and Intrauterine Fetal Death Caused by Seatbelt Injury

Junsuke Muraoka, Teruo Otsuka, Aya Yamauchi, and Kiminari Terao

Department of Obstetrics and Gynecology, Perinatal Medicine, Miyazaki Prefectural Nobeoka Hospital, 2-1-10 Shinkoji, Nobeoka, Miyazaki 882-0835, Japan

Correspondence should be addressed to Junsuke Muraoka; jyunsuke_muraoka@med.miyazaki-u.ac.jp

Academic Editor: Erich Cosmi

We present a case of uterine trauma and intrauterine fetal death caused by seatbelt injury. A 37-year-old primigravida at gestational week 24 was involved in a single-car accident when traveling as a front-seat passenger and wearing a three-point seatbelt. Fetal heart rate monitoring patterns revealed fetal demise, and computed tomography revealed intraperitoneal bleeding due to damage to the uterine vessels and placental lacerations across the seatbelt-compressed region. Intensive treatment, including transfusion therapy and surgical laparotomy, prevented the loss of her life but not that of the fetus. Seatbelt use can reduce the overall mortality associated with motor vehicle crashes. Pregnant women must be educated on the proper use of restraints while traveling in motor vehicles.

1. Introduction

Motor vehicle crashes account for >50% of all traumas incurred during pregnancy, with 82% of fetal deaths occurring during those crashes [1]. Organ damage, fracture, and hemorrhage can cause maternal and fetal morbidity and mortality. Wearing a properly adjusted and positioned seatbelt in a motor vehicle during pregnancy is effective at reducing the risk of adverse pregnancy outcomes [2–4]. Here, we describe an educational case of uterine trauma and intrauterine fetal death caused by an incorrectly positioned seatbelt; we also present characteristic images of uterine bleeding and placental lacerations.

2. Case Presentation

A 37-year-old primigravida at 24 + 0/7 gestational weeks was involved a single-car accident at a speed of approximately 50 km/h. She was traveling in the left front passenger seat, had worn a three-point seatbelt restraint, and had the supplemental restraints and airbag system deployed. She was transported to our hospital by ambulance 1 h after the event. On examination, her vital signs were as follows: Glasgow Coma Scale, E4V5M6; blood pressure level, 90/50 mmHg; and heart rate, 90 beats/min. She suffered seatbelt injuries to her right thorax and entire lower abdomen and presented such severe pain to her lower abdomen that she was unable to move her body. Fetal heart rate monitoring indicated bradycardia of 80–90 beats/min with loss of variability that led to rapid demise. Whole-body computed tomography revealed intraperitoneal bleeding due to vessel injury around the uterus and placental lacerations over the seatbelt-compressed region (Figure 1). Blood tests revealed D-dimer coagulopathy of 31.7 μg/mL (normal level, <1 μg/mL) and fibrinogen degradation product of 58.0 μg/mL (normal level, <10 μg/mL). Rapid and massive blood transfusion therapy, insertion of an intra-aortic balloon occlusion catheter, and emergency laparotomy under the stabilization of maternal hemodynamics were immediately performed. Bleeding occurred all across the uterine surface during the operation (Figure 2). After delivery of a deceased male baby weighing 640 g via uterine incision, the extensive bleeding surrounding the uterine vessels was stopped using sutures. The total intraoperative hemorrhage was 2500 mL, and total 12 units of red blood cells, 12 units of fresh frozen plasma, and 20 units of platelets were transfused. The mother was admitted to the intensive care unit and discharged after 2 weeks of hospitalization. The placenta was macroscopically lacerated into several parts (Figure 3), and

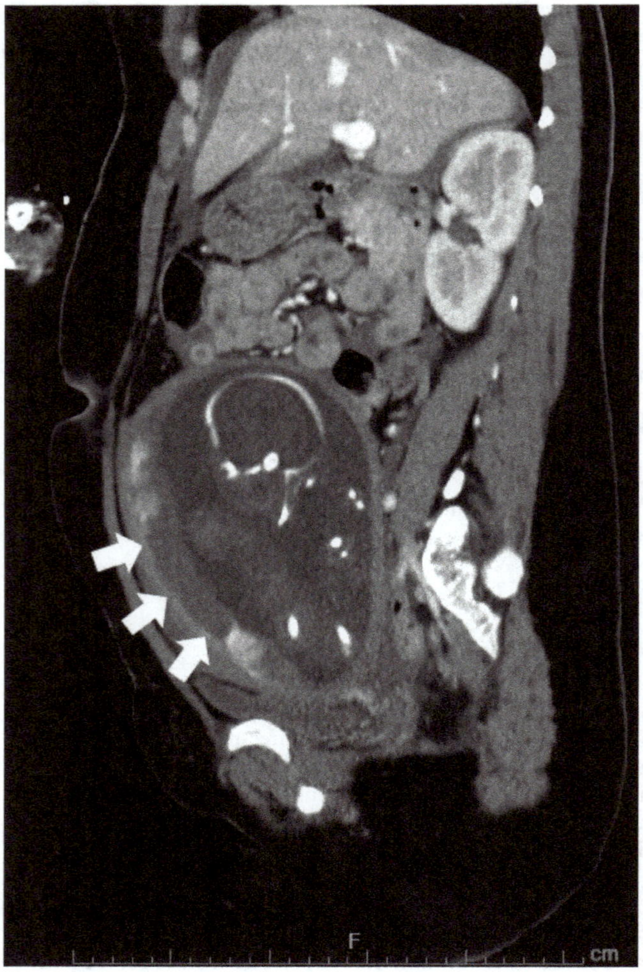

Figure 1: Computed tomography of the abdominopelvic region shows placental damage over the seatbelt-compressed area with a well-circumscribed low-density area (white arrows).

ischemic changes were microscopically noted. Written informed consent was obtained from the patient prior to publication of this case report and the accompanying images.

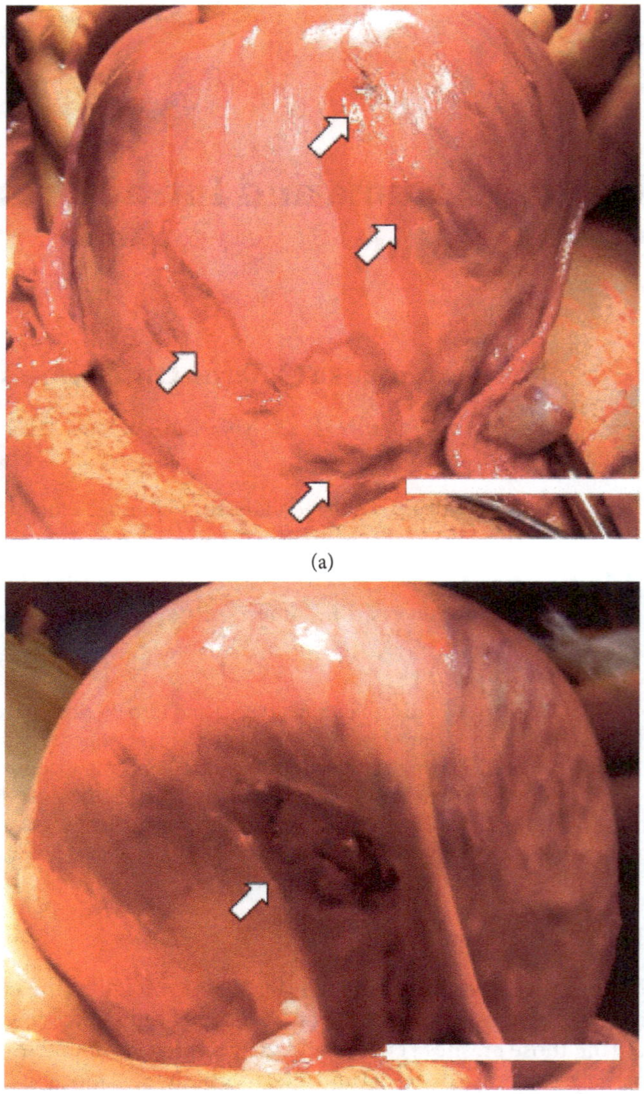

(a)

(b)

Figure 2: White arrows indicate uterine bleeding of the anterior surface (a) and right-side of wounds (b) during the operation prior to uterine incision.

3. Discussion

Obstetric complications occurring due to trauma include placental abruption, uterine rupture, preterm labor, and direct fetal injury [5]. Examination techniques are available for the assessment of both maternal and fetal conditions following motor vehicle injuries. In urgent situations, computed tomography is helpful for the rapid evaluation of maternal general conditions. In our patient, a notable low-density area of the placenta indicated placental laceration along the seatbelt-compressed area. This condition was clinically similar to placental abruption and led to subsequent intrauterine fetal death. In addition to this placental damage, numerous hemorrhages from the uterine surface were found. Bleeding from the right lateral aspect of the uterus persisted despite uterine involution after cesarean delivery. We speculated that the seatbelt caused the uterine hemorrhages and placental lacerations.

Motor vehicle crashes during pregnancy require rapid clinical judgment to assess the extent of the maternal and fetal damages. The indication for urgent surgical treatment would depend on maternal circulatory condition, blood coagulability, gestational age, and fetal well-being assessment. In cases of maternal cardiac arrest, perimortem cesarean section should be considered early in the resuscitation of the trauma victim when fetal viability is a concern and the pregnancy has extended beyond 23–24 weeks of gestation [6]. Emptying the uterus may improve maternal cardiac output and increase the likelihood of successful maternal resuscitation [7]. In the present case, the fetal heart rate patterns on admission implied an impending fetal demise and the mother remained in a critical but stable condition under transfusion therapy. Therefore, emergency laparotomy was performed after systemic workup of the source of bleeding and other organ damage. Because uterine injuries with coagulopathy were obvious

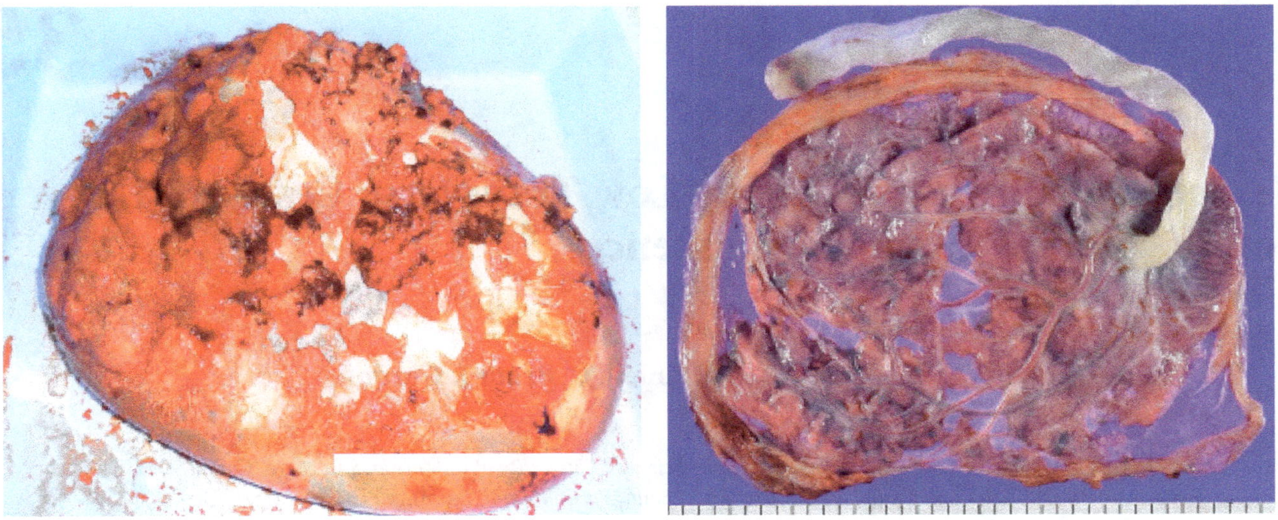

(a) (b)

FIGURE 3: Findings of the placenta on the maternal aspect just after en caul delivery (a). The fetal aspect (b) indicating placental lacerations.

from the operative findings, cesarean section was more favorable for delivery of the deceased neonate than labor induction was.

The use of three-point seatbelt restraints during pregnancy is highly recommended to reduce both maternal and fetal morbidity and mortality [8]. When women were properly restrained, adverse fetal outcomes occurred in 29% of motor vehicle crashes, whereas in women who were improperly restrained, adverse fetal outcomes occurred in 50% of motor vehicle crashes [2]. Early in mid-gestation, the pregnant abdomen may not be large enough to place the lap seatbelt below the abdominal dome. As in the present case, placement of the lap seatbelt over the dome of the uterus increases pressure transmission and uterine injury risk during a significant crash. Therefore, pregnant women should appropriately position seatbelts throughout gestation.

In summary, appropriate and prompt evaluation of maternal and fetal injuries is essential for subsequent intervention in cases of blunt trauma during pregnancy. Pregnant women should be educated on the proper use of seatbelt restraints while traveling in motor vehicles.

Acknowledgments

The authors would like to thank Enago (https://www.enago.jp/) for the English language review.

References

[1] K. L. Mattox and L. Goetzl, "Trauma in pregnancy," *Critical Care Medicine*, vol. 33, no. 10, pp. S385–S389, 2005.

[2] K. D. Klinich, C. A. Flannagan, J. D. Rupp, M. Sochor, L. W. Schneider, and M. D. Pearlman, "Fetal outcome in motor-vehicle crashes: effects of crash characteristics and maternal restraint," *American Journal of Obstetrics & Gynecology*, vol. 198, no. 4, pp. 450.e1–450.e9, 2008.

[3] K. F. Brookfield, V. H. Gonzalez-Quintero, J. S. Davis, and C. I. Schulman, "Maternal death in the emergency department from trauma," *Archives of Gynecology and Obstetrics*, vol. 288, no. 3, pp. 507–512, 2013.

[4] K. H. Hyde, L. J. Cook, L. M. Olson, H. B. Weiss, and J. M. Dean, "Effect of motor vehicle crashes on adverse fetal outcomes," *Obstetrics & Gynecology*, vol. 102, no. 2, pp. 279–286, 2003.

[5] V. Jain, R. Chari, S. Maslovitz et al., "Guidelines for the management of a pregnant trauma patient," *Journal of Obstetrics and Gynaecology Canada*, vol. 37, no. 6, pp. 553–571, 2015.

[6] V. L. Katz, D. J. Dotters, and W. Droegemueller, "Perimortem cesarean delivery," *Obstetrics & Gynecology*, vol. 68, no. 4, pp. 571–576, 1986.

[7] F. M. Jeejeebhoy, C. M. Zelop, and R. Windrim, "Management of cardiac arrest in pregnancy: a systematic review," *Resuscitation*, vol. 82, no. 7, pp. 801–809, 2011.

[8] H. C. Johnson and D. W. Pring, "Car seatbelts in pregnancy: the practice and knowledge of pregnant women remain causes for concern," *British Journal of Obstetrics and Gynaecology*, vol. 107, no. 5, pp. 644–647, 2000.

35

Hematometrocolpos following Low Transverse Cesarean Delivery Complicated by Uterine Dehiscence

Lauryn C. Gabby,[1] **Katherine E. McDaniel**,[2] **Brian J. Gordon**,[2] **and Laila A. Al-Marayati**[2]

[1]*Department of Obstetrics, Gynecology, & Reproductive Sciences, University of California, San Diego, California, USA*
[2]*Department of Obstetrics and Gynecology, University of Southern California, Los Angeles, California, USA*

Correspondence should be addressed to Laila A. Al-Marayati; laila.almarayati@med.usc.edu

Academic Editor: Seung-Yup Ku

Background. Hematometrocolpos is a rare complication following procedures performed on the female genital tract. While usually seen in adolescents with congenital anomalies including imperforate hymen and vaginal stenosis, it has also been described following obstetric vaginal lacerations. The incidence following cesarean delivery is unknown. *Case.* This is a 43-year-old multigravida who underwent a low transverse cesarean delivery complicated by uterine dehiscence, as well as cervical and vaginal lacerations. The repair resulted in lower genital tract obstruction. She presented seven months afterwards with severe abdominopelvic pain and secondary amenorrhea, which resolved after vaginal dilation and excision of the vaginal scar. *Conclusion.* Systematic inspection of the upper vagina should be undertaken following complicated cesarean delivery with vaginal extension. Hematometrocolpos after cesarean delivery should be managed similar to a transverse vaginal septum.

1. Introduction

Iatrogenic cases of hematometrocolpos are rare but have been reported after radiation therapy [1, 2] and vaginal deliveries causing obstetric trauma resulting in vaginal/labial adhesions [1–3]. Few cases of hematometra following cesarean section have been reported in the literature [4–7]; however, hematometrocolpos following cesarean section has not been yet been described, and the incidence is unknown. Most cases of hematometrocolpos are seen in adolescents, as a result of abnormal development of the lower genital tract. The most common congenital anomaly resulting in hematometrocolopos is imperforate hymen; however, transverse vaginal septum and agenesis of the lower vagina may also be etiologies of this pathology. Amenorrhea in the postpartum period is common, occurring most frequently secondary to lactation. Rarely, postpartum amenorrhea may be associated with pituitary dysfunction following postpartum hemorrhage or intrauterine adhesions secondary to pregnancy-related curettage. Here, we describe a case of postpartum amenorrhea and severe hematometrocolpos as a result of vaginal and cervical laceration repair during a low transverse cesarean delivery.

2. Case

This patient is a 43-year-old gravida 5, para 4, and abortus 1 with a history of uterine fibroids and two prior cesarean sections. The patient was referred by her obstetrician to Los Angeles County-University of Southern California (LAC +USC) Medical Center in 2019 for increasing pelvic pain and amenorrhea for seven months after her second cesarean delivery. Upon presenting to our institution, she reported that her pain was severe and had been gradually worsening over time with increasing intensity five weeks prior to presentation. The patient described the pain as constant and dull, localized to the pelvis and radiating to the lower back. Her pain was initially controlled with ibuprofen; more recently, she had required opioid medications for adequate pain control. Prior to receiving care at LAC+USC, the patient was initially evaluated for pelvic pain five months following her cesarean delivery in an emergency department. No imaging was performed at that time, and the provided diagnoses were uterine fibroids and incisional scarring. The patient then presented to other urgent care settings for worsening pain. At her first urgent care visit, she was treated empirically for endometritis without improvement in her symptoms. At another urgent care visit, a computed tomography (CT) scan of the abdomen and pelvis was performed and revealed an enlarged uterus with multiple fibroids and an enlarged cavity with suspicion of hematometra. She then presented to an outside outpatient clinic for follow-up and a stenotic cervical os was visualized on exam; she was subsequently referred to our institution.

The cesarean delivery operative report was obtained and revealed that the cesarean delivery was performed for persistent category two fetal heart rate tracing in the setting of one prior cesarean delivery. Upon entry into the abdomen, the surgeon documented a uterine scar dehiscence and multiple fibroids. The location and size of the fibroids were not described. After delivery of the infant, multiple supracervical and vaginal sulcal lacerations were encountered. These were repaired abdominally with a running 0-vicryl suture, beginning at the apex of the tear and suturing towards the hysterotomy. No other complications were noted. The patient was subsequently discharged home on postoperative day number two after meeting all postoperative milestones. At her postpartum visit, her provider documented her exam as limited due to an enlarged uterus and uterine fibroids. She ceased breastfeeding after two months and had not been using any hormonal or other methods of contraception at the time she was first seen at our institution.

Upon presentation to LAC+USC Medical Center, she had no urinary symptoms, and urinalysis was negative. A pelvic exam revealed an enlarged and tender uterus, approximately 22 weeks in size. Digital exam revealed a likely blind ending of the vaginal canal. The cervix was not palpated on exam nor clearly visualized on speculum exam. Transvaginal and transabdominal ultrasound were performed. The uterus measured 21.8 cm × 9.4 cm × 1.3 cm (Figure 1). The ultrasound showed a heterogeneous fluid-filled upper vagina and endometrial canal (Figure 2), as well as hypoechoic structures in the adnexa suggestive of hydro/hematosalpinges (Figure 3). Overall, the ultrasound findings were concerning for hematometrocolpos.

Due to her severe pain and suspected outflow tract obstruction, the patient was taken urgently to the operating room. During exam under anesthesia (EUA), a bulging obstruction was visualized within the upper vagina. An indentation was identified and a small opening created with a scalpel. This opening was then expanded using Hegar dilators under transabdominal ultrasound guidance with efflux of a large volume of old blood. Transabdominal ultrasound then revealed a persistent fluid collection above the level of dissection. A vaginoscopy was performed with passage of the hysteroscope through the narrow opening that had been entered with the Hegar dilators. Multiple pockets of fluid were serially identified, probed gently with the Hegar dilators, and then drained. Although visualization of the portio vaginalis was suboptimal, the cervix was deemed to be dilated and without stenosis. Vaginoscopy and ultrasound revealed that there was a small fluid collection contiguous with the uterine cavity above the level of the cervix, but no further blood was noted to be draining. The procedure was then terminated. Immediately postoperatively, the patient reported

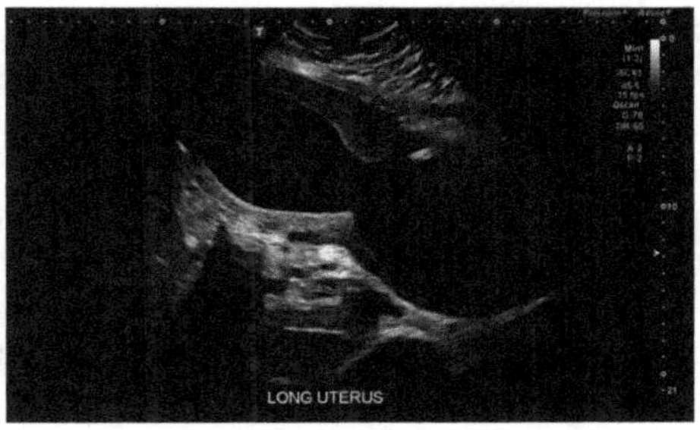

FIGURE 1: Transabdominal sagittal view of the uterus and vagina. The vagina, cervix, and uterus are distended with heterogeneous fluid.

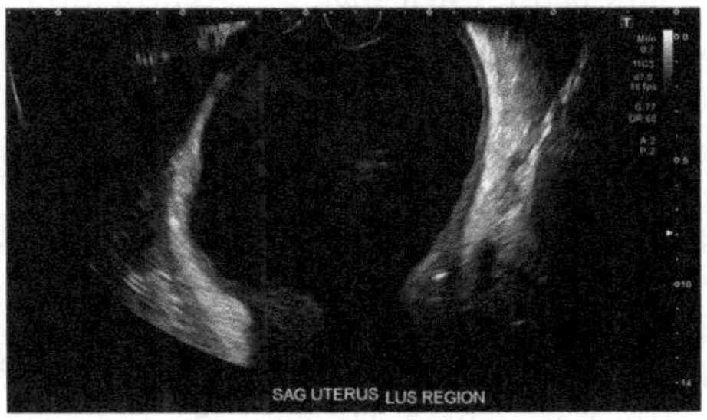

FIGURE 2: Transvaginal sagittal view of the vagina, cervix, and lower uterine segment.

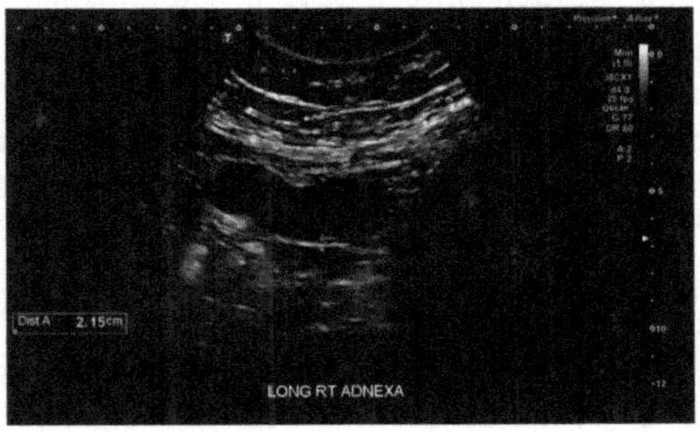

FIGURE 3: Transabdominal coronal view of the right adnexa showing a hypoechoic structure, suggestive of hydrosalpinx or hematosalpinx.

improvement in her pain and was discharged home the same day. She was seen in clinic two weeks later, where she reported improvement in her symptoms. However, on sterile speculum exam, she was again noted to have a bulge in the upper vagina. Ultrasound confirmed a persistence of her hematometrocolpos. She was therefore offered planned repeat vaginal exploration with scar excision versus hysterectomy and upper vaginectomy. She elected for scar excision.

The patient subsequently returned to the operating room and underwent an EUA, cystoscopy, vaginoscopy, and excision of vaginal scar. EUA and cystoscopy were performed first for surgical planning. The cystoscopy showed no fistulae or masses. Attention was then turned to the vagina, where the vaginal scar was palpated, and a small cruciate incision was made in the midline with a scalpel with efflux of a moderate volume of old blood products. This opening was serially expanded with Hegar dilators followed by placement of a 30 cc Foley balloon over a catheter guide. The scar was then placed on tension and estimated to be about 2 cm in thickness. The vaginal epithelium proximal to the scar was undermined, and the scar tissue was removed circumferentially by dividing it into quadrants, until the dilated cervix was visible. The denuded vaginal tissue at the base of the scar was covered by reapproximating the distal vaginal epithelium to the proximal vaginal epithelium in a circumferential fashion with 2-0 polyglactin suture. Intraoperative ultrasound showed complete resolution of the hematometrocolpos, and the procedure was terminated. The patient was then discharged home the same day.

She was subsequently followed in the outpatient setting. The patient had return of regular menses and complete resolution of her pain within two months of the surgery. She reported continued normal menses seven months after the scar revision.

3. Discussion

Hematometrocolpos is a very rare complication following cesarean delivery, with only a few reports of hematometra existing in the literature [4–7]. Our patient experienced cervical and vaginal lacerations during the cesarean procedure, which were repaired abdominally. She subsequently experienced months of amenorrhea and worsening abdominopelvic pain. Our investigations led to a diagnosis of hematometrocolpos, which was surgically corrected with scar revision. She subsequently had return of normal monthly menses and resolution of abdominal pain.

Cases of postcesarean hematometra identified in the literature were the result of a variety of causes. One reported case of hematometra after a cesarean delivery resulted after the placement of hemostatic sutures in the lower uterine segment following delivery of a placenta previa [4]. This led to uterine synechiae which required hysteroscopic adhesiolysis. A separate case likely resulted from inadvertent suturing of the anterior and posterior uterine walls during hysterotomy repair, which created a uterine pouch that did not communicate with the vagina [5]. Uterine compression sutures and postoperative endometritis have also been associated with postcesarean hematometra [6, 7].

Our patient's main risk factors for this outcome were a history of prior cesarean delivery, uterine dehiscence, and extensions of the hysterotomy into the vagina. The complex nature of the initial vaginal lacerations may have led to inadvertent closure of the vagina and/or the formation of significant scar tissue resulting in hematometrocolpos. In order to reduce the risk of postoperative persistent lower genital tract obstruction after extensive vaginal laceration repair at the time of delivery, the patency of the vagina may be assessed either by speculum exam or with digital palpation of the uterine cervix. Intraoperative assessment of the upper vagina at the time of cesarean delivery could reduce the risk of iatrogenic occlusion, though the chance of upper vaginal scarring may not be completely eliminated. Additionally, a thorough pelvic exam at the time of the postpartum visit following a cesarean delivery may be performed for complete evaluation of the lower genital tract. Heightened awareness of this potential postoperative complication and prompt investigation with imaging may lead to earlier recognition and surgical correction, which could greatly reduce morbidity. Furthermore, lower genital tract obstruction should always be included in the differential for postpartum amenorrhea, especially in patients that are no longer breastfeeding. Lastly, it is important to note that our initial surgical approach—vaginal dilation of the patient's genital tract obstruction—was not successful. As a result, we suggest first attempting surgical correction with scar excision in a manner similar to the approach for a transverse vaginal septum.

Although hematometrocolpos is a rare complication of cesarean delivery, it is important to identify potential risk factors for lower genital tract obstruction during and after the delivery and to treat with prompt surgical excision of the obstruction.

References

[1] S. C. Kaste, S. A. Gronemeyer, and D. Muram, "Vaginal occlusion induced by cancer therapy," *Pediatric Radiology*, vol. 23, no. 5, pp. 369-370, 1993.

[2] P. Gaillard, M. J. Krasin, F. H. Laningham et al., "Hematometrocolpos in an adolescent female treated for pelvic Ewing sarcoma," *Pediatric Blood & Cancer*, vol. 50, no. 1, pp. 157–160, 2008.

[3] S. Ghazizadeh and H. Rahmanpour, "Hematometrocolpos after failed vacuum delivery," *International Journal of Gynaecology and Obstetrics*, vol. 115, no. 1, pp. 69-70, 2011.

[4] M. B. Poothavelil, I. Hamdi, and G. Zunjurwad, "Occlusion of upper genital tract following lower segment caesarean section for placenta praevia," *Sultan Qaboos University Medical Journal*, vol. 8, no. 2, pp. 215–218, 2008.

[5] G. A. Saeed, "Case of postoperative haematometra in a 40-year-old woman," *Eastern Mediterranean Health Journal*, vol. 16, no. 2, pp. 237–239, 2010.

[6] V. Dadhwal, G. Sumana, and S. Mittal, "Hematometra following uterine compression sutures," *International Journal of Gynaecology and Obstetrics*, vol. 99, no. 3, pp. 255-256, 2007.

[7] G. Kaur, S. Jain, A. Sharma, and N. B. Vaid, "Hematometra formation- a rare complication of cesarean delivery," *Journal of Clinical and Diagnostic Research*, vol. 8, no. 8, pp. OD03–OD04, 2014.

Spontaneous Bilateral Tubal Ectopic Pregnancy in a Low-Risk Patient: A Case Report with Implications for Preoperative Patient Counseling

Josephine Eva Gathura, Amro Elfeky, Rodney McLaren Jr., David Herzog, and Richard Grazi

Department of Obstetrics and Gynecology, Maimonides Medical Center, Brooklyn, New York, USA

Correspondence should be addressed to Josephine Eva Gathura; ejg212@gmail.com

Academic Editor: Akihide Ohkuchi

Bilateral tubal ectopic pregnancies (BTP) are the rarest form of ectopic pregnancy. They are difficult to diagnose preoperatively, and an evidence-based guideline for management does not exist. In this report, we discuss a 35-year-old patient who presented with suspected right tubal ectopic pregnancy. BTP was diagnosed intraoperatively, and a laparoscopic bilateral salpingectomy was performed without complication. The diagnosis was subsequently confirmed by pathology. This case highlights the importance of patient counseling and comprehensive preoperative planning. Due to the poor presurgical diagnosis of BTP, patient counseling should include the possibility of BTP, appropriate options for management, and potential loss of fertility following treatment. In addition, all cases of suspected ectopic pregnancy necessitate a thorough preoperative investigation of bilateral adnexa and intraoperative inspection of the pelvis.

1. Introduction

Ectopic pregnancies account for approximately two percent of all reported pregnancies and are most commonly found in a unilateral fallopian tube [1]. Bilateral tubal ectopic pregnancy (BTP) is extremely rare, commonly followed by assisted reproductive technology (ART). The estimated incidence of BTP is 1 in 725 to 1 in 1580 of all ectopic pregnancies [2]. This corresponds to an occurrence of 1 per 200,000 live births [3]. The true incidence of BTP, however, may be higher as many cases can go unrecognized secondary to spontaneous resolution or successful medical management of presumed unilateral tubal ectopic pregnancies. BTP is clinically indistinguishable from a unilateral tubal ectopic pregnancy, and most cases are incidentally diagnosed at the time of surgery. An evidence-based guideline for management does not exist.

2. Case Report

A 35-year-old woman G4P0030 at 5 weeks and 6 days based on the last menstrual period initially presented to a reproductive endocrinologist (REI) for recurrent pregnancy loss. Past medical history was significant for three prior spontaneous abortions, the last of which was noted to be a pregnancy of unknown location, and was managed expectantly with spontaneous resolution. Past surgical history was unremarkable. Prior to starting any intervention, the patient was found to be pregnant. The beta-human chorionic gonadotropin (β-hCG) trend revealed the following values: 776 mIU/mL (day 1), 1203 mIU/mL (day 3), 2211 mIU/mL (day 7), and 2669 mIU/mL (day 9). A transvaginal ultrasound performed on day 9 showed a lack of an identifiable intrauterine pregnancy (IUP), a right adnexal mass measuring 33×17 mm, and a moderate amount of free fluid in the pelvis. No left adnexal mass was reported (Figure 1).

The patient was subsequently referred to the emergency room for complaints of moderate right lower quadrant pain in the setting of a pregnancy of unknown location with abnormally rising β-hCG. In the emergency room, the patient was hemodynamically stable with blood pressures 120 s/80 s mmHg and heart rate 70 s beats per minute. On physical exam, the abdomen was soft, nondistended, and

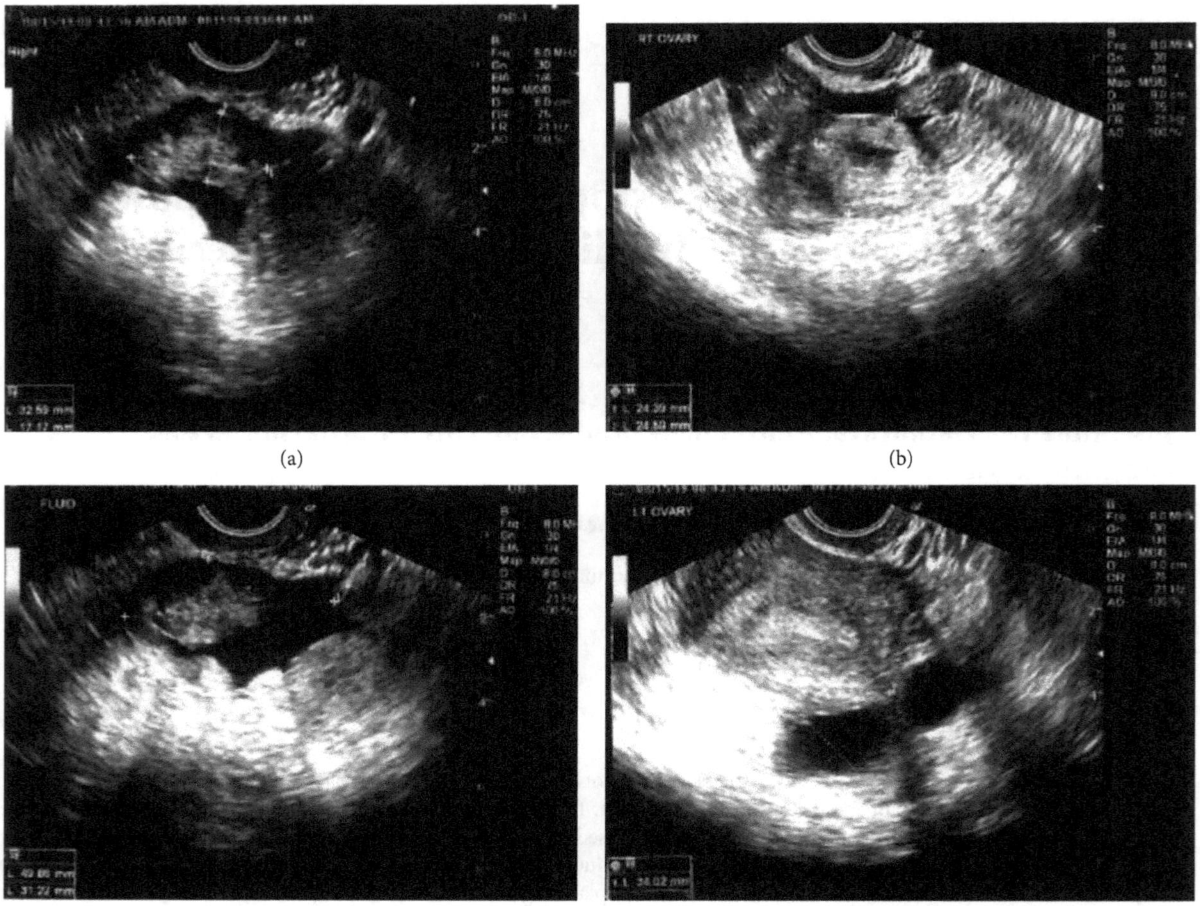

(a) (b) (c) (d)

FIGURE 1: Transvaginal ultrasound findings. (a) Right adnexa. (b) Right ovary. (c) Pelvic fluid. (d) Left ovary.

nontender without rebound or guarding. β-hCG was obtained and found to be 5454 mIU/mL. The repeat transvaginal ultrasound revealed the same findings as the ultrasound performed at the REI office. The patient was made aware of the concern for a ruptured ectopic pregnancy due to physical exam findings and free fluid on transvaginal ultrasound evaluation, without evidence of an IUP. Surgical management of ectopic pregnancy was advised, and consent was obtained for a diagnostic laparoscopy and possible salpingectomy or salpingostomy.

Intraoperatively, the uterus and ovaries were within normal limits. Approximately 100 mL of dark blood was present and evacuated from the cul de sac. A large, right ampullary ectopic pregnancy with damaged fimbria and fallopian tube was appreciated. The isthmic portion of the left fallopian tube was noted to have a blue-purple bulge suspicious for ectopic pregnancy versus a hemorrhagic or necrotic process (Figure 2). Due to the patient's history of infertility and desire to undergo in vitro fertilization, the REI and the family were contacted intraoperatively to discuss the findings of suspected BTP and to formulate a surgical plan that aligned with the patient's goals. The decision for definitive management was made, and bilateral salpingectomy was performed without complication.

The final diagnosis of bilateral tubal ectopic pregnancy was confirmed on pathology. The pathology report demonstrated chorionic villi within the right fallopian tube consistent with right intratubal ectopic pregnancy. The left fallopian tube demonstrated focal decidua and few trophoblast-like cells, which were positive for placental alkaline phosphatase suggestive of left tubal ectopic pregnancy. The patient's postoperative course was uneventful, and the β-hCG decreased appropriately following the procedure.

3. Discussion

BTP is a rare form of ectopic pregnancy, and BTP in the absence of preceding use of ART, as seen in this case, is considered to be the rarest form. The clinical presentation of unilateral versus bilateral tubal ectopic pregnancy is indistinguishable. Patients will often present with the classic triad of symptoms of amenorrhea, vaginal bleeding, and abdominal pain. Further investigation may reveal an inappropriately rising β-hCG level with or without sonographic evidence of tubal ectopic pregnancy. Ultrasonography is capable of diagnosing ectopic pregnancy when a gestational sac with a yolk sac or embryo is present within the tube, with a positive predictive value of 80 percent [1]. Most ectopic pregnancies do

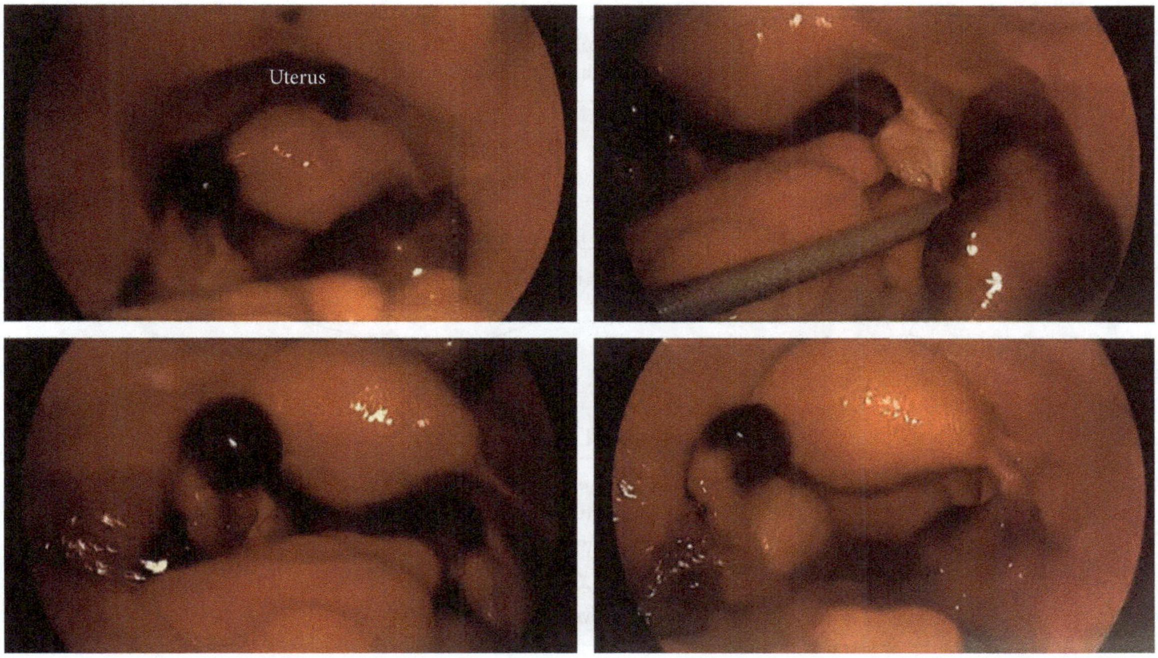

FIGURE 2: Intraoperative photos of the uterus and bilateral adnexal masses.

not advance to reach this stage, and the evaluation of the contralateral tube does not guarantee proper identification of BTP. Thus, due to the overlap of symptoms and the limitation of ultrasonography in the diagnosis of ectopic pregnancy, BTP is oftentimes diagnosed at the time of surgery rather than accurate preoperative diagnosis. To date, more than 200 cases have been reported in the literature, with only three cases of BTP diagnosed preoperatively by ultrasound [3–5]. There is a lack of data to support the use of additional imaging modalities for the diagnosis of BTP. Consequently, it is important to consider BTP in the preoperative planning period when investigating the adnexa and providing preoperative counseling, especially with patients who desire future fertility. The patient in our reported case would have had the opportunity to take part in the surgical planning after being aware of the possibility of BTP and the potential outcomes, which included bilateral salpingectomy. This would have also eliminated the need to contact the REI specialist and family intraoperatively to formulate a surgical plan.

Typically, for patients with a suspected unilateral tubal ectopic pregnancy to be considered for medical management, they must meet eligibility criteria for methotrexate administration and be monitored closely with serial β-hCG until resolution of pregnancy is confirmed. However, it is unknown whether medical management is an acceptable option for BTP because ultrasonography remains an unreliable method for the diagnosis of BTP. Furthermore, no studies address the dosing regimen and efficacy of methotrexate when treating BTP. Accurate diagnosis is an essential prerequisite to medical management, as failed medical management for BTP has been reported after the administration of a single dose injection of methotrexate for presumed unilateral tubal ectopic pregnancy [2]. To date, only one case of a spontaneous BTP was reported that was diagnosed by ultrasonography and successfully treated by two consecutive intratubal methotrexate injections under vaginal ultrasonographic guidance without complications [4]. The patient discussed in our case, however, was not eligible for medical management due to clinical signs consistent with ruptured ectopic pregnancy.

Patients who are hemodynamically unstable or symptomatic, have findings concerning for rupture, or have any contraindication to medical management should be managed surgically. It is important to note that surgical intervention does not guarantee the detection of BTP. As such, a thorough inspection of the pelvis is required to avoid missed intraoperative diagnosis which may lead to unnecessary repetitive procedures and rupture of the undetected ectopic pregnancy [2].

The question remains whether salpingostomy is a conservative surgical option for eligible patients with BTP given the possible risk of recurrent ectopic pregnancy and the possible need for additional medical or surgical management in the event of persistent ectopic pregnancy, while considering fertility preservation as compared to definitive radical surgical treatment with bilateral salpingectomy. There are two reported cases of intraoperatively diagnosed BTP treated with bilateral salpingostomy, one of which required a dose of intramuscular methotrexate for persistent ectopic pregnancy [2, 6]. There are a few reported cases of intrauterine conception following surgical management of BTP with unilateral salpingectomy and contralateral salpingostomy, the most recent of which was reported in 2013 [2, 4]. Nonetheless, the majority of BTP cases undergo bilateral salpingectomy, as did our patient.

In this case, our patient will need ART to achieve pregnancy. To date, the IVF success rate is approximately 27% [7]. For patients who undergo unilateral salpingostomy or unilateral salpingectomy with a contralateral healthy tube, the spontaneous pregnancy rate is approximately 56-60%

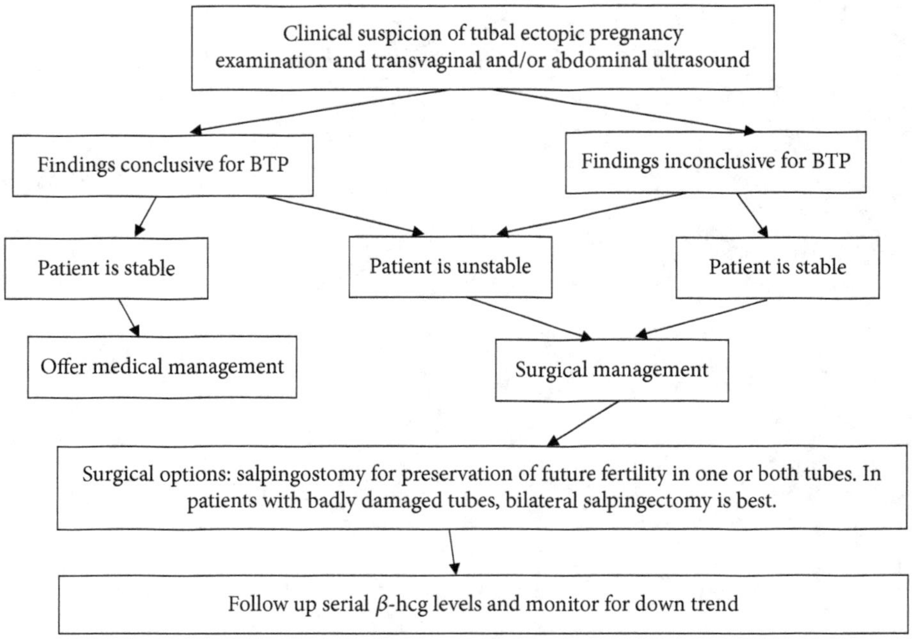

FIGURE 3: Algorithm for management of suspected bilateral tubal ectopic pregnancy (BTP). Modified from Jena SK, et al. Bilateral Simultaneous Tubal Ectopic Pregnancy: A Case Report, Review of Literature and a Proposed Management Algorithm. J Clin Diagn Res. 2016; 10(3).

[8]. This should be considered alongside accessibility of fertility services when pursuing surgical management. Fertility services are readily available in the United States. However, access to ART can be limited and should not be assumed to be a viable option for all patients [9].

4. Conclusion

Ectopic pregnancy still remains the leading cause of maternal mortality in the first trimester, accounting for 4 to 10 percent of all pregnancy-related deaths, making timely diagnosis and appropriate management of the utmost importance. [3]. An algorithm for the management of suspected BTP has been proposed by Jena et al. to address this concern and decrease the chances of missed or delayed diagnosis (Figure 3) [2]. Ideally, an evidence-based protocol would guide the management of BTP; however, given the low incidence and poor presurgical diagnosis of BTP, such a protocol has to be extrapolated from current case reports in the literature and individualized for each case.

Although rare, BTP can be a life-threatening condition if misdiagnosed and should be considered in all cases of suspected ectopic pregnancy. The case described highlights the importance of patient counseling and comprehensive preoperative planning. Patient counseling should include the possibility of BTP, appropriate options for management, and the potential loss of fertility following surgical management. This approach promotes both shared-decision making and preparedness which are needed to provide patient-centered and comprehensive care. Lastly, a thorough preoperative investigation of the bilateral adnexa and inspection of the pelvis intraoperatively may mitigate the risk of persistent ectopic pregnancy and resulting sequelae.

References

[1] Tubal ectopic pregnancy, "ACOG Practice Bulletin No. 193. Obstet Gynecol [Internet]," 2018 Mar [cited 2021 Jan 18]; 131: e91–103. Available from: https://www.acog.org/clinical/clinical-guidance/practice-bulletin/articles/2018/03/tubal-ectopic-pregnancy.

[2] S. K. Jena, S. Singh, M. Nayak, L. Das, and S. Senapati, "Bilateral Simultaneous Tubal Ectopic Pregnancy: Bilateral simultaneous tubal ectopic pregnancy: a case report, review of literature and a proposed management algorithm," *Journal of Clinical and Diagnostic Research*, vol. 10, no. 3, pp. QD01–QQD3, 2016.

[3] M. Othman, S. Karali, K. Badawi, and H. Mossa, "Bilateral ectopic pregnancy: case report," *WebmedCentra Obstet and Gynaecol*, vol. 4, no. 7), article WMC00435, 2013.

[4] V. R. S. Rani and G. Puliyath, "Viable intrauterine pregnancy after spontaneous bilateral tubal ectopics in a multiparous woman: a case report," *J Med Case*, vol. 7, p. 159, 2013.

[5] H. Xu, "A spontaneous bilateral tubal pregnancy," *Medicine*, vol. 97, no. 38, article e12365, 2018.

[6] S. Hoffmann, H. Abele, and C. Bachmann, "Spontaneous Bilateral Tubal Ectopic Pregnancy: Incidental finding during laparoscopy - brief report and review of literature," *Geburtshilfe und Frauenheilkunde*, vol. 76, no. 4, pp. 413–416, 2016.

[7] Assisted Reproductive Technology (ART) Data; National Data, "Centers for Disease Control and Prevention [Internet]," 2018 [cited 2021 May 4]. Available from: Assisted Reproductive Technology (ART) DataAssisted Reproductive Health Data: Clinic | DRH | CDC.

[8] F. Mol, N. M. van Mello, A. Strandell et al., "Salpingotomy versus salpingectomy in women with tubal pregnancy (ESEP study): an open-label, multicentre, randomised controlled trial," *Lancet*, vol. 383, no. 9927, pp. 1483–1489, 2014.

[9] G. Weigel, U. Ranji, M. Long, and A. Salganicoff, "Coverage and Use of Fertility Services in the U.S. Kaiser Family Foundation Women's Health Policy Brief [Internet]," 2020 September 15 [cited 2021 May 4]. Available from: https://www.kff.org/womens-health-policy/issue-brief/coverage-and-use-of-fertility-services-in-the-u-s/.

Treatment of a Chronic Vulvar Wound by Hyperbaric Oxygen Therapy (HBOT)

D. Ricard-Gauthier,[1] **M.-A. Panchard,**[2] **and D. E. Huber**[1]

[1]*Department of Gynecology and Obstetrics, Valais Hospital, Sion, Switzerland*
[2]*Department of Underwater and Hyperbare, University Hospital of Geneva, Switzerland*

Correspondence should be addressed to D. Ricard-Gauthier; d.ricard.gauthier@gmail.com

Academic Editor: Seung-Yup Ku

We hereby report the case of a 66-year-old obese patient (BMI 30) with type 2 diabetes, who presented a chronic vulvar lesion on the left labia majora following surgical drainage of an abscess. After multiple unsuccessful treatments by antibiotics and local wound care, we proposed a trial of hyperbaric oxygen therapy (HBOT). The patient fully recovered after 54 sessions at 2.5 ATA, 95 minutes each. HBOT has been studied for perineal lesion such as skin atrophy or necrosis caused by irradiation but not for vulvar nonhealing chronic lesions in the case of impaired vascularization caused by diabetes. This case is, to our knowledge, one of the first publications about the healing boost of HBOT in chronic vulvar wounds due to vascular impairment.

1. Background

Impaired healing causing chronic wounds is a constant and increasing challenge for the medical society with an estimation of 6.5 million cases per year [1]. Patient's quality of life is particularly compromised by this affliction which demands a lot of care and long-term treatments. During the past years, numerous techniques have been developed such as skin substitutes, wound dressing, injection of growth factors, negative pressure wound therapy, and hyperbaric oxygen therapy (HBOT) [1, 2]. HBOT is an established treatment for chronic nonhealing wounds of different origins: due to arterial insufficiency and mucosal ulcers postradiotherapy [3]. The treatment consists in breathing 100% oxygen in ambient pressure greater than 1 atmosphere absolute (ATA) in a chamber. At 2.5 ATA 100% O_2, the total content is 24.2 ml O_2/100 ml blood instead of 19.2 ml O_2/100 ml at 1 ATA room air. Consequently, it saturates the blood with oxygen causing hyperoxia of the lesions and massively increases the blood oxygen content. The mechanisms of action for improving wound healing are numerous and varied: fibroblast proliferation, induction of collagen synthesis, neoangiogenesis, and antimicrobial defense [4]. Most of the studies focused their research on chronic wounds occurring after an oncological surgery or radiation and only a few on lesions caused by other origins [5–8].

In this case report, we describe the successful healing of a vulvar chronic wound using HBOT after numerous treatment failures.

2. Case Presentation

A 66-year-old obese patient (BMI 30) was referred to our department for vulvar pain and redness. The patient's medical history revealed type 2 diabetes treated by insulin aspart 30 U, insulin degludec 60 U, liraglutide 1-8 mg, hypertension treated by metoprolol 100 mg, cilazapril 5 mg, and finally atrial fibrillation with intake of rivaroxaban 20 mg. In 1992, she underwent a hysterectomy with bilateral salpingectomy. In March 2020, a perianal abscess, far from the vulva, was treated surgically with good skin healing. The patient had no arterial insufficiency or diabetic vasculopathy history.

In July 2020, the patient consulted in our department due to an increasing and painful swelling which appeared within two weeks. At examination, we observed a unilateral swelling with redness of the left labia majora. We diagnosed a vulvar abscess of 5 × 3 cm and proposed a conservative treatment with local application of Ichtyol. After two days

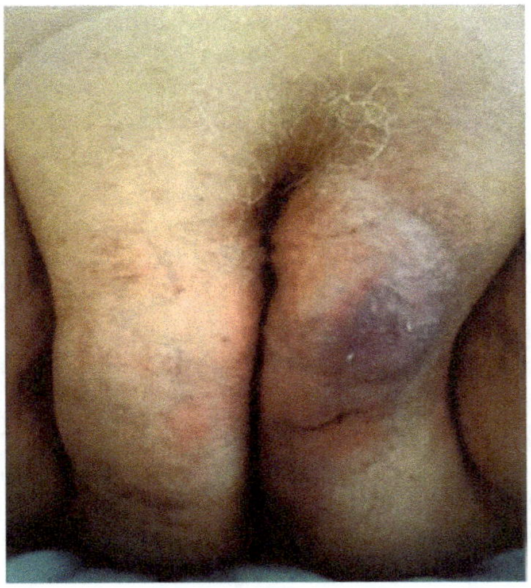

FIGURE 1: Incision site of the labia majora with an impaired healing and suspicion of cellulitis.

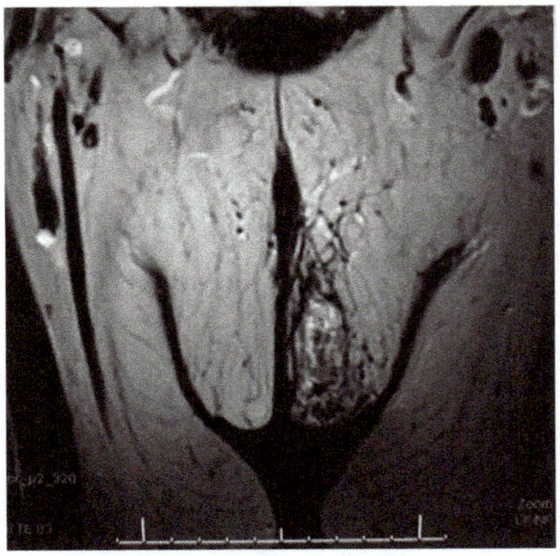

FIGURE 2: MRI showing an empty cavity without any collection. Skin infiltration with suspicion of a cellulitis. Absence of fistula.

of treatment, no improvement was observed and surgical treatment of the abscess by incision with drainage was decided. We made a 2 cm incision on a 1 cm depth and 5 cm length collection. Local swab of a brownish and odorous liquid considered as pus remained negative for any pathogen. Biopsies showed inflammatory change but no malignant signs.

After surgery, we observed impaired wound healing with the development of severe skin swelling and redness of the labia (Figure 1). We suspected a cellulitis and decided to treat the patient with clindamycin 600 mg per os two times per day for seven days. No improvement was noted, and new swabs showed the presence of *E. faecalis*. We decided to introduce a treatment of cotrimoxazole two times per day for 10 days. Even after this second treatment, there was still no healing, and as a result, the patient was hospitalized for IV treatment with vancomycin 1.5 g two times per day and ciprofloxacin 500 mg two times per day for 18 days.

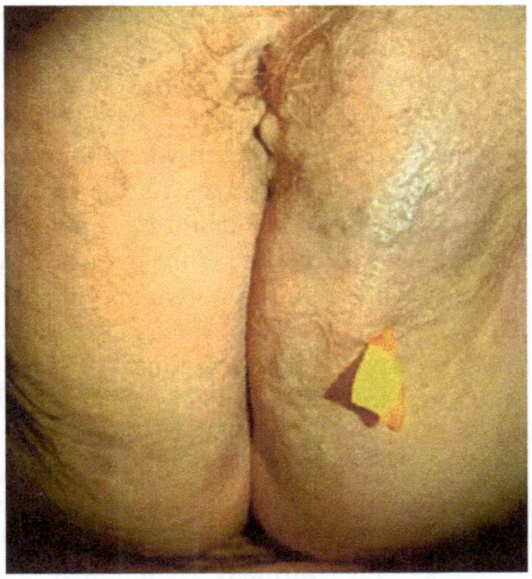

FIGURE 3: Image of the labia majora after the first session of HBOT.

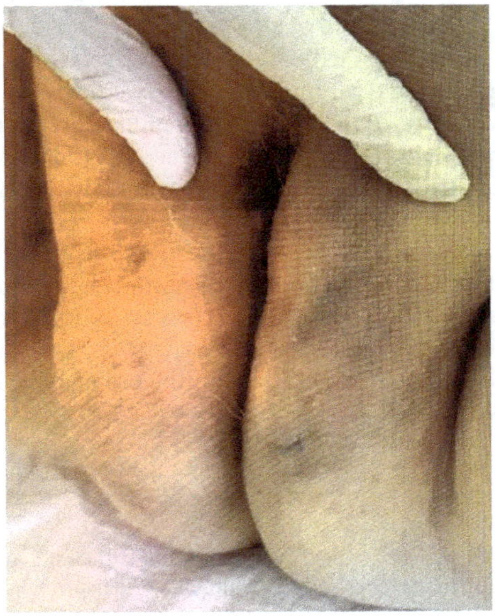

FIGURE 4: Image of the labia majora at the end of the treatment with complete healing of the incision site.

MRI confirmed vulvar cellulitis as well as the remnants of a 2.8 cm over 2.1 cm cavity without any new abscess or fistula (Figure 2). A swab of the lesion was negative for bacteria following antibiotic therapy. Following these multiple unsuccessful treatments during 4 weeks, we proposed HBOT. The patient did not present any contraindications for this therapy.

For the HBOT, the patient was hospitalized in the Department of Underwater and Hypercare Medicine, at the University Hospital of Geneva. Two sessions at 2.5 ATA, 95 minutes each, were done from Monday to Friday and one session every Saturday. Local treatment of the lesion was done with disinfection by aqueous chlorhexidine once a day. After 54 sessions, the patient presented full recovery with only a small skin lesion with no remaining cavity (Figures 3 and 4).

3. Discussion

For vulvar chronic wounds, negative pressure therapy, application of platelet gel, and growth factors have been used with good healing results [2, 9]. However, when lesions are small with cutaneous fistula, these options can be laborious with limited access. As such, HBOT could be a new option for those specific cases. Moreover, healing requires oxygen in order to be used by the immune system and new proliferating cells [1]. Wounds with low oxygen saturation are more at risk of necrosis and impaired healing [10]. In our case, the patient suffered from diabetes causing impaired wound healing due to a multifactorial origin (vascular, neuropathic, immune, and biochemical disturbance). In consequence, with difficult access of the wound and probable low oxygen saturation in the context of diabetes, we think this case is perfect for HBOT. This treatment has minimal side effects, is unpainful, and is easy to apply. There are only few absolute contraindications such as untreated pneumothorax, decompensated pulmonary obstructive disease, or decompensated cardiac failure [11]. On the other hand, the treatment can be long with the need of repeated sessions requiring organization. In our case, we were able to observe, full recovery after HBOT and minimal local treatment. The patient complained about the time needed for this method with long-lasting hospitalization; however, she was very satisfied with the final result.

In our knowledge, this case is the first to report an efficient treatment by HBOT of a nonhealing chronic lesion not caused by irradiation. This supports HBOT as an optional treatment for impaired vulvar wound healing. As such, we believe that more studies should concentrate on the use of HBOT for the healing of chronic vulvar lesions.

References

[1] G. Han and R. Ceilley, "Chronic wound healing: a review of current management and treatments," *Advances in Therapy*, vol. 34, no. 3, pp. 599–610, 2017.

[2] P. J. Stanirowski, A. Wnuk, K. Cendrowski, and W. Sawicki, "Growth factors, silver dressings and negative pressure wound therapy in the management of hard-to-heal postoperative wounds in obstetrics and gynecology: a review," *Archives of Gynecology and Obstetrics*, vol. 292, no. 4, pp. 757–775, 2015.

[3] Z. Borab, M. D. Mirmanesh, M. Gantz, A. Cusano, and L. L. Q. Pu, "Systematic review of hyperbaric oxygen therapy for the treatment of radiation- induced skin necrosis," *Journal of Plastic, Reconstructive & Aesthetic Surgery*, vol. 70, no. 4, pp. 529–538, 2017.

[4] M. Y. Memar, M. Yekani, N. Alizadeh, and H. B. Baghi, "Hyperbaric oxygen therapy: Antimicrobial mechanisms and clinical application for infections," *Biomedicine & Pharmacotherapy*, vol. 109, pp. 440–447, 2019.

[5] A. D. Altman, G. Nelson, J. Nation, P. Chu, and P. Ghatage, "Vacuum assisted wound closures in gynaecologic surgery," *J Obstet Gynaecol Can*, vol. 33, no. 10, pp. 1031–1037, 2011.

[6] N. Wahab, F. A. Saadeh, A. Wong, and N. Gleeson, "Negative pressure wound treatment (NPWT) in vulva and groin wounds in gynaecologic oncology," *European Journal of Gynaecological Oncology*, vol. 37, no. 5, pp. 632–637, 2016.

[7] M. Morelli, M. L. Rocca, R. Venturella et al., "Adjuvant use of platelet gel for wound breakdown prevention in advanced vulvar cancer surgery: a retrospective study," *International Journal of Gynecological Cancer*, vol. 23, no. 8, pp. 1490–1494, 2013.

[8] L. A. Dainty, J. J. Bosco, J. W. McBroom, W. E. Winter III, G. S. Rose, and J. C. Elkas, "Novel techniques to improve split-thickness skin graft viability during vulvo- vaginal reconstruction," *Gynecologic Oncology*, vol. 97, no. 3, pp. 949–952, 2005.

[9] A. Llueca, J. L. Herraiz, R. del Moral et al., "Use of negative pressure wound therapy after infection and flap dehiscence in radical vulvectomy: a case report," *International Journal of Surgery Case Reports*, vol. 41, no. 41, pp. 370–372, 2017.

[10] P. J. Sheffield, "Measuring tissue oxygen tension: a review," *Undersea & Hyperbaric Medicine*, vol. 25, no. 3, pp. 179–188, 1998.

[11] R. Gawdi and J. S. Cooper, "Hyperbaric contraindications," in *StatPearls*, StatPearls Publishing, Treasure Island (FL), 2021, http://www.ncbi.nlm.nih.gov/books/NBK557661/.

38

Mixed Intervillositis in SARS-CoV-2 Infection Associated with Fetal Death: A Case Report

Boban Gjakov,[1] Darja Kopač,[2] Mateja Vukmanič Pohar,[1] and Miha Lučovnik[2,3]

[1]*Department of Gynecology and Obstetrics, Brežice General Hospital, Černelčeva cesta 15, 8250, Brežice, Slovenia*
[2]*Division of Obstetrics and Gynecology, University Medical Center Ljubljana, Šlajmerjeva 3, 1000 Ljubljana, Slovenia*
[3]*Medical Faculty, University of Ljubljana, Vrazov trg 2, 1000 Ljubljana, Slovenia*

Correspondence should be addressed to Miha Lučovnik; miha.lucovnik@kclj.si

Academic Editor: Maria Grazia Porpora

Maternal severe acute respiratory syndrome coronavirus 2 (SARS-CoV-2) infection has been shown in epidemiological studies to be associated with an increased risk of stillbirth. Several histopathologic features of placental SARS-CoV-2 infection have been proposed as potential causes of fetal death. We present a case of an otherwise healthy G3P1 women with mild symptoms of SARS-CoV-2 infection at 23 6/7 weeks of gestation. At 25 2/7 weeks, she presented with signs and symptoms of preterm labor and decreased fetal movements. Fetal death was diagnosed at admission. Placental pathology showed pronounced placental mixed intervillositis. Inflammatory infiltrate caused extreme narrowing of intervillous space leading to placental malfunction and fetal death. Placental tissue SARS-CoV-2 infection was confirmed by positive immunohistochemistry staining of syncytiotrophoblasts with spike protein antibody. The case presented suggests that SARS-CoV-2 associated inflammatory placental changes pose an elevated risk for the fetus.

1. Introduction

Pregnant women are at increased risk of severe and critical coronavirus disease 2019 (COVID-19) due to immunological and cardiopulmonary changes related to pregnancy [1, 2]. They are more likely to require intensive care unit admission, invasive mechanical ventilation, and extracorporeal membrane oxygenation than nonpregnant severe acute respiratory syndrome coronavirus 2 (SARS-CoV-2) positive women of reproductive age [1–5]. COVID-19 has also been associated with increased risk of maternal mortality [1, 6].

In addition to the impact of pregnancy on COVID-19 severity, there are also concerns of adverse effects of SARS-CoV-2 infection during pregnancy on the fetus. Maternal COVID-19 has been shown to be associated with an increased incidence of small-for-gestational age neonatal birth weight, preterm birth, and approximately doubled risk of stillbirth [1, 7–10]. Neonatal infections due to vertical SARS-CoV-2 transmission have been infrequently reported, but they can occur under certain biologic conditions [11–13]. Several potential mechanisms that could cause impairment of placental function from COVID-19 infection have been proposed so far. Placental pathology studies have reported increased rates of features associated with maternal and fetal vascular malperfusion in COVID-19 [14–17]. However, most of these were not significantly associated with severity of maternal illness nor with fetal or neonatal outcomes [14–17]. More recently, placental inflammatory infiltrates have been proposed as a feature of acute placental SARS-CoV-2 infection, which could lead to adverse perinatal outcomes [17, 18]. We present a case of fetal death following SARS-CoV-2 infection in the second trimester of pregnancy with pronounced mixed intervillositis seen on placental histopathologic examination. Consent to publish this case report was obtained from the patient.

2. Case Presentation

25-year-old G3P1 was diagnosed with SARS-CoV-2 infection (by reverse-transcription polymerase chain reaction test) at 23 6/7 weeks of gestation. She had mild COVID-19 symptoms, i.e., cough, sore throat, and fever (up to 38.5°C)

with no dyspnea. She had not been vaccinated against COVID-19 and was otherwise healthy, not taking any medications, with a body-mass-index of 23 kg/m2. She attended regular prenatal visits, had normal first trimester genetic screening, normal second trimester anatomy scan, no signs of gestational diabetes mellitus or hypertensive disorders in pregnancy, and negative toxoplasmosis, hepatitis B, and syphilis screening. Her first trimester indirect Coombs' test was also negative. In her previous pregnancy in 2020, she delivered a 2480 g neonate at 35 weeks of gestation. She had a medical termination of pregnancy at 8 weeks in her second pregnancy.

Ten days after confirmed SARS-CoV-2 infection (at 25 2/7 weeks), she presented at obstetrical triage because she could not feel fetal movements for the last 12 hours. She also reported uterine contractions and vaginal bleeding at that time. Intrauterine fetal death was confirmed by ultrasound. The cervix was 5 cm dilated, and she was admitted to labor and delivery unit, where she delivered a 680 g stillborn neonate. The fetus, umbilical cord, and placenta were send for histopathologic examination.

Fetal autopsy found no congenital malformations and no signs of fetal viral infection. There were also no macroscopic signs of acute inflammation in the umbilical cord, which had two arteries and one vein. Placenta weighted 270 g (75 centile for gestational age). On histologic examination, diffuse villous agglutination could be seen accompanied by massive trophoblast necrosis (highlighted by homogenized, hyperchromatic and dusky nuclei that were pycnotic and karyorrhectic at late stages with an often persistent cytoplasmatic clearing). Heavy intervillous acute and chronic inflammatory infiltrates could be observed (Figure 1), admixed with variable amounts of increased perivillous fibrinoid deposition, highlighted by special phosphotungstic acid haematoxylin (PTAH) stain (Figure 2). Extreme narrowing of already collapsing intervillous space by inflammatory infiltrates was seen (Figure 1).

The inflammatory infiltrate was composed predominantly of hystiocytes highlighted by immunohistochemistry with strongly positive CD 68 (Figure 3) and neutrophils and positively stained with CD 15 (Figure 4).

Positive immunohistochemistry staining of syncytiotrophoblasts with spike protein antibody showed a granular binding pattern in syncytiotrophoblasts (Figure 5). Villous stroma remained unaffected with a well-preserved capillary network and sporadic local placed nodular intravillous fibrinoid.

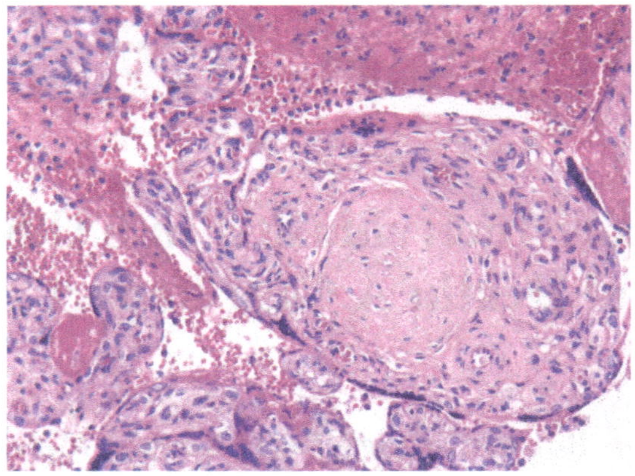

FIGURE 1: Placental pathology in SARS-CoV-2 infection; haematoxylin and eosin staining. Heavy intervillous acute and chronic inflammatory infiltrates narrow a collapsing intervillous space.

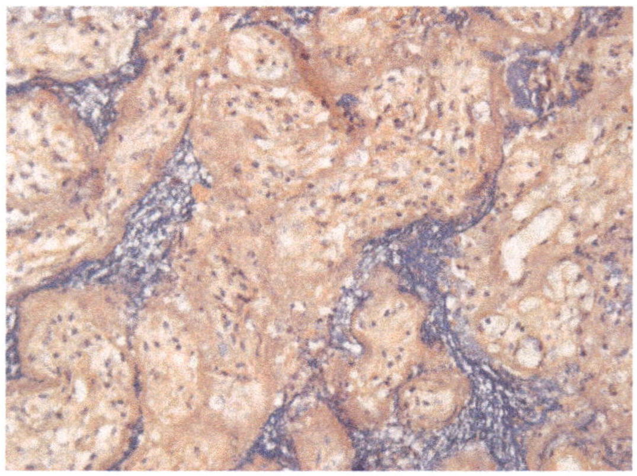

FIGURE 2: Increased perivillous fibrinoid deposition, phosphotungstic acid haematoxylin (PTAH) stain.

3. Discussion

We present a case of an intrauterine fetal death at 25 weeks of pregnancy complicated by SARS-CoV-2 infection associated with prominent mixed intervillositis. Reporting placental pathology findings in pregnancies with adverse fetal/neonatal outcomes after maternal COVID-19 is essential to elucidate potential mechanisms that could explain increased rates of perinatal complications reported with this disease, such as fetal growth restriction and stillbirth [1, 7–10].

Placental tissue has already been described to be the target of several viral infections, such as Cytomegalovirus, Herpes simplex virus, Rubella, and more recently Zika, leading to a wide range of placental histopathologic changes [19, 20]. COVID-19 has also been associated with a variegated spectrum of placental pathology. Most early studies reported features of maternal and fetal malperfusion that could result from placental SARS-CoV-2 infection [14–17]. Such features included increase in intervillous fibrin and decidual vasculopathy, thrombosis of fetal microvasculature, delayed villous maturation, and chorangiosis [17]. However, more recent studies did not confirm a significant causal correlation between SARS-CoV-2 infection in pregnancy and an increased incidence of histologic features of malperfusion [21–24]. Moreover, most studies did not explore associations between placental pathology findings and COVID-19 severity, time from infection to delivery, and pregnancy outcomes.

Inflammatory response, such as villitis and intervillositis, was observed much less frequently in placentas following SARS-CoV-2 infection [14–16]. It was mostly seen in cases of acute and severe COVID-19 [17]. Menter et al. described placental pathology findings in five SARS-CoV-2 positive women delivering at term. They found features of malperfusion in all of the placentas examined, while villitis and

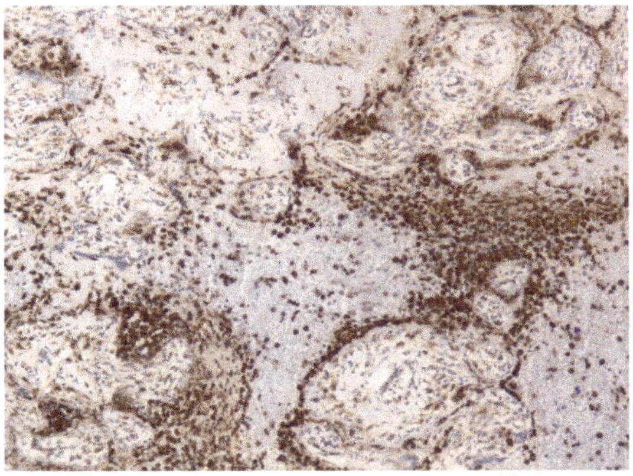

FIGURE 3: Inflammatory intervillous infiltrate; CD68 positive hystiocytes.

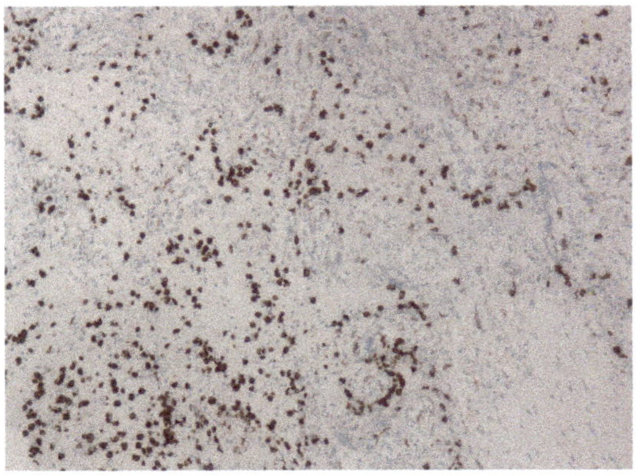

FIGURE 4: Inflammatory intervillous infiltrate; CD15 positive neutrophils.

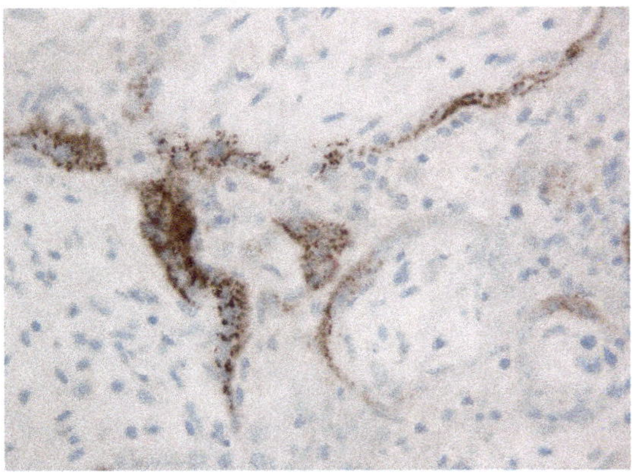

FIGURE 5: Positive immunohistochemistry staining of syncytiotrophoblasts with spike protein antibody.

intervillositis only in one case of acute maternal infection at the time of delivery [17]. Therefore, pregnant women with SARS-CoV-2 infection are not a homogenous group in terms of placental pathology. Placental changes associated with this infection differ depending on severity and timing of infection. Moreover, some placental changes may be associated with increased fetal risks as compared to others. The case presented suggests that SARS-CoV-2 associated inflammatory placental changes pose an especially elevated risk for the fetus. Maternal and fetal blood samples were not examined for the presence of anti SARS-CoV-2 antibodies or SARS-CoV-2 viral RNA. Vertical transmission can, therefore, not be entirely excluded as the cause of fetal death [11–13]. This should certainly be viewed as a limitation of this report despite postmortem fetal evaluation revealing no sign of fetal viral infection.

Histopathologic changes associated with SARS-CoV-2 infection of the placenta described in our case report would seriously hinder intervillous blood flow, disrupt the placental barrier, and cause inadequate exchange of nutrients, gases, and metabolic end products. These changes could explain the increased risks of fetal death described with maternal SARS-CoV-2 infection in several cohort studies [1, 7–10]. A single case does not allow drawing definitive conclusions on causality. It does, however, emphasize the need for larger prospective placental studies in SARS-CoV-2 infection during pregnancy which will eventually help to identify features of this infection that pose particularly increased risks to the developing fetus.

Disclosure

This study was performed as part of the employment of the authors (Brežice General Hospital and University Medical Center Ljubljana).

References

[1] J. Allotey, E. Stallings, M. Bonet et al., "Clinical manifestations, risk factors, and maternal and perinatal outcomes of coronavirus disease 2019 in pregnancy: living systematic review and meta-analysis," *BMJ*, vol. 370, article m3320, 2020.

[2] K. S. Jering, B. L. Claggett, J. W. Cunningham et al., "Clinical characteristics and outcomes of hospitalized women giving birth with and without COVID-19," *JAMA Internal Medicine*, vol. 181, no. 5, pp. 714–717, 2021.

[3] M. Andrikopoulou, N. Madden, T. Wen et al., "Symptoms and critical illness among obstetric patients with coronavirus disease 2019 (COVID-19) infection," *Obstetrics and Gynecology*, vol. 136, no. 2, pp. 291–299, 2020.

[4] M. J. Blitz, B. Rochelson, H. Minkoff et al., "Maternal mortality among women with coronavirus disease 2019 admitted to the intensive care unit," *American Journal of Obstetrics and Gynecology*, vol. 223, no. 4, pp. 595–599., 2020.

[5] R. J. Martinez-Portilla, A. Sotiriadis, C. Chatzakis et al., "Pregnant women with SARS-CoV-2 infection are at higher risk of death and pneumonia: propensity score matched analysis of a nationwide prospective cohort (COV19Mx)," *Ultrasound in Obstetrics & Gynecology*, vol. 57, no. 2, pp. 224–231, 2021.

[6] The WAPM (World Association of Perinatal Medicine) Working Group on COVID-19, G. Saccone, C. Sen et al., "Maternal and perinatal outcomes of pregnant women with SARS-CoV-2 infection," *Ultrasound in Obstetrics & Gynecology*, vol. 57, no. 2, pp. 232–241, 2021.

[7] PAN-COVID investigators and the National Perinatal COVID-19 Registry Study Group, "Pregnancy and neonatal

outcomes of COVID-19: coreporting of common outcomes from PAN-COVID and AAP-SONPM registries," *Ultrasound Obstetrics Gynecol*, vol. 57, no. 4, pp. 573–581, 2021.

[8] I. Gurol-Urganci, J. E. Jardine, F. Carroll et al., "Maternal and perinatal outcomes of pregnant women with SARS-CoV-2 infection at the time of birth in England: national cohort study," *American Journal of Obstetrics and Gynecology*, vol. 225, no. 5, pp. 522.e1–522.e11, 2021.

[9] J. Villar, S. Ariff, R. B. Gunier et al., "Maternal and neonatal morbidity and mortality among pregnant women with and without COVID-19 infection," *JAMA Pediatrics*, vol. 175, no. 8, pp. 817–826, 2021.

[10] S. Q. Wei, M. Bilodeau-Bertrand, S. Liu, and N. Auger, "The impact of COVID-19 on pregnancy outcomes: a systematic review and meta-analysis," *CMAJ*, vol. 193, no. 16, pp. E540–E548, 2021.

[11] R. Sessa, E. Anastasi, G. Brandolino et al., "What is the hidden biological mechanism underlying the possible SARS-CoV-2 vertical transmission? A mini review," *A Mini Review. Front Physiol*, vol. 13, article 875806, 2022.

[12] S. Sinaci, D. F. Ocal, B. Seven et al., "Vertical transmission of SARS-CoV-2: a prospective cross-sectional study from a tertiary center," *Journal of Medical Virology*, vol. 93, no. 10, pp. 5864–5872, 2021.

[13] R. Sessa, L. Masciullo, S. Filardo et al., "SARS-CoV-2 vertical transmission in a twin-pregnant woman: a case report," *International Journal of Infectious Diseases*, vol. 125, no. 22, pp. 192–194, 2022.

[14] R. N. Baergen and D. S. Heller, "Placental pathology in covid-19 positive mothers: preliminary findings," *Pediatric and Developmental Pathology*, vol. 23, no. 3, pp. 177–180, 2020.

[15] E. D. Shanes, L. B. Mithal, S. Otero, H. A. Azad, E. S. Miller, and J. A. Goldstein, "Placental pathology in COVID-19," *American Journal of Clinical Pathology*, vol. 154, no. 1, pp. 23–32, 2020.

[16] M. C. Smithgall, X. Liu-Jarin, D. Hamele-Bena et al., "Third-trimester placentas of severe acute respiratory syndrome coronavirus 2 (SARS-CoV-2)-positive women: histomorphology, including viral immunohistochemistry and in-situ hybridization," *Histopathology*, vol. 77, no. 6, pp. 994–999, 2020.

[17] T. Menter, K. D. Mertz, S. Jiang et al., "Placental pathology findings during and after SARS-CoV-2 infection: features of villitis and malperfusion," *Pathobiology*, vol. 88, no. 1, pp. 69–77, 2021.

[18] L. Debelenko, I. Katsyv, A. M. Chong, L. Peruyero, M. Szabolcs, and A. C. Uhlemann, "Trophoblast damage with acute and chronic intervillositis: disruption of the placental barrier by severe acute respiratory syndrome coronavirus 2," *Human Pathology*, vol. 109, pp. 69–79, 2021.

[19] J. K. Lee, S. J. Oh, H. Park, and O. S. Shin, "Recent updates on research models and tools to study virus-host interactions at the placenta," *Viruses*, vol. 12, p. E5, 2020.

[20] D. A. Schwartz, "Viral infection, proliferation, and hyperplasia of Hofbauer cells and absence of inflammation characterize the placental pathology of fetuses with congenital Zika virus infection," *Archives of Gynecology and Obstetrics*, vol. 295, no. 6, pp. 1361–1368, 2017.

[21] M. He, P. Skaria, K. Kreutz et al., "Histopathology of third trimester placenta from SARS-CoV-2-positive women," *Fetal and pediatric pathology*, vol. 41, no. 3, pp. 403–412, 2020.

[22] J. L. Hecht, B. Quade, and V. Deshpande, "SARS-CoV-2 can infect the placenta and is not associated with specific placental histopathology: a series of 19 placentas from COVID-19-positive mothers," *Modern Pathology*, vol. 2, pp. 1–12, 2020.

[23] M. Gulersen, L. Prasannan, and H. T. Tam, "Histopathologic evaluation of placentas after diagnosis of maternal severe acute respiratory syndrome coronavirus 2 infection," *American journal of obstetrics & gynecology MFM*, vol. 2, no. 4, article 100211, 2020.

[24] P. Zhang, C. Salafia, T. Heyman, C. Salafia, S. Lederman, and B. Dygulska, "Detection of severe acute respiratory syndrome coronavirus 2 in placentas with pathology and vertical transmission," *Am J Obstet Gynecol MFM.*, vol. 2, no. 4, article 100197, 2020.

39

Cultivating the Apprentice-Mentor Model for Minimally Invasive Gynaecology in the Era of Surgically Scarce Training: A Case Report of Laparoscopic Cornuostomy for Interstitial Ectopic Pregnancy by a Trainee

Dave R. Listijono,[1,2] David M. B. Rosen,[1] Sarah Choi,[1] Mujahid Bukhari,[1] Gregory M. Cario,[1] and Danny Chou[1]

[1]*Sydney Women's Endosurgery Centre (SWEC), Sydney, Australia*
[2]*IVF Australia, Sydney, Australia*

Correspondence should be addressed to Dave R. Listijono; d.listijono@unsw.edu.au

Academic Editor: Maria Grazia Porpora

Over the last few years, there is an apparent growing concern amongst O&G trainees of the inadequacy in exposure to minimally invasive gynaecology surgical training, which has been inadvertently compounded by the more stringent working hour regulations and disproportionately increasing number of trainees relative to surgical volume. Therefore, it is vitally important for trainees to maximise opportunities in the operating theatre and develop autonomy in carrying out more complex surgical procedures. This case report outlines the step-by-step approach of laparoscopic excision of a cornual ectopic pregnancy performed by a trainee under the supervision of a surgical mentor. This manuscript highlights key characteristic traits of a trainee that serve to foster surgical trust and simple but effective steps to foster surgical preparedness.

1. Introduction

With the rapidly increasing number of trainees in the specialty of Obstetrics and Gynaecology (O&G) and ongoing restrictions in working hours which, while beneficial from a lifestyle perspective, ultimately limits the volume of surgical procedures and overall experience, the issue of suboptimal surgical exposure amongst trainees is quickly becoming a widespread problem in our specialty, particularly in developed countries [1]. In attempts to overcome this limitation of surgical exposure, trainees have increasingly utilised "lap box trainers" to practice and more recently adapted virtual reality training simulation programs [2, 3], with good effect [4]. Nonetheless, given inadequate allocated time and lack of available curricula, few trainees have truly benefited from this proxy-style practice [5]. Further, a clear disadvantage of simulation training is its deficiency in fostering teamwork and situational decision-making skills [6]. It would therefore seem apparent that real-time primary operation with appropriate guidance remains the most effective form of training to develop surgical competency and autonomy [7, 8]. We hereby present a case report of laparoscopic cornuostomy performed by an O&G trainee, under direct supervision by a gynaecological surgeon consultant, to exemplify the applicability of the apprentice-mentor tenet of surgical education.

Cornual pregnancy (CP) represents a minority (2-4%) of the overall incidence, while carrying the bulk of the morbidity and mortality risk (up to 7 times greater), of ectopic pregnancies [9]. This is in part associated with the anatomical location of the ectopic gestational sac, often proximal to (or within) the interstitial portion of the fallopian tube as it traverses through the muscular wall of the uterus [10] which, in addition to the rich vascular supply of the uterine and ovarian arteries, allows for the tendency to expand prior to rupture, compared to the ampulla segment of the tube, which is commonplace for ectopic pregnancy [9]. With the increasing availability of state-of-the-art equipment and expertise, laparoscopic excision has of late become the first-line approach to surgical management of CP [11]. Compared to conventional laparotomy, laparoscopy has the advantages of improved visualisation, reduced risk of wound dehiscence and blood loss, shorter hospital stay, and faster recovery [12]. Nonetheless, a clear barrier against the uptake of laparoscopic removal of CP remains the technical proficiency required to carry out the procedure [9]. Often touted as a notoriously risky and technically challenging procedure, we present a step-by-step approach to a simple cornuostomy procedure undertaken by an O&G *apprentice* with guidance from a surgical *mentor*.

2. Case

2.1. History, Examination, and Investigations. A 32-year-old woman presented with an ultrasound-confirmed right cornual ectopic pregnancy (Figures 1 and 2) to the emergency department of a tertiary referral hospital. The patient was haemodynamically stable and opted for surgical removal of the ectopic pregnancy via laparoscopy.

2.2. Intraoperative Course. Following general anaesthesia, laparoscopic entry was carried out using the Hasson open technique with a 10 mm umbilical port. Two 5 mm lateral ports and a 10 mm suprapubic port were introduced under direct vision. The right uterine cornua was notably distended by a 4 × 4 cm mass. Following administration of vasopressin (20 IU in 100 mL normal saline) along the base (Figure 3), a single 3 cm curvilinear incision was made on the serosal surface of the mass using monopolar scissors, exposing the underlying gestational sac (Figure 4). The trophoblastic tissue was evacuated, and the specimen was removed via a 10 mm Endo Catch™ bag. Bipolar diathermy was used to obtain haemostasis along the base of the ectopic site. The incision was closed continuously using a V-Loc™ absorbable barbed monofilament suture (Figure 5). The procedure was completed in 45 minutes with an estimated blood loss of 20 mL.

2.3. Postoperative Course. The patient was discharged the following day. Histopathology of the specimen confirmed trophoblastic tissue.

3. Discussion

Anecdotally, most surgeons would agree that laparoscopic management of cornual ectopic pregnancy is considerably complex and challenging; therefore, it would have been plausible for the consultant to opt as the primary operator in most such cases. The above was performed by a 3rd-year O&G trainee for the first time in their career, having previously only seen videos of similar procedures. This case exemplifies the "see one, do one" mantra of traditional surgical education. In the current era, where most O&G trainees are facing unrelenting reduction in surgical volume and exposure, such opportunities are rare and should indeed be cultivated wherever possible. At the heart of surgical training, apprentice-mentor trust is arguably the most important factor in consultants granting trainees increasing levels of autonomy [8, 13]. While *trusting* a trainee to carry out a straightforward low-risk procedure independently may be commonplace amongst supervisors, the extent of supervisor involvement would likely escalate in more complex cases, considering patient safety as the ultimate priority [14]; however, it is in fact in being allowed the opportunity to "safely struggle" that trainees would achieve maximal benefit [13]. To this end, it is imperative for trainees to foster *trustworthiness* and *reliability*.

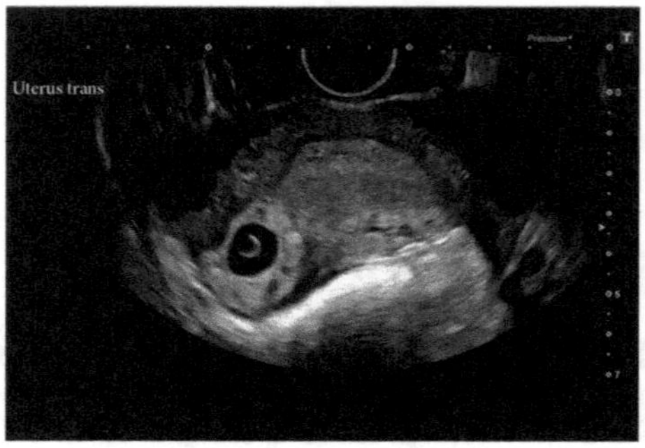

FIGURE 1: Ultrasound image of a right-sided cornual ectopic pregnancy.

3.1. Construct Surgical Trust through Consistent Display of Ownership and Humility. A recent survey of general surgeons on how they judge a trainee's readiness for operative independence revealed that, aside from the perceived risk of the case itself, the trainee's trustworthiness most likely determines a surgeon's decision to entrust the trainee to do the procedure [8]. However, surgeons rarely referred to trust directly, instead, by observation through a variety of actions and behaviours over time. Survey responses obtained from 120 surgeons identified "integrity," along with professionalism and work ethic, as the most important attribute they value in trainees [15]. With increasing concern of litigation and fear of criticism, there is a clear shift in surgical trainees away from taking ownership of their decision-making and inevitable mistakes; instead, shifting the focus more towards promotion-associated behaviours [16]. Such etiquette is in fact counterproductive in instilling a sense of integrity [13]. To this end, trainees ought not to fear committing mistakes but rather cultivate the humility to own, and learn from, their mistakes. Anecdotally, there seems to be a tendency, especially within surgical specialties, for humility to be perceived as a form of weakness or lack of self-confidence; however, it would appear that such view is predominantly held by trainees and more junior surgeons [17]. So, make no mistake, humility in medicine implies maturity and emotional resilience—traits that are highly prized amongst surgeons. If only for the development of their character as human beings, trainees should always strive to cultivate these qualities.

3.2. I Will Prepare and Someday My Chance Will Come. Be that as it may, a trainee's personality trait would likely only serve in the "initiation of trust" where they are allowed to begin the procedure; ultimately, it is their surgical skills and ability to follow intricate instructions that determine whether the *teacher* adopts the "hands-off" or "takes over completely"

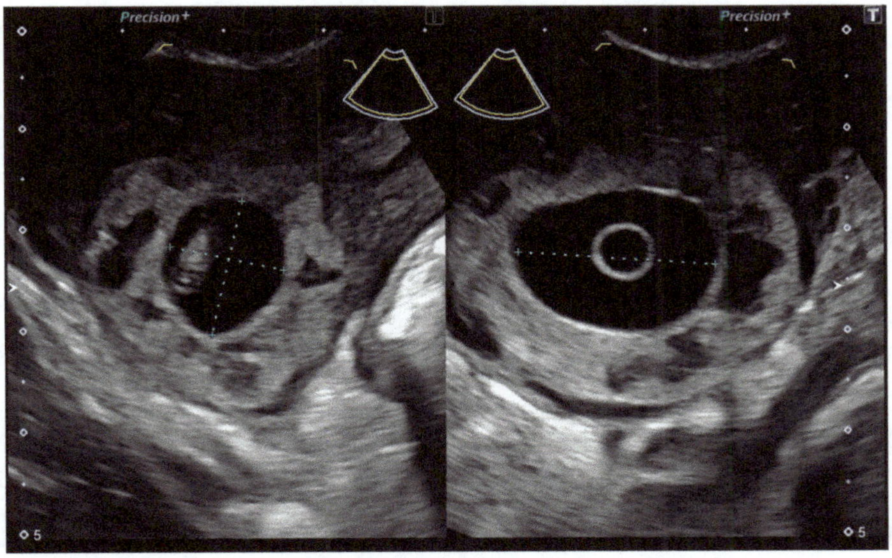

Fetus A		
GA (EDD)	6w4d EDD	15/03/2021
U/S GA	6w4d U/S EDD	15/03/2021
GS	14.9 mm (Rempen) 6w1d	30% title

FIGURE 2: Ultrasound image of the ectopic gestational sac.

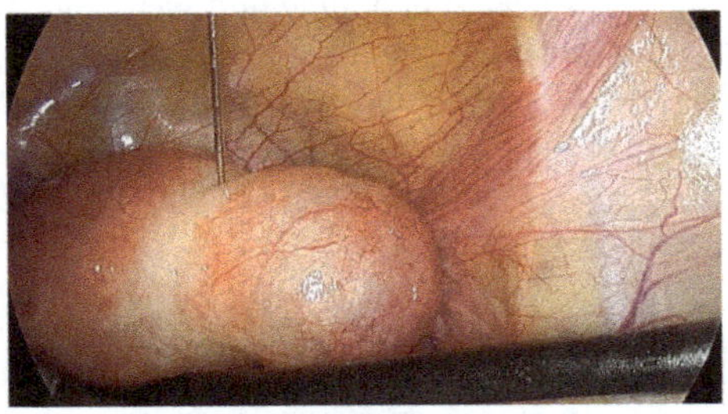

FIGURE 3: Administration of vasopressin at base of ectopic mass, with good vasoconstrictive effect.

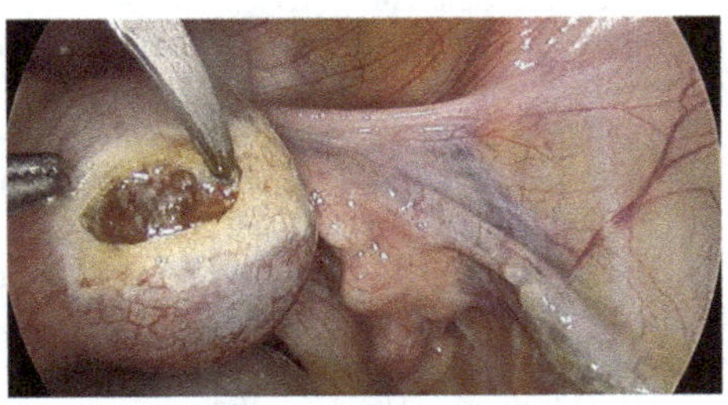

FIGURE 4: Curvilinear incision to the surface of ectopic mass, exposing underlying trophoblastic tissue.

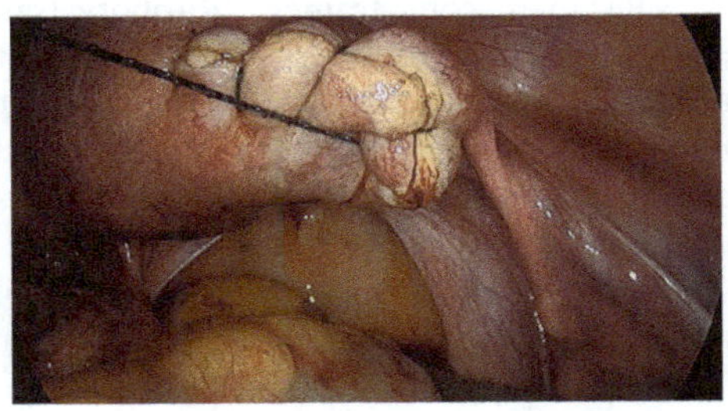

FIGURE 5: Incision was closed using continuous barbed monofilament suture.

approach to supervision [18]. In the operating room (OR), the surgeon educator is constantly faced with the critical balance between supervision, appropriate trainee autonomy, and most importantly patient safety. Studies on factors influencing the level of trainee autonomy in the operating theatre have consistently ranked surgical competency and perception as a "safe proceduralist" as features that would garner sufficient trust for the surgeon to allow the resident to continue with the procedure [8, 19–21]. Therefore, the onus lies on the trainee to place themselves in such favourable positions.

Three fundamental principles that are readily achievable for the trainee include basic understanding of surgical anatomy, familiarity with basic steps of a procedure, and core laparoscopic skills such as knot tying, suturing, and surgical dissection [6]. With working hour restrictions, lack of protected training time, and merciless struggle for operating time amongst trainees, the bulk of these preparations needs to be done outside of working hours and the OR. A simple initial step would be to develop a solid grasp of surgical anatomy through textbooks or focused workshops [22]; indeed, a recent survey of Australian O&G trainees revealed a clear dearth of structured anatomy curricula in the training program [23]. Further, regular review of laparoscopic videos, either open-source or those manually recorded, has also been shown to be useful for skill acquisition amongst gynaecologic residents, particularly in junior learners [24]. However, caution should be exercised in the choice of videos, as there is a clear absence of peer-review process and quality control on most open-source video streaming sites [25]. Trainees should instead be directed towards instructional video

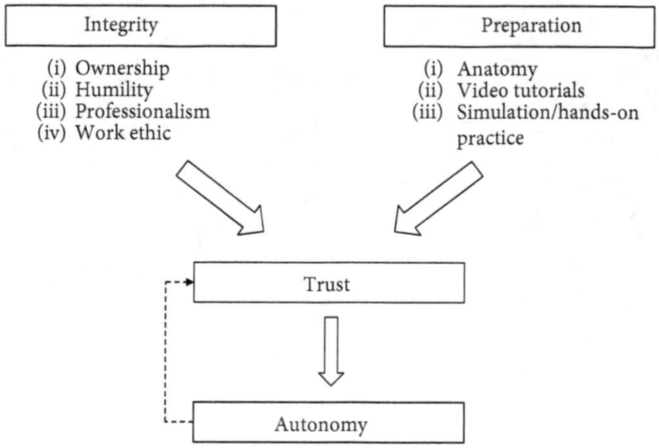

FIGURE 6: Flow chart of our proposed process towards surgical autonomy for trainees.

tutorials from accredited surgical societies [21]. Finally, to develop psychomotor and visuospatial skills involved in core laparoscopic skills, hands-on *deliberate* practice is indispensable; short of being in the OR and "practicing" on patients, this can be achieved through simulation training [26]. Over the past decade, gynaecological surgical simulation has evolved rapidly, offering a myriad of options, including a virtual reality (VR) laparoscopic trainer, VR robotic trainer, and high-fidelity mannequin simulators [26]. However, the simple and inexpensive laparoscopic box trainer has been shown to be noninferior to more costly options and may be the more worthwhile simulation training of choice for trainees [27].

Indeed, the trainee who carried out the above laparoscopic cornuostomy was, from a surgical case logbook standpoint, no more than *average* compared to other trainees of their level, but what separates them from the *average trainee* was their personal dedication to minimally invasive gynaecological surgery (MIGS). This drive resulted in them taking initiative in acquiring a basic laparoscopic box trainer as a junior trainee and consistently practiced core laparoscopic skills in their own time, mostly at home. The trainee also undertook surgical anatomy courses from early on in their residency and a Master's degree to further develop relevant theoretical knowledge. To compensate for limited OT time, the trainee obtained laparoscopic videos from MIGS mentors and regularly study the clips and simulate specific movements (e.g., intracorporeal suturing and needle handling) with the box trainer. To maximise OT exposure, they routinely stayed back following their shift *unpaid*, for the opportunity to observe cases by the hospital's dedicated MIGS team. These actions, as summarised in Figure 6, have effectively placed the trainee-in-question in a far more favourable position than their peers, not only from a theoretical knowledge and surgical skills perspective but more importantly, by demonstrating outstanding work ethic and professionalism to prospective MIGS *mentors*—one of whom happen to be the supervising surgeon in the above case.

4. Conclusion

The concepts described in this manuscript are by no means groundbreaking, neither is it particularly unique for an O&G trainee to perform laparoscopic cornuostomy. In reporting this case, we endeavour to highlight firstly a relatively *uncomplicated* step-by-step approach to managing a potentially *complicated* surgical case and, in addition, key strategies for current trainees to draw on every opportunity as they navigate through this era of surgically scarce O&G training. The age-old apprenticeship model of gynaecological surgical training is very much alive and well, and it is up to trainees to utilise available tools to optimise training outside of the OR and align themselves with character traits to engender trust in their surgeon mentors.

References

[1] E. L. Moss, F. E. Bredaki, P. W. Jones, J. Hollingworth, D. M. Luesley, and K. K. Chan, "Is gynaecological surgical training a cause for concern? A questionnaire survey of trainees and trainers," *BMC Medical Education*, vol. 11, no. 1, pp. 1–7, 2011.

[2] D. L. Diesen, L. Erhunmwunsee, K. M. Bennett et al., "Effectiveness of laparoscopic computer simulator versus usage of box trainer for endoscopic surgery training of novices," *Journal of Surgical Education*, vol. 68, no. 4, pp. 282–289, 2011.

[3] B. H. Van Duren and G. I. van Boxel, "Use your phone to build a simple laparoscopic trainer," *Journal of Minimal Access Surgery*, vol. 10, no. 4, pp. 219-220, 2014.

[4] E. Wilson, S. Janssens, L. A. McLindon, D. G. Hewett, B. Jolly, and M. Beckmann, "Improved laparoscopic skills in gynaecology trainees following a simulation-training program using take-home box trainers," *The Australian & New Zealand Journal of Obstetrics & Gynaecology*, vol. 59, no. 1, pp. 110–116, 2019.

[5] E. Wilson, S. Janssens, D. Hewett, B. Jolly, and M. Beckmann, "Simulation training in obstetrics and gynaecology: what's happening on the frontline?," *The Australian & New Zealand Journal of Obstetrics & Gynaecology*, vol. 56, no. 5, pp. 496–502, 2016.

[6] S. V. Kotsis and K. C. Chung, "Application of the "see one, do one, teach one" concept in surgical training," *Plastic and Reconstructive Surgery*, vol. 131, no. 5, pp. 1194–1201, 2013.

[7] D. J. Cassidy, S. K. McKinley, J. Ogunmuyiwa et al., "Surgical autonomy: a resident perspective and the balance of teacher development with operative independence," *American Journal of Surgery*, vol. S0002-9610, no. 20, p. 30664, 2020.

[8] S. Y. Salim, M. Govaerts, and J. White, "The construction of surgical trust," *Annals of Surgery*, vol. 271, no. 2, pp. 391–398, 2020.

[9] N. S. Moawad, S. T. Mahajan, M. H. Moniz, S. E. Taylor, and W. W. Hurd, "Current diagnosis and treatment of interstitial pregnancy," *American Journal of Obstetrics and Gynecology*, vol. 202, no. 1, pp. 15–29, 2010.

[10] T. Tulandi and D. Al-Jaroudi, "Interstitial pregnancy: results generated from the Society of Reproductive Surgeons Registry," *Obstetrics and Gynecology*, vol. 103, no. 1, pp. 47–50, 2004.

[11] V. B. Bayyarapu and S. R. Gundabattula, "Diagnosis and management of 'cornual' pregnancies from 2002 to 2015 at a tertiary referral centre in South India: insights from introspection," *Journal of Obstetrics and Gynaecology of India*, vol. 67, no. 6, pp. 414–420, 2017.

[12] R. Baumann, A. L. Magos, and A. Turnbull, "Prospective comparison of videopelviscopy with laparotomy for ectopic pregnancy," *BJOG*, vol. 98, no. 8, pp. 765–771, 1991.

[13] G. Sandhu, C. P. Magas, A. B. Robinson, C. P. Scally, and R. M. Minter, "Progressive entrustment to achieve resident autonomy in the operating room," *Annals of Surgery*, vol. 265, no. 6, pp. 1134–1140, 2017.

[14] L. Torbeck, A. Wilson, J. Choi, and G. L. Dunnington, "Identification of behaviors and techniques for promoting autonomy in the operating room," *Surgery*, vol. 158, no. 4, pp. 1102–1112, 2015.

[15] P. Mankowski, D. Demsey, E. Brown, and A. Knox, "Resident behaviours to prioritize according to Canadian plastic surgeons," *Plastic Surgery*, vol. 28, no. 3, pp. 148–155, 2020.

[16] A. Nishii, J. Burdine, N. Matusko et al., "Identification of promotion and prevention associated surgeon behaviors in the operating room to facilitate resident self-regulated learning," *American Journal of Surgery*, 2020.

[17] D. M. Elfenbein, "Confidence crisis among general surgery residents," *JAMA Surgery*, vol. 151, no. 12, pp. 1166–1175, 2016.

[18] C. A. Moulton, G. Regehr, L. Lingard, C. Merritt, and H. MacRae, "Operating from the other side of the table: control dynamics and the surgeon educator," *Journal of the American College of Surgeons*, vol. 210, no. 1, pp. 79–86, 2010.

[19] B. Q. Smith, I. Woelfel, R. Salani, A. Harzman, and X. Chen, "Resident self-entrustment and expectations of autonomy: OB>GYN?," *Journal of Surgical Education*, vol. 78, no. 1, pp. 275–281, 2020.

[20] G. J. Kim, M. J. Clark, S. L. Meyerson et al., "Mind the gap: the autonomy perception gap in the operating room by surgical residents and faculty," *Journal of Surgical Education*, vol. 77, no. 6, pp. 1522–1527, 2020.

[21] H. E. Hoops, C. Haley, M. R. Cook, and O. Lopez, "Factors influencing amount of guidance in the operating room during laparoscopic cases," *American Journal of Surgery*, vol. 217, no. 5, pp. 979–985, 2019.

[22] D. M. Koppes, C. P. R. Triepels, A. N. Schepens-Franke et al., "What do we need to know about anatomy in gynaecology: a Delphi consensus study," *European Journal of Obstetrics, Gynecology, and Reproductive Biology*, vol. 245, pp. 56–63, 2020.

[23] J. Sgroi and J. Abbott, "Surgical anatomy in obstetrics and gynaecology: the trainee's perspective," *The Australian & New Zealand Journal of Obstetrics & Gynaecology*, vol. 54, no. 2, pp. 172–176, 2014.

[24] N. B. Rindos, M. Wroble-Biglan, A. Ecker, T. T. Lee, and N. M. Donnellan, "Impact of video coaching on gynecologic resident laparoscopic suturing: a randomized controlled trial," *Journal of Minimally Invasive Gynecology*, vol. 24, no. 3, pp. 426–431, 2017.

[25] H. A. Rodriguez, M. T. Young, H. T. Jackson, B. K. Oelschlager, and A. S. Wright, "Viewer discretion advised: is YouTube a friend or foe in surgical education?," *Surgical Endoscopy*, vol. 32, no. 4, pp. 1724–1728, 2018.

[26] K. Wohlrab, E. Jelovsek, and D. Myers, "Incorporating simulation into gynecologic surgical training," *American Journal of Obstetrics and Gynecology*, vol. 217, no. 5, pp. 522–526, 2017.

[27] M. M. Li and J. George, "A systematic review of low-cost laparoscopic simulators," *Surgical Endoscopy*, vol. 31, no. 1, pp. 38–48, 2017.

40

Treatment of Cervical Pregnancy with Ultrasound-Guided Intragestational Injection of Methotrexate: A Case Report

Angeliki Rouvali,[1] Panagiotis Vlastarakos,[1] Sofoklis Stavros,[1] Maria Giourga,[1] Kalliopi Pappa,[1] Angeliki Gerede,[2] Alexandros Rodolakis,[1] and Ekaterini Domali[1]

[1] *1st Department of Obstetrics and Gynaecology, Alexandra Hospital, National and Kapodistrian University of Athens, Athens, Greece*
[2] *Department of Obstetrics and Gynecology Democritus, University of Thrace Alexandroupolis, Greece*

Correspondence should be addressed to Panagiotis Vlastarakos; pan.vlastarakos@gmail.com

Academic Editor: Maria Grazia Piccioni

This study is aimed at describing a noninvasive conservative strategy to the treatment of cervical pregnancy and highlighting the success of ultrasound-guided therapeutic techniques. A 43-year-old woman with a history of one previous cesarean section presented in our unit with vaginal spotting and a positive urine pregnancy test. She was diagnosed with a cervical pregnancy, and she was successfully treated conservatively with the administration of intragestational sac methotrexate under ultrasound guidance. Cervical pregnancy is a rare form of ectopic pregnancy that results from conceptus implantation in the cervical canal. The main concern is the associated life-threatening hemorrhage and subsequent need for urgent hysterectomy. The evolution of ultrasound over the past decades has enabled early diagnosis and has shifted the management from a radical surgical approach towards a stepwise conservative therapeutic approach, when possible.

1. Introduction

A cervical ectopic pregnancy occurs when a blastocyst implant in the endocervical canal. Cervical pregnancies are relatively uncommon, and it is estimated that they account for less than one percent of all ectopic pregnancies [1]. Although this condition is rare, it has been associated with high morbidity due to the risk of major fatal hemorrhage. Early diagnosis of cervical implantation is crucial for the subsequent management that should minimize the risk of hemorrhage, eliminate the gestational tissue, and spare fertility. Nowadays, transvaginal ultrasound allows the diagnosis of cervical ectopic pregnancies at early stages, thus increasing the chances of success with medical treatment.

Although there is no consensus about the appropriate treatment of cervical pregnancies, conservative management is preferred [2, 3] in asymptomatic or minimally symptomatic and hemodynamically stable patients, leaving more radical surgical approaches such as hysterectomy for unstable patients with life-threatening symptoms and/or failure of a conservative approach. In this paper, we describe a case of cervical pregnancy which was successfully treated with ultrasound-guided intragestational sac methotrexate injection in our unit.

2. Case Presentation

A 43-year-old woman (gravida 2, para 1, cesarean section 1) presented in the Early Pregnancy Unit (EPU) with nausea and one-day history of painless vaginal spotting. Her last menstrual period was five weeks before admission, and she had a positive urine pregnancy test. She reported regular menstrual cycles, and she was not using any contraception. Her past medical history was unremarkable, and she had a cesarean section 13 years ago from her surgical history. She was a non-smoker, and her body mass index was (BMI) was 20.9 kg/m^2. Upon arrival, she was hemodynamically stable with hemoglobin of 11.2 g/dL. White blood count, platelets, liver,

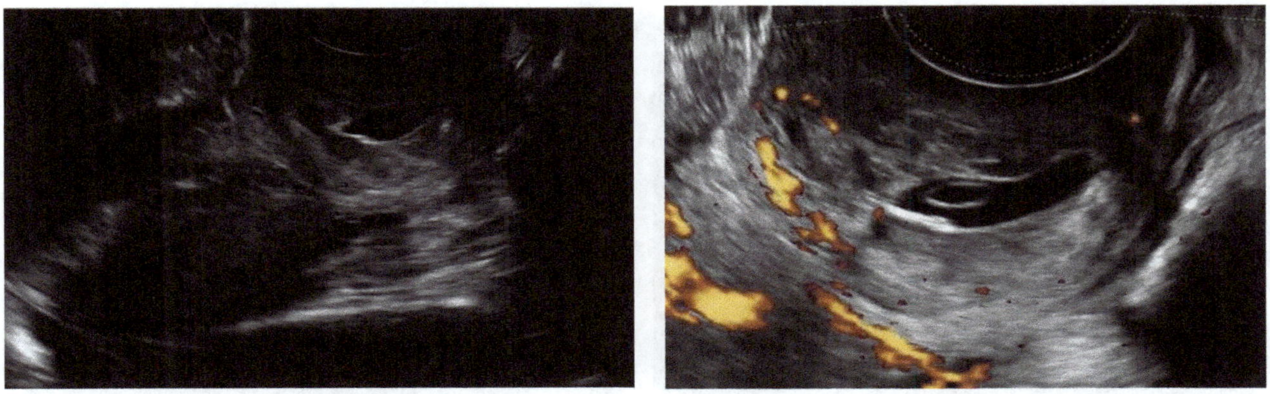

(a) (b)

FIGURE 1: Cervical pregnancy at presentation (a) 2D transvaginal sonography in sagittal view shows an empty uterine cavity and closed internal os with ballooned cervical canal containing gestational tissue with (b) evidence of peritrophoblastic vascularity.

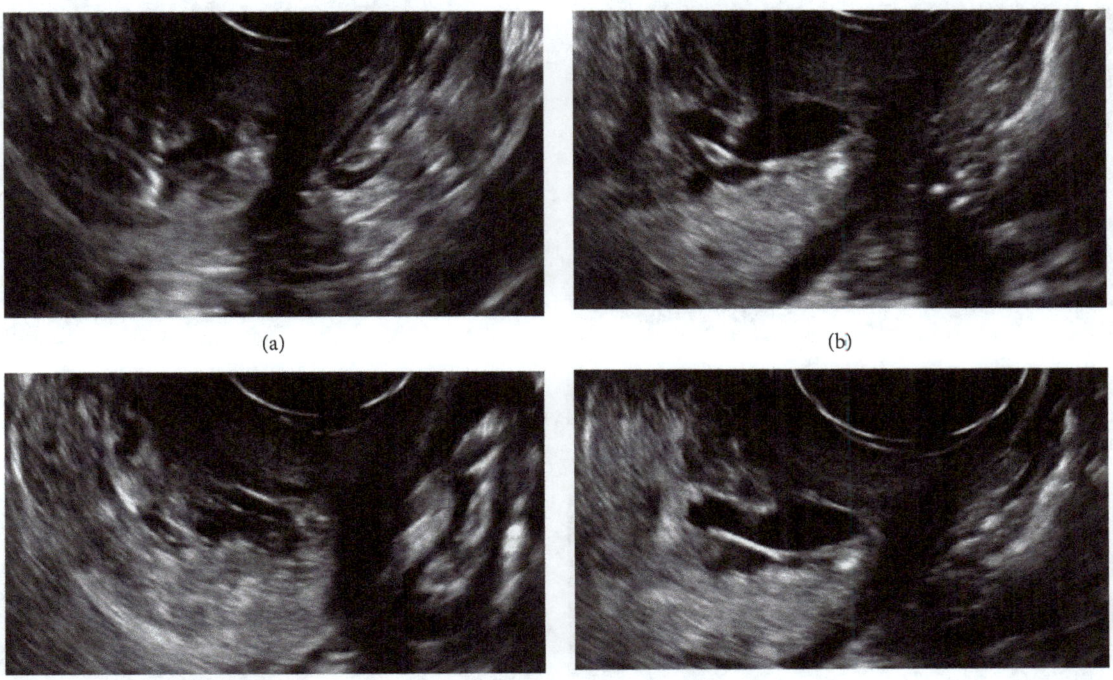

(a) (b) (c) (d)

FIGURE 2: Transabdominal puncture using a 17-gauge needle under transvaginal ultrasound guidance. Aspiration of (a, b) gestational content followed by (c, d) local methotrexate administration.

and renal function tests were all normal. The initial serum beta chorionic gonadotropin (β-hCG) level was 25.270 mIU/mL.

On physical examination, her abdomen was soft and nontender. A gentle speculum examination revealed a hyperemic cervix with gestational tissue on the anterior lip of the external cervical os and no active bleeding. Transvaginal ultrasound showed an empty uterine cavity with thick endometrial lining and a ballooned cervical canal with a gestational sac containing a yolk sac in the lower portion of the cervix and an absent "sliding sign" (Figure 1(a)). The use of Color Doppler studies showed extensive blood flow to the gestational sac (Figure 1(b)). Both ovaries were normal, and there was no evidence of free fluid. Thus, a diagnosis of cervical pregnancy was established.

Following a thorough discussion with the patient, informed consent was obtained to treat with ultrasound-guided methotrexate injection at the implantation site. Under general anesthesia, a local 75 mg dose of methotrexate was injected into the gestational sac using a 17-gauge needle (Chiba Needle, Cook Medical) under transvaginal ultrasound guidance with

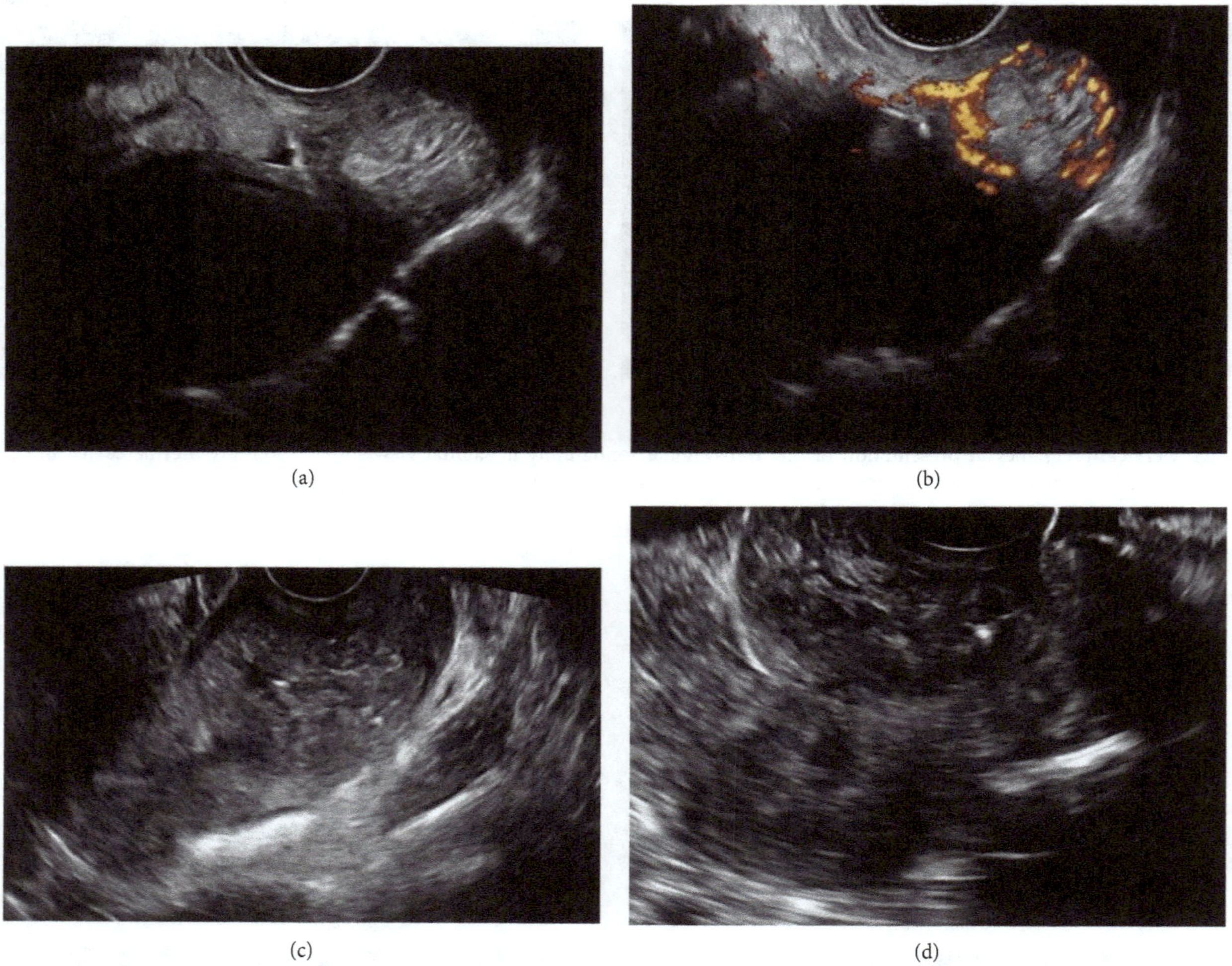

Figure 3: (a, b) 16 days posttreatment, β-hCG levels 3.689 mIU/mL, (c) 28 days posttreatment, β-hCG levels 305.7 mIU/mL, and (d) 31 days posttreatment, β-hCG levels 86.4 mIU/mL.

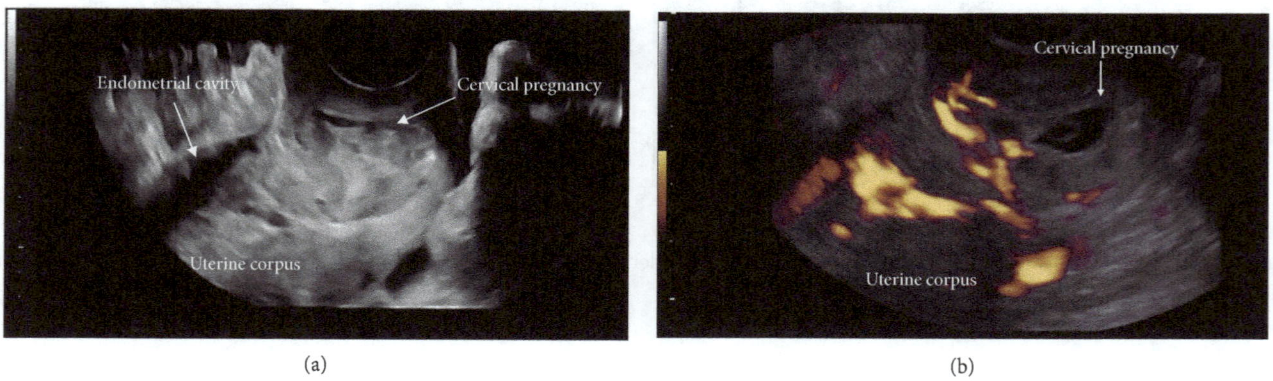

Figure 4: Cervical ectopic pregnancy in (a) 2D and (b) 3D transvaginal ultrasound.

a prior aspiration of the gestational sac's fluid content to reduce pregnancy volume (Figure 2).

The therapeutic effect was assessed by serial monitoring of β-hCG levels on days one, four, and seven and transvaginal ultrasound. Posttreatment, the patient remained clinically stable, and the spotting subsided. There were no side effects associated with methotrexate administration. There was a slight decrease of β-hCG levels on day one and a plateau on day four, 22.605 mIU/mL and 23.136 mIU/mL, respectively. On day seven, β-hCG dropped to 20.075 mIU/mL and the patient was discharged. A weekly follow-up was arranged in the Early Pregnancy Unit (EPU) on an outpatient basis.

During four weeks of follow-up (EPU), the patient remained asymptomatic and serum β-hCG levels decreased steadily from 3.689 mIU/mL on day 16 (Figures 3(a) and

3(b)) to 4 mIU/mL on day 46. Transvaginal ultrasound findings were suggestive of gestational sac regression (Figure 3).

3. Discussion

Cervical ectopic pregnancy is a rare entity that accounts for a small proportion of all ectopic pregnancies, and the reported incidence is approximately one per 10.000 live births [4]. It occurs when a fertilized ovum implants in the lining of the endocervix below the internal os level. Cervical pregnancy can be a life-threatening condition, and early diagnosis and treatment are essential to preserve fertility and avoid the need for hysterectomy.

The pathogenesis of ectopic pregnancy remains unclear. Prior dilatation and curettage and cesarean section have been reported as predisposing factors, possibly causing damage to the endometrial lining and the cervix [4]. Another theory suggests a rapid crossing of the fertilized ovum to the cervical canal before it is capable of implantation [5]. Cervical ectopic pregnancies have also been associated with assisted reproductive techniques [6].

Most commonly, patients with cervical ectopic pregnancy present with painless vaginal bleeding, and less than one-third of them experience lower abdominal pain [6].

Diagnosis of cervical ectopic pregnancy is based on clinical examination and ultrasound findings in a patient with a positive pregnancy test. Differential diagnosis, especially from an incomplete miscarriage or a cesarean section scar pregnancy, can be challenging. Ultrasound diagnostic criteria include (a) empty uterine cavity, (b) hourglass uterine shape with ballooned cervical canal, (c) the presence of gestational sac or placental tissue within the cervical canal, (d) absent "sliding sign," and (e) high peritrophoblastic vascularity on Doppler examination [7].

Also, the use of three-dimensional (3D) ultrasound imaging in addition to two-dimensional (2D) scan (Figure 4) may provide additional information from the coronal section and help towards the correct diagnosis of cervical pregnancy [8, 9].

There is a wide array of therapeutic options for cervical ectopic pregnancy, varying from conservative drug therapies to radical surgical procedures. The optimal treatment method depends on the gestational age at the time of diagnosis, the clinical manifestation and its severity, the presence of coexisting viable intrauterine pregnancy, and clinician's experience.

Among the conservative management options, the use of methotrexate has revolutionized the treatment of cervical ectopic pregnancies. In cervical pregnancies, methotrexate can be administered systemically (single- or multidose regimen) with high treatment success; however, if gestational age is >9weeks, $\beta-\mathrm{hCG}$ levels > 10.000 IU/L, fetal cardiac activity is present, and failure rates are higher [10]. Local methotrexate injection has also been proved successful and is the proposed first-line option in cervical ectopic pregnancies with fetal cardiac activity [2]. Alternatively, potassium chloride (KCL) injection can be used as a first step [11]. Some authors suggest that curettage is necessary to reduce severe hemorrhage associated with trophoblastic shedding from the atonic cervix that occurs as a metabolic effect of methotrexate [10, 12].

Other approaches that can be used in conjunction with drug therapies or if medical treatments fail to reduce the risk of bleeding include uterine artery embolization, Foley catheter balloon tamponade [13], suction evacuation, high cervical cerclage, dilatation and curettage, and ligation of cervicovaginal branches of the uterine arteries at third and ninth o'clock positions of the cervix [14].

4. Conclusion

Although cervical ectopic pregnancy is a rare event, delay in diagnosis or misdiagnosis can be detrimental for the patient with life-threatening consequences. The introduction of EPUs and the widespread use of transvaginal ultrasound means that recognizing this condition is feasible early in pregnancy. Early detection enables the use of conservative therapeutic options. Intragestational injection of methotrexate with posttreatment surveillance in clinically stable patients is an effective and safe approach that preserves fertility.

Consent

Written informed consent was obtained from the patient for publication of this case report and accompanying images. A copy of the written consent is available for review by the Editor-in-Chief of this journal on request.

References

[1] J. Bouyer, J. Coste, H. Fernandez, J. L. Pouly, and N. Job-Spira, "Sites of ectopic pregnancy: a 10 year population-based study of 1800 cases," *Human Reproduction*, vol. 17, no. 12, pp. 3224–3230, 2002.

[2] E. Kirk, G. Condous, Z. Haider, A. Syed, K. Ojha, and T. Bourne, "The conservative management of cervical ectopic pregnancies," *Ultrasound in Obstetrics & Gynecology*, vol. 27, no. 4, pp. 430–437, 2006.

[3] S. H. Bakour, P. K. Thompson, and K. S. Khan, "Successful conservative management of cervical ectopic pregnancy with combination of methotrexate, mifepristone, surgical evacuation and tamponade using a double balloon three-way catheter," *Journal of Obstetrics and Gynaecology*, vol. 25, no. 6, pp. 616–618, 2005.

[4] G. Vela and T. Tulandi, "Cervical pregnancy: the importance of early diagnosis and treatment," *Journal of Minimally Invasive Gynecology*, vol. 14, no. 4, pp. 481–484, 2007.

[5] W. Studdiford, "Cervical pregnancy: a partial review of the literature and a report of two probable cases," *American Journal of Obstetrics and Gynecology*, vol. 49, no. 2, pp. 169–185, 1945.

[6] E. S. Ginsburg, M. C. Frates, M. S. Rein, J. H. Fox, M. D. Hornstein, and A. J. Friedman, "Early diagnosis and treatment of cervical pregnancy in an in vitro fertilization program," *Fertility and Sterility*, vol. 61, no. 5, pp. 966–969, 1994.

[7] D. Jurkovic, E. Hacket, and S. Campbell, "Diagnosis and treatment of early cervical pregnancy: a review and a report of two cases treated conservatively," *Ultrasound in Obstetrics & Gynecology*, vol. 8, no. 6, pp. 373–380, 1996.

[8] R. Ruano, F. Reya, O. Picone et al., "Three-dimensional ultrasonographic diagnosis of a cervical pregnancy," *Clinics (São Paulo, Brazil)*, vol. 61, no. 4, pp. 355–358, 2006.

[9] D. Jurkovic, A. Geipel, K. Gruboeck, E. Jauniaux, M. Natucci, and S. Campbell, "Three-dimensional ultrasound for the assessment of uterine anatomy and detection of congenital anomalies: a comparison with hysterosalpingography and two-dimensional sonography," *Ultrasound in Obstetrics & Gynecology*, vol. 5, no. 4, pp. 233–237, 1995.

[10] T. H. Hung, W. Y. Shau, T. T. Hsieh, J. J. Hsu, Y. K. Soong, and C. J. Jeng, "Prognostic factors for an unsatisfactory primary methotrexate treatment of cervical pregnancy: a quantitative review," *Human Reproduction*, vol. 13, no. 9, pp. 2636–2642, 1998.

[11] C. J. Jeng, M. L. Ko, and J. Shen, "Transvaginal ultrasound-guided treatment of cervical pregnancy," *Obstetrics and Gynecology*, vol. 109, no. 5, pp. 1076–1082, 2007.

[12] S. Mesogitis, A. Pilalis, G. Daskalakis, N. Papantoniou, and A. Antsaklis, "Management of early viable cervical pregnancy," *BJOG : An International Journal of Obstetrics and Gynaecology*, vol. 112, no. 4, pp. 409–411, 2005.

[13] D. L. Fylstra, "Cervical pregnancy: 13 cases treated with suction curettage and balloon tamponade," *American Journal of Obstetrics and Gynecology*, vol. 210, no. 6, pp. 581.e1–581.e5, 2014.

[14] E. S. Saygili Yilmaz, D. Aydin, and Z. Yilmaz, "Conservative treatment of cervical pregnancy by evacuation after transvaginal suture ligation of the cervicovaginal branches of uterine arteries," *Acta Obstetricia et Gynecologica Scandinavica*, vol. 81, no. 10, pp. 988–990, 2002.

41

Monochorionic Diamniotic Vasa Previa Pregnancy: A Medical Student Perspective

Joshua M. Samuel, Fatima Ali, Jonathan Faro, and Jonathan D. Baum

Department of Obstetrics and Gynecology, Jersey Shore Medical Center, Neptune, NJ 07754, USA

Correspondence should be addressed to Joshua M. Samuel; jsamuel5@sgu.edu

Academic Editor: Maria Grazia Porpora

Monochorionic diamniotic twins and vasa previa are uncommon. We present a case that was followed from ultrasound diagnosis to delivery.

1. Introduction

Vasa previa is a vascular pathology of the placenta where unprotected fetal vessels are in close proximity to the cervix. Labor is avoided as cervical dilation with rupture of membranes can lead to disruption of these vessels and rapid exsanguination of the fetus. The first report of this rare condition dates back to 1801, while diagnosis via ultrasound was first reported in 1987 [1].

Although uncommon, the incidence of vasa previa may be increasing due to the availability of high-quality ultrasonography [2]. Vasa previa affects up to 1 : 2500 pregnancies [3]. Twin gestation, specifically monochorionic diamniotic twins, occurs in 1 : 300 pregnancies [4]. This case is presented from a medical student perspective during subinternship at a community teaching hospital.

2. Case

The patient is a 29-year-old G3P0111 with monochorionic diamniotic twins diagnosed with vasa previa by transvaginal ultrasound at 16-week gestation (Figure 1). Her prior pregnancy was complicated by preterm labor and delivery at 36-week gestation. The current pregnancy was otherwise uneventful, and the plan was for inpatient observation starting at 30 weeks with planned cesarean delivery to avoid labor.

At 29-week gestation, the patient presented with preterm contractions. Betamethasone was administered for fetal organ maturation, and magnesium sulfate was given for neuroprotection. She had persistent preterm contractions with cervical effacement, and therefore, cesarean delivery was indicated. During the low transverse hysterotomy, unprotected umbilical vessels were visualized. Amniotomy was performed while avoiding these vessels, and clear amniotic fluid was noted. Twin male neonates were delivered with Apgar scores 8/8 and birth weights of 1.26 kg and 1.33 kg for A and B, respectively. Both twins were evaluated and admitted to the NICU. Cord gases and hemoglobin for both twins were normal.

The remainder of the surgery was uncomplicated. Gross inspection of the placenta and membranes confirmed vasa previa affecting both fetuses (see Figures 2 and 3). Placental pathology confirmed membranous insertion of the umbilical cord for twin A and twin B. The postpartum course was unremarkable, and NICU courses for infants were typical for gestational age. At the time of this writing, both twins are doing well and meeting appropriate milestones.

3. Discussion

Early anatomy ultrasound at 16-week gestation showed abnormal fetal vessels in relation to the placenta, consistent

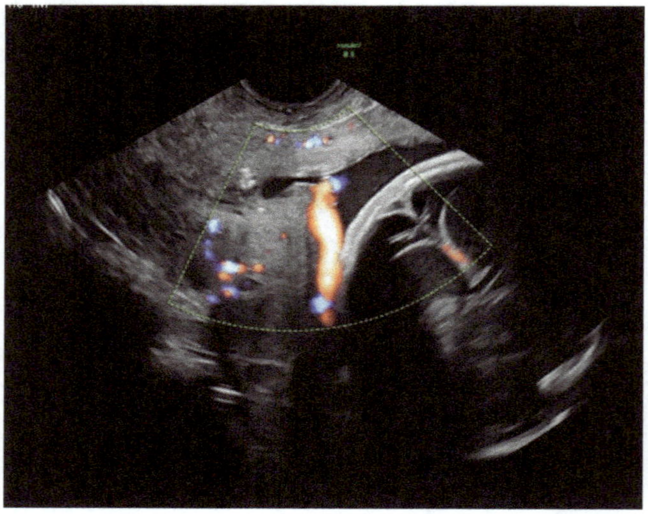

Figure 1: Transvaginal ultrasound image at 16 weeks showing vasa previa.

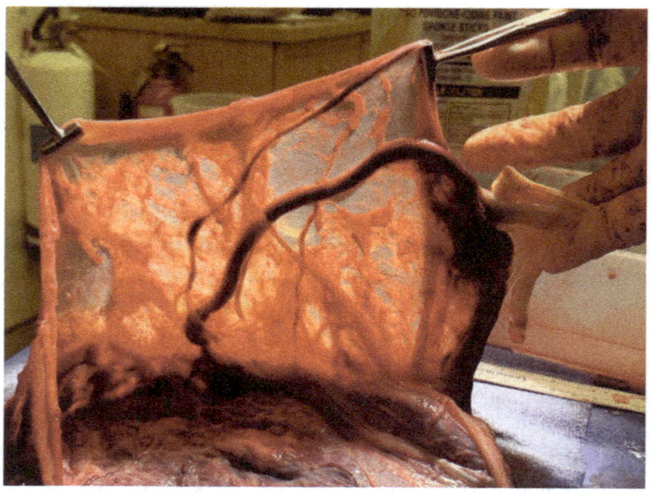

Figure 2: Gross specimen showing vasa previa affecting twin A.

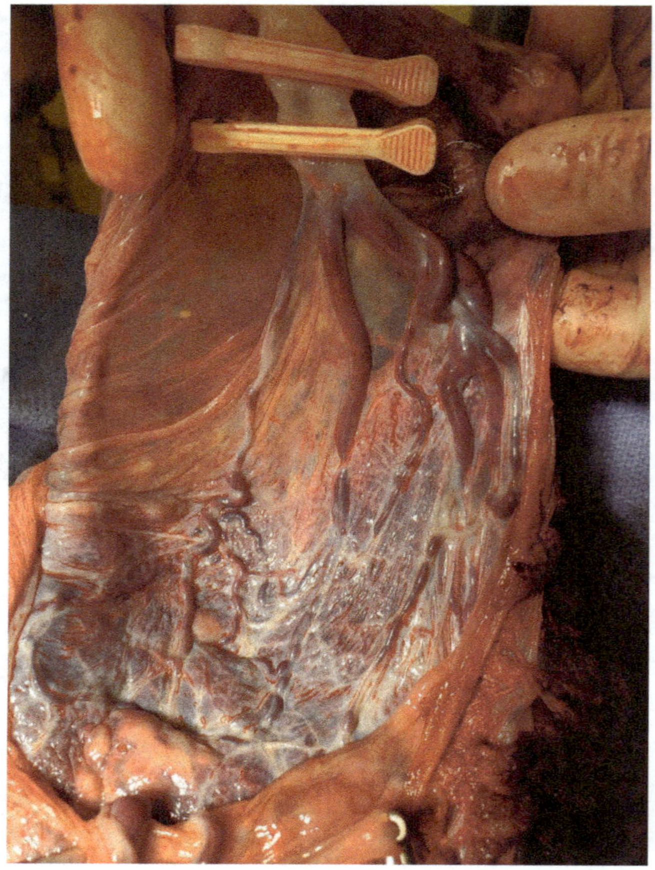

Figure 3: Gross specimen showing vasa previa affecting twin B.

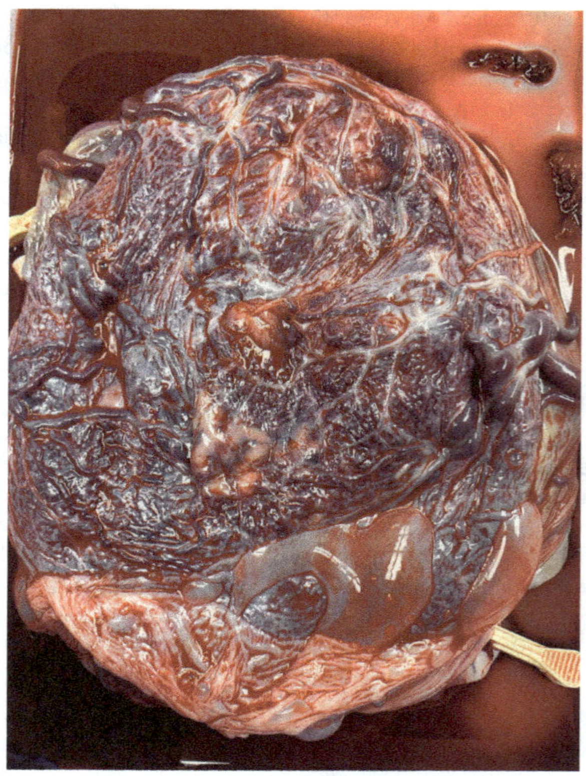

Figure 4: The placenta of the monochorionic diamniotic twins.

with vasa previa. Fetal anatomy was normal. The findings were discussed with the patient, highlighting the proximity of the fetal vessels to her cervix.

While vasa previa remains uncommon, the rate of diagnosis has increased due to the availability of high-quality ultrasonography. Furthermore, 10% of vasa previa cases are diagnosed in twin pregnancies [5].

This placental abnormality is problematic because of the location of the unprotected vessels. If the fetal head compresses these vessels, it can result in fetal hypoperfusion and acidemia [6]. Vessel rupture will lead to fetal hemorrhage, and therefore, early diagnosis is critical, highlighting the importance of ultrasound [7]. The Society of Maternal-Fetal Medicine (SMFM) recommends routine ultrasound of the lower uterine segment and the placenta during the second trimester. If vasa previa is suspected, transvaginal ultrasound with color Doppler is performed. Pulsations consistent with the fetal heart rate confirm the diagnosis [8]. Prenatal diagnosis improves outcome with neonatal survival rates up to

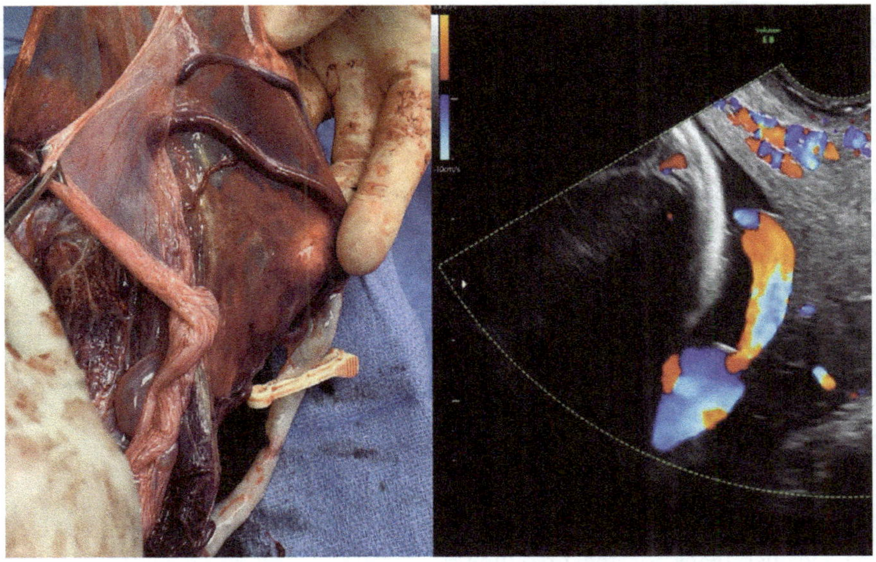

Figure 5: Gross image of the placenta with corresponding ultrasound. Ultrasound image shows proximity of fetal vessel to cervix.

97%. With a postnatal diagnosis, neonatal survival decreases to less than 50% [9].

There are no guidelines on elective hospitalization for vasa previa. A recent case series showed it might be lifesaving [10]. Delivery for pregnancies complicated by vasa previa is recommended between 34 and 37 weeks to balance the risk of premature rupture of membranes, fetal hemorrhage, and death versus the risks of prematurity [11]. Given our patient's history of preterm labor and current monochorionic/diamniotic twin pregnancy, she was at increased risk for preterm delivery. Therefore, intervention on the earlier part of the recommended range was advised. The initial plan was in-hospital observation at 30-week gestation with cesarean delivery at 34 weeks.

Usually, a twin pregnancy is more than enough to excite any medical student. I remember the night this patient with twins was admitted in preterm labor. She had monochorionic diamniotic twins with vasa previa that was diagnosed in her second trimester. To the patient, everything was going as planned. To the medical student, she was a rare case that turned into a great learning opportunity. So many thoughts ran through my mind: will her contractions stop, would she hemorrhage, would the twins be okay?

Labor rooms were full, and I had "magnesium notes" to write—one of the few responsibilities delegated to medical students. I will never forget the emergency cesarean delivery that was suddenly necessary. I recalled how quickly everyone worked to get this patient into the operating room. I was immediately told to scrub in, with no time to prepare. Within a few minutes, the twins were delivered almost three months before their due date and were given immediately to the pediatric team.

While the twins were tended to, we delivered the placenta, which appeared strikingly different from the other placentas. "Why does the placenta look like this?" I asked the attending as I continued to stare at the spongy vascular mass (Figure 4). "What you see here is called vasa previa, and this is why this patient needed surgery right away," stated my attending (coauthor). He put the specimen in a bucket and handed it to the surgical tech, who placed it on a nearby table. As the attending started the process of "closing," I stepped away from the operating table to take a closer look.

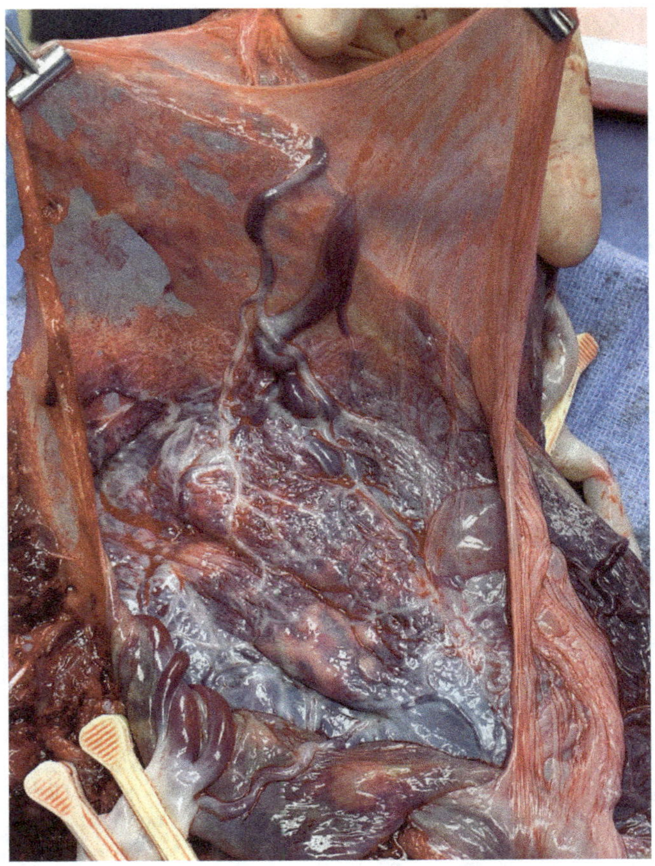

Figure 6: Gross image of the specimen showing vessels passing through the amnion as well as the unprotected insertion of umbilical cord.

The vessels were large, engorged, and unprotected. It was unusual; even the OBGYN residents were fascinated. While they examined the specimen, I heard the two babies cry—a reassuring sound in any delivery room. I looked towards the warmer, where a team of pediatric residents and attendings were assessing the babies. Now, I understood why this patient needed an emergent cesarean delivery.

This case highlighted the importance of ultrasound played in this patient's management. The transvaginal ultrasound with Doppler at 16-week gestation (Figure 5) illustrated the proximity of fetal vessels to the cervix. This information complicated an already high-risk pregnancy and determined the route and timing of delivery. The gross specimen shows the vessels coursing through the amnion and the unprotected insertion of the umbilical cord (Figure 6).

Reflecting on my third- and fourth-year rotations, this is the most exciting case I was a part of. The look of joy on the patient's face when she saw her twins for the first time inspired me to write this medical student perspective.

4. Conclusion

This paper discusses a clinical case observed during a fourth-year subinternship rotation, focusing primarily on how this patient was diagnosed with vasa previa via ultrasound, the management, and the final clinical outcome.

References

[1] K. Norvilaitė, A. Peštenytė, D. Bužinskienė et al., "Vasa praevia: a case report and literature review," *Acta Medica Lituanica*, vol. 23, no. 1, pp. 11–16, 2016.

[2] N. Donnolley, L. E. Halliday, and Y. Oyelese, "Vasa praevia: a descriptive review of existing literature and the evolving role of ultrasound in prenatal screening," *Australasian Journal of Ultrasound in Medicine*, vol. 16, no. 2, pp. 71–76, 2013.

[3] G. Coleman and H. Venables, "Is ultrasound screening for vasa praevia clinically justified and a financially viable screening test? A literature review," *Ultrasound (Leeds, England)*, vol. 26, no. 1, pp. 6–15, 2018.

[4] L. Lewi, "Monochorionic diamniotic twins: what do I tell the prospective parents?," *Prenatal Diagnosis*, vol. 40, no. 7, pp. 766–775, 2020.

[5] T. Y. Fung and T. K. Lau, "Poor perinatal outcome associated with vasa previa: is it preventable? A report of three cases and review of the literature," *Ultrasound in Obstetrics & Gynecology: the official journal of the International Society of Ultrasound in Obstetrics and Gynecology*, vol. 12, no. 6, pp. 430–433, 1998.

[6] Y. Amo, T. K. Adu-Bredu, K. Appiah-Denkyira, and C. M. Senaya, "Antenatal diagnosis of vasa previa: report of three cases in an African setting," *The Pan African Medical Journal*, vol. 37, p. 24, 2020.

[7] A. Kulkarni, J. Powel, M. Aziz et al., "Vasa previa: prenatal diagnosis and outcomes: thirty-five cases from a single maternal-fetal medicine practice," *Journal of Ultrasound in Medicine: official journal of the American Institute of Ultrasound in Medicine*, vol. 37, no. 4, pp. 1017–1024, 2018.

[8] Society of Maternal-Fetal (SMFM) Publications Committee, R. G. Sinkey, A. O. Odibo, and J. S. Dashe, "37: diagnosis and management of vasa previa," *American Journal of Obstetrics and Gynecology*, vol. 213, no. 5, pp. 615–619, 2015.

[9] Y. Oyelese, V. Catanzarite, F. Prefumo et al., "Vasa previa: the impact of prenatal diagnosis on outcomes," *Obstetrics and Gynecology*, vol. 103, 5, Part 1, pp. 937–942, 2004.

[10] V. Catanzarite, L. Cousins, S. Daneshmand et al., "Prenatally diagnosed vasa previa: a single-institution series of 96 cases," *Obstetrics and Gynecology*, vol. 128, no. 5, pp. 1153–1161, 2016.

[11] B. K. Robinson and W. A. Grobman, "Effectiveness of timing strategies for delivery of individuals with vasa previa," *Obstetrics and Gynecology*, vol. 117, no. 3, pp. 542–549, 2011.

42

Aplastic Anemia Treated with Eltrombopag during Pregnancy

Yuri Suminaga,[1] Yoshitsugu Chigusa,[1] Tadakazu Kondo,[2] Haruko Okamoto,[1] Yosuke Kawamura,[1] Mana Taki,[1] Masaki Mandai,[1] and Haruta Mogami[1]

[1]*Department of Gynecology and Obstetrics, Kyoto University, 54 Shogoin Kawahara-cho, Sakyo-ku, Kyoto 606-8507, Japan*
[2]*Department of Hematology and Oncology, Kyoto University, 54 Shogoin Kawahara-cho, Sakyo-ku, Kyoto 606-8507, Japan*

Correspondence should be addressed to Yoshitsugu Chigusa; chigusa@kuhp.kyoto-u.ac.jp

Academic Editor: Seung-Yup Ku

Aplastic anemia is a rare blood disorder characterized by pancytopenia and hypocellular bone marrow. In patients with aplastic anemia, pancytopenia sometimes worsens during pregnancy, and relapse of aplastic anemia in pregnancy is common. Nevertheless, only supportive care with blood products is the mainstay of treatment of aplastic anemia in pregnancy. Thus, the obstetric management and treatment of aplastic anemia in pregnancy is extremely challenging. We herein report the first case of a pregnant woman complicated with aplastic anemia who was successfully treated with eltrombopag, a thrombopoietin receptor agonist. A 27-year-old primigravida woman who had a history of aplastic anemia refractory to immunosuppressive therapy and was treated with eltrombopag became pregnant. Eltrombopag treatment was continued after weighing the benefits and potential risks. Throughout pregnancy, the woman's pancytopenia did not progress, and she delivered a 2336 g baby vaginally at 38 weeks of gestation. Her postpartum outcome was uneventful, and the neonate did not develop thrombocytosis. Since the efficacy and safety of eltrombopag in pregnancy has not yet been established, its routine use should be avoided. However, if limited to refractory cases and with adequate maternal and fetal monitoring, including neonatal blood examinations, the use of eltrombopag for patients with aplastic anemia during pregnancy may be acceptable and result in favorable maternal and fetal outcomes.

1. Introduction

Aplastic anemia is a rare and heterogeneous blood disorder characterized by pancytopenia and hypocellular bone marrow [1]. Aplastic anemia causes anemia, bleeding, and infection due to associated cytopenia, and these complications can sometimes be life-threatening, especially during pregnancy. Generally, pancytopenia can often progress during pregnancy [1], and relapse of aplastic anemia is common in pregnancy in patients previously treated with immunosuppressive therapy [2]. Therefore, together with the paucity of cases and limited treatment choices, it remains challenging to manage a pregnancy complicated by aplastic anemia.

Eltrombopag, a thrombopoietin receptor agonist, acts as a thrombopoietin mimetic and leads to increased platelet counts in patients with immune thrombocytopenia (ITP). In a phase 2 study involving patients with refracted aplastic anemia, eltrombopag produced a hematologic response in at least one lineage in 11 of 25 patients (44%) [3]. Moreover, in its follow-up study, eltrombopag eventually increased in neutrophil, red blood cell, and platelet lineages in 7 of 43 patients (16%) [4]. Thus, eltrombopag is a promising option for the treatment of aplastic anemia. However, thus far, there have been no reports in which patients with aplastic anemia were treated with eltrombopag during pregnancy, although it has been used in limited cases for patients with ITP in pregnancy [5, 6].

We herein show the case of a pregnant woman with aplastic anemia who continued eltrombopag treatment throughout pregnancy, and maternal and neonatal outcomes were favorable.

2. Case Report

The patient was a 27-year-old primigravida woman. She was diagnosed with aplastic anemia by bone marrow examination at the age of 20. She had been in remission with the treatment of antithymocyte globulin (ATG) and cyclosporine. At the age

Table 1: The changes in maternal complete blood counts.

Timing	At the age of 24	Just before conception	11w5d	13w4d	27w2d	37w2d	38w5d	PPD 32
WBC (10^9/L)	2.88	4.64	4.97	5.84	4.89	4.72	5.32	4.04
Neut (10^9/L)	1.73	2.74	3.71	4.45	3.75	3.56	3.72	2.30
Hb (g/dL)	7.8	12.9	12.4	13.4	10.1	10.4	10.0	11.6
Ht (%)	23.3	40.3	36.7	39.1	30.9	33.8	33.1	36.4
Reti (10^{12}/L)	0.04	0.08	0.07	0.08	0.06	0.10	0.14	0.07
Plt (10^9/L)	18	98	66	73	65	72	57	125

WBC: white blood cells. Neut: neutrophils. Hb: hemoglobin. Ht: hematocrit. Reti: reticulocytes. Plt: platelets. w: weeks. d: days. PPD: postpartum day.

Table 2: The changes in neonatal complete blood counts.

Timing	Day 0*	Day 2	Day 4	Day 95
WBC (10^9/L)	4.77	6.95	4.67	4.97
Hb (g/dL)	10.9	14.9	14.3	10.2
Ht (%)	32.4	42.0	39.6	30.1
Plt (10^9/L)	237	197	179	237

WBC: white blood cells. Hb: hemoglobin. Ht: hematocrit. Plt: platelets. * umbilical vein data.

of 24, however, pancytopenia progressed (Table 1), and eltrombopag was introduced at 25 mg/day and soon increased to 50 mg/day, in addition to cyclosporine at 50 mg/day. She achieved a trilineage response, and she continued to show hematologic improvement. At the age of 27, she became pregnant, and cyclosporine treatment was ceased at her request. Her hematologist explained that the usage of eltrombopag during pregnancy was limited, but the treatment of ITP with eltrombopag during pregnancy showed no maternal complications or fetal abnormalities, and the benefits of using eltrombopag would overcome the disadvantages. She decided to continue taking eltrombopag, and the dose was reduced to 25 mg/day because her condition was stable. In the first trimester of pregnancy, she could not take eltrombopag for three weeks due to hyperemesis gravidarum, and her platelet count slightly decreased (Table 1). After the improvement of hyperemesis gravidarum, she was able to resume taking eltrombopag, her platelet count recovered, and her pregnancy course was stable thereafter. At 37^{+2} weeks of gestation, her systolic blood pressure rose to 130 mmHg, and a urinalysis showed proteinuria (+). In addition, a fetal ultrasound showed mild fetal growth restriction: the baby's estimated body weight was less than the 10th percentile. Thus, the patient was admitted to the hospital for enhanced monitoring of the mother and baby. Although there was no increase in her blood pressure after admission, her platelet count at 38^{+5} weeks of gestation was 57×10^9/L with a downward trend. Due to the indications of mild fetal growth restriction, comparably high blood pressure, and maternal thrombocytopenia, we decided to induce labor. She vaginally delivered a mature female infant weighing 2336 g (5.4^{th} percentile) with an Apgar score of 9 at 1 minute and 5 minutes. The blood loss at delivery was 680 grams, the delivery was uneventful, and no blood transfusion was required. The infant was formula-fed. The results of the newborn's blood tests were all normal (Table 2). Pathological examination of the placenta revealed one small infarction in the villi. Microscopically, perivillous fibrin deposition was prominent. In addition, fibrous thickening and obliteration at stem vessels were observed, which indicated fetal vascular malperfusion. These pathological findings are consistent with fetal growth restriction. The mother's postpartum course was uneventful, and her remission was maintained by 25 mg of eltrombopag alone.

3. Discussion

The first case of aplastic anemia described in the literature was a pregnant woman who died of postpartum hemorrhage in 1888. Although there has been no proven causal association between pregnancy and aplastic anemia, it cannot be ruled out that pregnancy may have some influence on the disease [7]. In some cases, women with aplastic anemia experience worsening symptoms or relapse during pregnancy [1, 2], and marked thrombocytopenia is often observed with advancing gestation. However, available treatment options during pregnancy are limited; hematopoietic stem-cell transplantation or the use of ATG is generally contraindicated in pregnancy [1, 8], and only cyclosporin, whether it is effective or not, is thought to be safe. Ultimately, supportive care with blood products is the mainstay of treatment of aplastic anemia in pregnancy. Thus, an effective treatment that can be used during pregnancy is needed.

Eltrombopag is a relatively new drug for the treatment of steroid-refractory ITP and severe aplastic anemia that is refractory to immunosuppressive therapy. Eltrombopag binds to the thrombopoietin receptor on megakaryocytes and hematopoietic stem cells, which results in platelet production and overcoming the depletion of hematopoietic stem cells in aplastic anemia [3]. The Food and Drug Administration assigned eltrombopag to pregnancy risk category C. This means that eltrombopag, although its use is not contraindicated, should be administered very carefully during pregnancy, only when its benefits outweigh its potential risks, because there are no adequate and well-controlled studies in humans, and eltrombopag is thought to cross the placenta. The patient in this case had been refractory to immunosuppressive therapy and achieved remission by eltrombopag. In other words, the risk of pancytopenia was extremely high if eltrombopag treatment was discontinued. Moreover, the worsening of aplastic anemia during pregnancy has been shown to be associated not only with disease complications but also with pregnancy-related complications [9]. Therefore, it was not advisable for her to discontinue the use of eltrombopag, and after obtaining her informed consent, eltrombopag treatment was continued during pregnancy.

At present, no marked maternal or fetal toxicity of eltrombopag has been reported in animal studies at drug doses equivalent to those given to humans [6]. Case series and case reports have been published in which eltrombopag was administered to pregnant women with ITP [5, 6]. According to these studies, the platelet response to eltrombopag was favorable in most cases, and significant maternal and neonatal complications that could be clearly attributed to eltrombopag were not reported. There have also been published case reports of the successful treatment of severe thrombocytopenia with eltrombopag during pregnancy in patient with systemic lupus erythematosus [10] or MYH9-related disease, an autosomal dominant thrombocytopenia [11]. In these literatures, no short-term adverse effects of eltrombopag on newborns have been reported. Nonetheless, eltrombopag could theoretically cross the placenta [12, 13], and potentially affect the fetus. In the present case, we assessed a complete blood count of the neonate for 3 months after birth and confirmed that there was no abnormal increase in trilineage. Michel et al. reported one neonate with thrombocytosis that was born to a mother taking 100 mg of eltrombopag due to ITP for 4 weeks beginning at 30 weeks of gestation [5]. Careful observation and blood examinations are necessary for neonates born to mothers who receive eltrombopag treatment during pregnancy.

Currently, there are no data on the safety of breastfeeding while taking eltrombopag, and the patient, in our case, discontinued breastfeeding. However, given that the molecular weight of eltrombopag is 445.2 [14] and its protein binding rate is more than 99% [15], the secretion of eltrombopag in the milk may be small. Furthermore, calcium in breast milk may attenuate the effect of eltrombopag because the bioavailability of eltrombopag is reduced by the chelation of calcium [16]. In this light, breastfeeding while receiving eltrombopag may not necessarily be contraindicated if the neonate's blood and symptoms such as vomiting, ecchymosis, hepatotoxicity, and conjunctival hemorrhage are adequately monitored, even though it is not recommended in principle.

It is not clear whether the fetal growth restriction seen in our case was directly associated with aplastic anemia or eltrombopag treatment. Other than postpartum hemorrhage, there are no known obstetrical complications that are specific to pregnancy in women with aplastic anemia. Remarkably, however, previous studies have reported that the rate of pregnancy complications in women with aplastic anemia, including preeclampsia, fetal growth restriction, and preterm delivery, were variable [8, 17, 18]. Interestingly, infarction in the placenta without fetal growth restriction has been reported previously in cases of ITP that were treated with the thrombopoietin receptor agonist romiplostim during pregnancy [19]. Given that the thrombopoietin receptor is only slightly expressed in cytotrophoblasts [20], it is unlikely that eltrombopag caused the pathological changes in the placenta, including in our case.

In conclusion, to the best of our knowledge, this is the first case report in which a patient with aplastic anemia was successfully treated with eltrombopag during pregnancy. Since the efficacy and safety of eltrombopag in pregnancy has not yet been established, its routine use should be avoided. However, if limited to refracted cases and with adequate maternal and fetal monitoring, including neonatal blood examinations, the use of eltrombopag for patients with aplastic anemia during pregnancy may be acceptable and result in favorable maternal and fetal outcomes.

Consent

Written informed consent was obtained from the patient for publication of this case report and accompanying images.

References

[1] S. B. Killick, N. Bown, J. Cavenagh et al., "Guidelines for the diagnosis and management of adult aplastic anaemia," *British Journal of Haematology*, vol. 172, no. 2, pp. 187–207, 2016.

[2] A. Tichelli, G. Socié, J. Marsh et al., "Outcome of pregnancy and disease course among women with aplastic anemia treated with immunosuppression," *Annals of Internal Medicine*, vol. 137, no. 3, pp. 164–172, 2002.

[3] M. J. Olnes, P. Scheinberg, K. R. Calvo et al., "Eltrombopag and improved hematopoiesis in refractory aplastic anemia," *The New England Journal of Medicine*, vol. 367, no. 1, pp. 11–19, 2012.

[4] R. Desmond, D. M. Townsley, B. Dumitriu et al., "Eltrombopag restores trilineage hematopoiesis in refractory severe aplastic anemia that can be sustained on discontinuation of drug," *Blood*, vol. 123, no. 12, pp. 1818–1825, 2014.

[5] M. Michel, M. Ruggeri, T. J. Gonzalez-Lopez et al., "Use of thrombopoietin receptor agonists for immune thrombocytopenia in pregnancy: results from a multicenter study," *Blood*, vol. 136, no. 26, pp. 3056–3061, 2020.

[6] N. Agarwal and A. Mangla, "Thrombopoietin receptor agonist for treatment of immune thrombocytopenia in pregnancy: a narrative review," *Therapeutic Advances in Hematology*, vol. 12, p. 204062072110011, 2021.

[7] N. S. Young and J. Maciejewski, "The pathophysiology of acquired aplastic anemia," *The New England Journal of Medicine*, vol. 336, no. 19, pp. 1365–1372, 1997.

[8] E. Riveros-Perez, A. C. Hermesch, L. A. Barbour, and J. L. Hawkins, "Aplastic anemia during pregnancy: a review of obstetric and anesthetic considerations," *International Journal of Women's Health*, vol. Volume 10, pp. 117–125, 2018.

[9] J. E. Shin, Y. Lee, S. J. Kim, and J. C. Shin, "Association of severe thrombocytopenia and poor prognosis in pregnancies with aplastic anemia," *PLoS One*, vol. 9, no. 7, article e103066, 2014.

[10] Q. Leng, W. Wang, Y. Wang, and L. Wu, "Treatment of severe thrombocytopenia associated with systemic lupus erythematosus in pregnancy with eltrombopag: a case report and literature review," *Journal of Clinical Pharmacy and Therapeutics*, vol. 46, no. 2, pp. 532–538, 2021.

[11] R. Favier, C. De Carne, E. Elefant, R. Lapusneanu, V. Gkalea, and A. Rigouzzo, "Eltrombopag to treat thrombocytopenia during last month of pregnancy in a woman with MYH9-related disease: a case report," *A A Pract.*, vol. 10, no. 1, pp. 10–12, 2018.

[12] P. Imbach and M. Crowther, "Thrombopoietin-receptor agonists for primary immune thrombocytopenia," *The New England Journal of Medicine*, vol. 365, no. 8, pp. 734–741, 2011.

[13] Z. Kong, P. Qin, S. Xiao et al., "A novel recombinant human thrombopoietin therapy for the management of immune thrombocytopenia in pregnancy," *Blood*, vol. 130, no. 9, pp. 1097–1103, 2017.

[14] D. J. Kuter, "Biology and chemistry of thrombopoietic agents," *Seminars in Hematology*, vol. 47, no. 3, pp. 243–248, 2010.

[15] G. Cheng, "Eltrombopag, a thrombopoietin- receptor agonist in the treatment of adult chronic immune thrombocytopenia: a review of the efficacy and safety profile," *Therapeutic Advances in Hematology*, vol. 3, no. 3, pp. 155–164, 2012.

[16] M. B. Wire, J. Bruce, J. Gauvin et al., "A randomized, open-label, 5-period, balanced crossover study to evaluate the relative bioavailability of eltrombopag powder for oral suspension (PfOS) and tablet formulations and the effect of a high-calcium meal on eltrombopag pharmacokinetics when administered with or 2 hours before or after PfOS," *Clinical Therapeutics*, vol. 34, no. 3, pp. 699–709, 2012.

[17] K. J. Chen, Y. L. Chang, H. Chang et al., "Long-term outcome of pregnancy complicating with severe aplastic anemia under supportive care," *Taiwanese Journal of Obstetrics & Gynecology*, vol. 56, no. 5, pp. 632–635, 2017.

[18] K. E. McGowan, A. K. Malinowski, A. C. Schuh, W. Whittle, and N. Shehata, "Aplastic anaemia in pregnancy-a single centre, North American series," *British Journal of Haematology*, vol. 184, no. 3, pp. 436–439, 2019.

[19] A. S. Patil, S. K. Dotters-Katz, A. D. Metjian, A. H. James, and G. K. Swamy, "Use of a thrombopoietin mimetic for chronic immune thrombocytopenic purpura in pregnancy," *Obstetrics and Gynecology*, vol. 122, no. 2, pp. 483–485, 2013.

[20] S. E. Segerer, F. Martignoni, A. Bogdan et al., "Thrombopoietin modulates the proliferation, migration and cytokine profile of decidual cell subsets during early gestation," *Molecular Human Reproduction*, vol. 19, no. 6, pp. 361–368, 2013.

43

Intravesicular Onabotulinumtoxin A Hemorrhage on Rivaroxaban

Allison Eubanks , Katherine Dengler, and Daniel Gruber

Department of Urogynecology in Obstetrics & Gynecology, Walter Reed National Military Medical Center, Bethesda, MD, USA

Correspondence should be addressed to Allison Eubanks; aac.eubanks@gmail.com

Academic Editor: Erich Cosmi

Overactive bladder (OAB) is urgency, with or without urgency incontinence. For OAB, an injection of onabotulinumtoxin A (BOTOX®) can be a low-risk outpatient procedure. We present a patient on a novel anticoagulant that experienced excessive bleeding after this procedure. This 80-year-old G2P2002 Caucasian female had a history of urge urinary incontinence. She presented for intravesicular onabotulinumtoxin A injection (150 units) after recent initiation of rivaroxaban (Xarelto®) for her atrial fibrillation. Several hours after an uncomplicated procedure, she presented with anuria and pain after gross hematuria earlier in the day. Her pain was immediately alleviated with bladder irrigation. She was discharged home and remained asymptomatic. With the popularity of the novel anticoagulants, new guidance on management of these medications during procedures is limited. When managing a patient on a novel anticoagulant before any procedure, even a low risk procedure, several factors should be considered to determine if the medication should be held, bridged, or continued. In sum, each patient on anticoagulation undergoing any procedure should be assessed individually for thrombotic risk, bleeding risk, and the procedural risk to best avoid postprocedural hemorrhage.

1. Introduction

The International Continence Society defines overactive bladder (OAB) as "urgency, with or without urgency incontinence usually with increased daytime frequency and nocturia" [1]. OAB often has a significant impact on quality of life.

Behavioral modifications are first-line treatment for OAB. The patient should focus on lifestyle changes, such as weight loss, caffeine and alcohol reduction, bladder control strategies, and fluid management. In addition, pelvic floor physical therapy can help with bladder retraining and pelvic floor muscle training. If these conservative measures fail then medication, nerve stimulation, and injection of bladder onabotulinumtoxin A (BOTOX®) can help relax detrusor muscles.

Intravesicular onabotulinumtoxin A injection is a quick, outpatient procedure that has been shown to be more effective than mirabegron in a large meta-analysis and, furthermore, without the invasiveness of sacral neuromodulation as shown in a randomized control trial [1, 2]. The risks of this procedure include urinary tract infections, elevated postvoid residual volumes requiring intermittent catheterization, and hematuria that can occur in 3.6-5.2% of patients [2, 3].

As the likelihood of overactive bladder increases with patient age along with other medical comorbidities, it is not uncommon for patients with OAB to be on blood thinners. Furthermore, patients are on newer, novel anticoagulants that do not have reversal agents. Given the small size of the needle and minimal bleeding expected, there is currently no guidance on stopping or bridging any anticoagulation medications for this same day procedure typically performed in the office setting.

2. Case

This is the case of an 80-year-old G2P2002 Caucasian female with a long history of urge urinary incontinence. She presented to clinic for intravesicular onabotulinumtoxin A injection (150 units). She had undergone this procedure seven times with six- to twelve-month intervals, depending on the return of symptoms, ranging from 50 to 150 units of onabotulinumtoxin A since March of 2011. These treatments have significantly improved her symptoms of urgency incontinence after previously trying several anticholinergic medications and sacral neuromodulation.

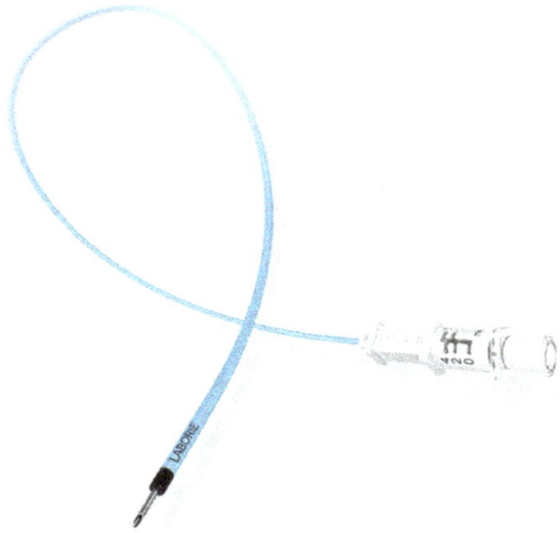

Figure 1: Laborie injeTAK® (Williston, VT) needle.

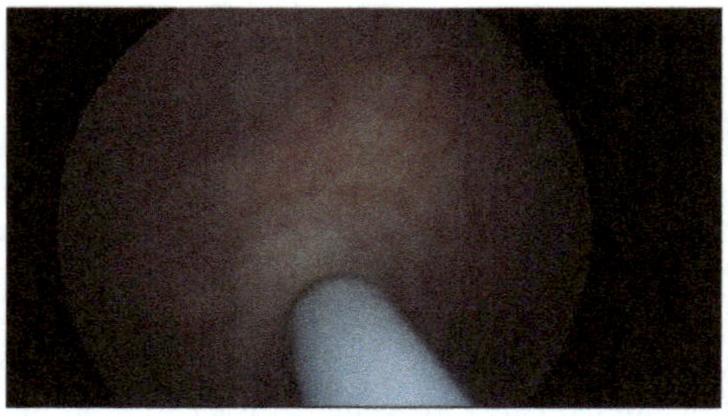

Figure 2: Injection of needle through uroepithelium.

Her other past medical history is significant for hypertension, peripheral vascular disease, scoliosis, hypothyroidism, diverticulosis, and open-angle glaucoma. She was diagnosed with paroxysmal atrial fibrillation in the beginning of 2016 and developed renal emboli prior to initiation of warfarin. She was transitioned to rivaroxaban (Xarelto®) in mid-2016 after struggling with frequent clinic visits and limited diet while on warfarin. She tolerated this medication transition well.

The patient had not undergone intravesicular onabotulinumtoxin A injections while on warfarin but however did have a single treatment just one month after initiating rivaroxaban without issues. She returned for the repeat procedure one year later. Using sterile technique, the bladder was filled with 20 mL of 1% lidocaine and 2% viscous lidocaine was administered to the urethra 15 minutes before the procedure. The onabotulinumtoxin A dose was reconstituted in 20 milliliters' saline solution. A 30-degree operative cystoscope was inserted into the bladder. A total of 150 units of onabotulinumtoxin A were injected into the bladder wall in 20 sites with one milliliter in each injection covering the posterior surface of the bladder wall and sparing the trigone. The depth of the injection was set at 3 mm under the urothelium layer with the Laborie injeTAK® (Williston, VT) needle; see Figures 1–6. The patient tolerated the procedure well. There was minor bleeding from a few needle injection sites, but not an atypical amount. She voided immediately after the procedure without difficulty and was sent home from the office feeling well.

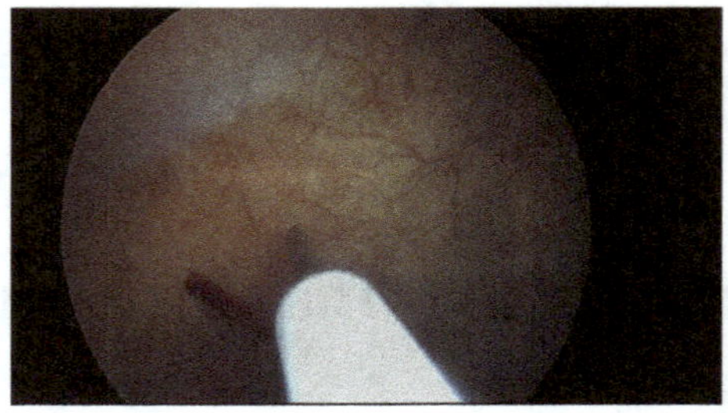

Figure 3: Needle retracting from uroepithelium, appropriate amount of bleeding noted.

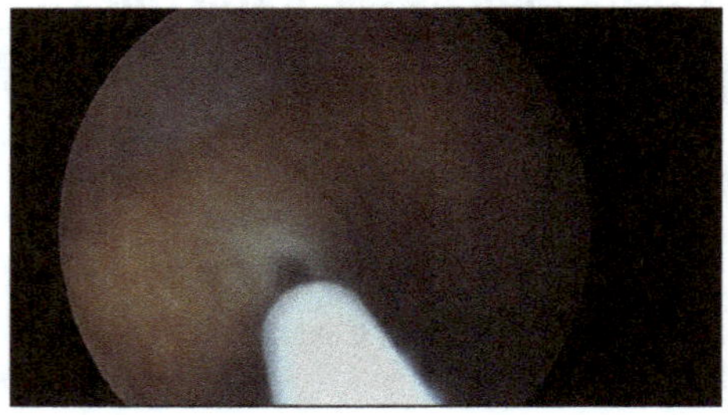

Figure 4: Needle replaced into uroepithelium.

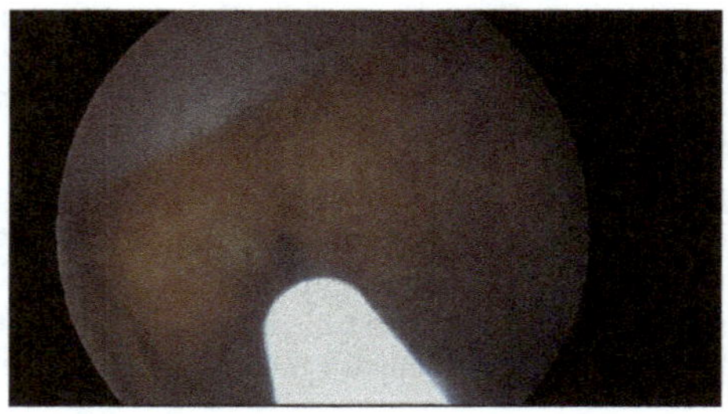

Figure 5: Needle removed completely with no bleeding noted from injection site.

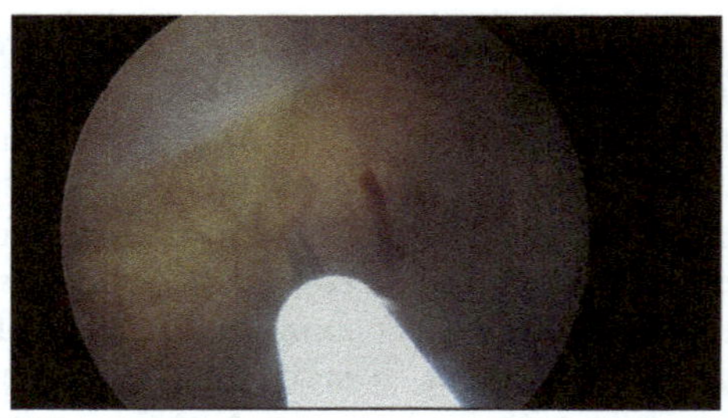

Figure 6: Needle replaced into uroepithelium, appropriate amount of bleeding noted.

Seven hours later, the patient called the clinic and reported two hours of frank blood in her urine with passage of several clots. She reported drinking large volumes of water and frequent voiding without improvement. She was encouraged to keep her bladder full to allow distension to tamponade the bleeding, rather than empty frequently. She was given strict return precautions to present to the emergency department if her bleeding persisted or for any retention symptoms. The following morning, the patient presented to the emergency department in pain with no urine output for the last several hours. She was given intravenous morphine, which alleviated her immediate pain.

A 14-French Foley catheter was placed and slowly drained dark red urine with clots. Only about 200 milliliters returned in the catheter. Several flushes were attempted to alleviate the blockage without success. Continuous bladder irrigation (CBI) was initiated which cleared the obstruction. The patient continued to put out frank blood with the CBI. Her complete blood cell count was normal and did not show a significant drop [15.2/45.8 to 14.0/43.5]. Her pain was completely alleviated with the CBI until new clots developed that caused a repeat obstruction two more times overnight requiring Foley adjustment.

Cardiology was consulted to aid with management of her anticoagulation in the setting of bleeding and her rivaroxaban was held for three days. Following 36 hours of CBI, her urine was lighter, indicating bleeding cessation. The CBI was stopped and the patient was taught to flush the catheter with normal saline.

The patient returned for a scheduled clinic appointment four days later and reported that she only had a few episodes of hematuria that resolved with minimal flushing. The bladder was back-filled with 400 milliliters and the Foley catheter removed. She voided 350 milliliters of clear yellow urine without difficulty. The patient continued on prophylactic nitrofurantoin for ten days. She followed up three weeks later without return of the hematuria. She reported some continued overactive bladder symptoms such as frequent voiding, some urgency incontinence upon standing, and nighttime voids up to four to five times per night; however the frequency of these symptoms was all decreased from prior to her procedure. She continues to find the best solution to manage her symptoms.

3. Discussion

Despite the resulting hemorrhage from this intravesicular onabotulinumtoxin A injection, bleeding with this procedure is rare. This case is significant in that bleeding is so rare and the injection sites are so small. The patient had additionally not bled during the procedure while previously on rivaroxaban, approximately one year priorly. She reported no tobacco or alcohol use, and her medications at the time of this procedure had not changed.

Antifactor Xa was not collected during or around the time of either procedure. Her weight and renal function remained unchanged and liver function was previously normal. However, it is important to consider any changes to these values in patients on novel anticoagulants as they can cause patients to be supratherapeutic and increase risk of bleeding with even minor procedures. There is only one case report that reviews the management of a patient using warfarin before intravesicular onabotulinumtoxin A injection [4]. The purpose of that publication was to simply demonstrate the proper discontinuation, bridging management, and reinitiation of warfarin to safely complete the procedure for a patient [4].

Allergan, the onabotulinumtoxin A manufacturer, does not list anticoagulation as a contraindication and suggests only managing patients on anticoagulant therapy appropriately to decrease the risk of bleeding [5]. It is at the clinician's discretion to determine the procedural bleeding risk and weigh the patient's thrombotic risk.

Spyropoulos et al. and the American College of Cardiology (ACC) both compiled a list of procedures and delineated their bleed risk level [6, 7]. According to the list from Spyropoulos et al., a bladder biopsy is considered a low procedural risk, with a 2-day risk of major bleed at 0% to 2%. According to the list from the ACC, as contributed by Dr. Bruce Jacobs and the American Urological Association, uncomplicated ureteral stenting and exchange is considered a low bleed risk. Intravesicular onabotulinumtoxin A injections are much less invasive than bladder biopsies and less invasive than ureteral stenting. ACCP gives 2C recommendations regarding continuing vitamin K antagonists (VKAs) in minor dermatologic procedures and cataract surgery. It is also recommended to discontinue VKAs for two to three days before the procedure or coadministration of an oral prohemostatic, a suggestion that may be applied to this situation [8].

The patient was taking rivaroxaban for paroxysmal atrial fibrillation, diagnosed in the wake of a renal infarct attributed to a cardioembolic source. Given the prior documented history of cardioembolic phenomenon to the kidneys, the patient's cardiologist determined that she requires lifelong anticoagulation. Her CHA_2DS_2-Vasc score of at least five points estimated her stroke risk at 7.2% per year. It was not unreasonable to continue anticoagulation during this minimal procedure for such a high-risk patient.

In future intravesicular onabotulinumtoxin A injections performed for this patient, and similar patients, it would be reasonable to consider discontinuing her anticoagulant for two to three days before procedure and bridging with low-molecular weight heparin or heparin. The physician could also consider coadministering an oral prohemostatic agent such as tranexamic acid. Working with the prescribing physician managing these medications and comorbidities may prove beneficial. However, for other intravesicular onabotulinumtoxin A procedures performed for OAB, we would continue to treat this as a low-risk procedure. Each patient on anticoagulation undergoing any procedure should be assessed individually for thrombotic risk, bleeding risk, and the procedural risk to best avoid postprocedural hemorrhage.

Consent

The involved patient has signed consent for publication.

Disclosure

The opinions or assertions contained herein are the private views of the authors and are not to be construed as official or as reflecting the views of the Departments of the Army, Navy, Air Force, or the Department of Defense.

References

[1] N. Freemantle, D. A. Ginsberg, R. McCool et al., "Comparative assessment of onabotulinumtoxinA and mirabegron for over-

active bladder: An indirect treatment comparison," *BMJ Open*, vol. 6, no. 2, Article ID e009122, 2016.

[2] C. Chapple, K.-D. Sievert, S. Macdiarmid et al., "OnabotulinumtoxinA 100 U significantly improves all idiopathic overactive bladder symptoms and quality of life in patients with overactive bladder and urinary incontinence: A randomised, double-blind, placebo-controlled trial," *European Urology*, vol. 64, no. 2, pp. 249–256, 2013.

[3] D. Ginsberg, A. Gousse, V. Keppenne et al., "Phase 3 efficacy and tolerability study of onabotulinumtoxinA for urinary incontinence from neurogenic detrusor overactivity," *The Journal of Urology*, vol. 187, no. 6, pp. 2131–2139, 2012.

[4] G. L. Peters and S. M. Vouri, "Use of onabotulinumtoxinA for overactive bladder with concomitant warfarin," *The Consultant Pharmacist: The Journal of the American Society of Consultant Pharmacists*, vol. 29, no. 7, pp. 480–486, 2014.

[5] *Botox (onabotulinumtoxinA) [package insert]*, Allergan, Irvine, CA, USA, 2017.

[6] A. C. Spyropoulos and J. D. Douketis, "How I treat anticoagulated patients undergoing an elective procedure or surgery," *Blood*, vol. 120, no. 15, pp. 2954–2962, 2012.

[7] *Common Procedures And Associated Procedural Bleed Risk*, American College of Cardiology, 2017, http://jaccjacc.acc.org/Clinical_Document/PMAC_Online_Appendix.pdf.

[8] J. D. Douketis, A. C. Spyropoulos, F. A. Spencer et al., "Perioperative management of antithrombotic therapy: antithrombotic therapy and prevention of thrombosis: American College of Chest Physicians evidence-based clinical practice guidelines," *Chest*, vol. 141, no. 2, pp. e326S–e350S, 2012.

C4d Deposition in Fetal Vessels of the Placenta in Neonatal Lupus Syndrome

Yuichiro Sato [1], Tomoko Yamaguchi,[2] Jyunsuke Muraoka,[2] Hajime Taniguchi,[2] Atsushi Kisanuki,[3] Kazunari Maekawa,[4] Atushi Yamashita,[4] Murasaki Aman,[1] Yuki Kodama,[5] Hiroshi Sameshima [5] and Yujiro Asada[4]

[1]*Department of Diagnostic Pathology, Faculty of Medicine, Miyazaki University Hospital, University of Miyazaki, 5200 Kihara, Kiyotake, Miyazaki 889-1692, Japan*
[2]*Department of Obstetrics and Gynecology, Miyazaki Prefectural Nichinan Hospital, 1-9-5, Kiyama, Nichinan, Miyazaki 887-0013, Japan*
[3]*Department of Diagnostic Pathology, Miyazaki Prefectural Nichinan Hospital, 1-9-5, Kiyama, Nichinan, Miyazaki 887-0013, Japan*
[4]*Department of Pathology, Faculty of Medicine, University of Miyazaki, 5200 Kihara, Kiyotake, Miyazaki 889-1692, Japan*
[5]*Department of Obstetrics and Gynecology, Faculty of Medicine, University of Miyazaki, 5200 Kihara, Kiyotake, Miyazaki 889-1692, Japan*

Correspondence should be addressed to Yuichiro Sato; yuichiro_sato@med.miyazaki-u.ac.jp

Academic Editor: Akihide Ohkuchi

Neonatal lupus syndrome (NLS) is a rare, passively acquired autoimmune syndrome caused by maternal autoantibodies. We describe a case of a newborn with NLS and the accompanying placental findings. A female neonate was born by emergency cesarean delivery due to non-reassuring fetal status at 35 weeks and 3 days. This neonate had congenital erythematous and scar lesions on the face, back, and upper and lower extremities. Maternal and fetal anti-SSA and SSB antibodies were elevated and this baby was diagnosed as NLS. Histologically, the chorionic villi demonstrated capillary shrinkage. An immunohistochemical study revealed complement deposition (C4d) in the capillaries of the villi and umbilical vessels. Our findings suggest that maternal autoantibodies affect the inflammatory response of the fetus through the placenta and that C4d deposition may be useful for diagnosing NLS.

1. Introduction

Neonatal lupus syndrome (NLS) is an acquired autoimmune disease caused by the transplacental passage of maternal anti-SSA/Ro and/or anti-SSB/La antibodies [1, 2]. However, the pathological findings in the placenta of neonates with NLS have not been documented.

Complement deposition (C4d) is a split product of C4b and C4d deposition in vascular endothelial cells with organ rejection, and it is generally considered evidence for classical complement pathway activity [3]. Recently, C4d deposition in the placenta was reported for systemic lupus erythematosus (SLE), preeclampsia, and miscarriage [4, 5]; however, the histological findings of NLS have not been documented. We describe a case of a newborn with NLS and the accompanying placental findings of C4d deposition.

2. Case Presentation

A 31-year-old woman (gravida 5, para 2) was referred to our hospital due to labor pain. She was suspected to have SLE because of facial erythema at age 29 years, but clinical and serological findings failed to satisfy the diagnosis criteria for SLE. She gave birth to two boys without any problems at age 23 years (birth weight, 2822 g) and 26 years (birth weight, 2946 g). The fetal heart monitor showed non-reassuring fetal status. A female neonate was born by emergency cesarean delivery at 35 weeks and 3 days. The neonate weight was 1,909 g. She had fetal growth restriction (FGR) and Apgar scores of 5 and 7 (1 minute and 5 minutes). Her skin was pale. She had congenital erythematous and scar lesions on the face, back, and upper and lower extremities (Figure 1). An examination revealed a slight elevation in hepatic

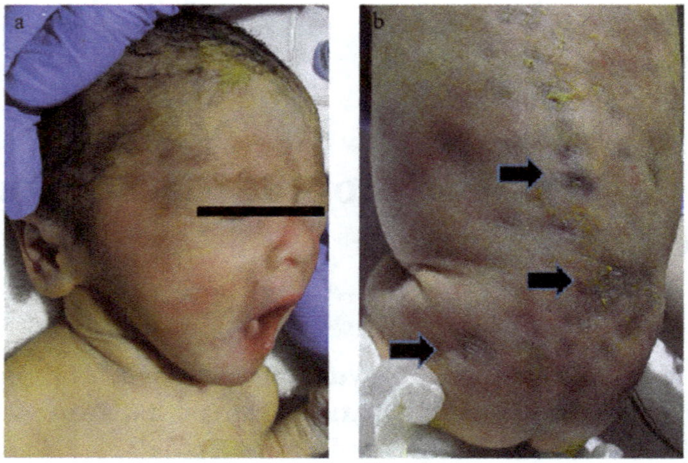

(a) (b)

FIGURE 1: Skin lesions. (a) Skin rash with annular erythematous lesions on the face. (b) Annular, erythematous, scaly, atrophic patches on the trunk and back (arrows).

transaminases, thrombocytopenia, and mild cardiac failure. No heart blockage was detected. The serological examination of the neonate showed elevated anti-SSA/Ro (281 U/mL) and anti-SSB/La antibodies (≧1000 U/mL). Other antibodies were normal range (anti-DNA antibody ≦2.0 IU/mL, anti-RNP antibody <2.0 U/mL), and complements were not reduced (C3; 92 mg/dl, C4; 22 mg/dl). The serological examination of the mother also showed elevation of these antibodies, and a histological examination demonstrated lymphocytic infiltration of the minor salivary gland; therefore, a diagnosis of Sjögren syndrome was made. The symptoms of the neonate had almost resolved by 7 months of age.

The placenta was 17 x 13.5 x 2 cm and weighed 285 g. The amnion color was green, and the cut surface showed anemia. Histological examination revealed collapsed capillaries in the terminal villi (Figure 2(e)). No apparent inflammatory cells or thrombus formation was found in the fetal vessels. Partial focal maternal vessel thrombosis was noted, but no apparent infarction was seen. A meconium stain with amnion degeneration was observed in the amnion. Focal maternal thrombosis and increased syncytial knots were also present.

Immunohistostaining of a normal placenta (Figure 2(b)), placenta with maternal SLE (Figure 2(d)), and the placenta involved in this case (Figure 2(f)) was performed using C4d (ABGENT, San Diego, CA, USA). In the normal placenta, focal or weak C4d deposits were present at the syncytiotrophoblasts, but not in the lumen of the vessels (Figure 2(b)). C4d deposits were strongly observed at the syncytiotrophoblasts in SLE cases (Figure 2(d)). The placenta with NLS showed C4d deposition in the lumen of the capillaries of the terminal villi (Figure 2(f)). C4d deposition was also seen in the stem vessels, chorionic vessels, and umbilical vessels in this case. C4d deposition was not detected in the maternal vessels.

3. Discussion

We found C4d depositions in the fetal endothelial cells of the NLS placenta. C4d is commonly referred to as the "footprint" of antibody-mediated tissue injury [6]. This report demonstrated the direct findings of antibody-mediated tissue injury by examining the placenta. Capillary collapse was also detected in the placenta, but apparent thrombus formation, massive inflammatory cell infiltration, and apoptotic cells were not found with hematoxylin and eosin (HE) staining. We found C4d deposition in fetal vessels in the placenta, but not in the maternal vessels in the decidua. Our findings suggest that maternal antibody reactions across the placenta induce fetal organ injury but do not attack the placenta or maternal vessels. We hypothesized that complement is activated by maternal antibodies in the fetal vessels, through the classical pathway, cleaved C4d bounds the surface of fetal endothelium.

Even though it is an inactive split product of the complement cascade, C4d is a biomarker. Covalently bound C4d anchors tightly to the tissue; therefore, it serves as a footprint of antibody-mediated tissue injury [6]. C4d deposits are now considered the gold standard for diagnosing renal graft acute humoral resection [3]. Furthermore, several groups have shown that C4d deposition in capillaries is a reliable and specific marker of antibody-mediated injury in other transplanted solid organs that are rejected [7, 8]. Interestingly, placental C4d detected in the majority of SLE and anti-phospholipid syndrome cases has a diffuse staining pattern at the syncytiotrophoblasts [4]. We have found C4d deposition in the lumen of placental fetal vessels; however, that deposition had patterns that were different from those of our case. We studied C4d deposition in normal placenta and SLE cases, but we could not detect the capillary deposition pattern in other cases. We speculate that antibodies in SLE or anti-phospholipid syndrome are activated by maternal inflammatory cells or cytokines in the intervillous space, and this induces the C4d binding at the syncytiotrophoblasts. In NLS, these antibodies are silent in the intervillous space, and then these become activated complement cascade in the fetal circulation. However, further examinations are needed because C4d deposits may be useful markers of NLS.

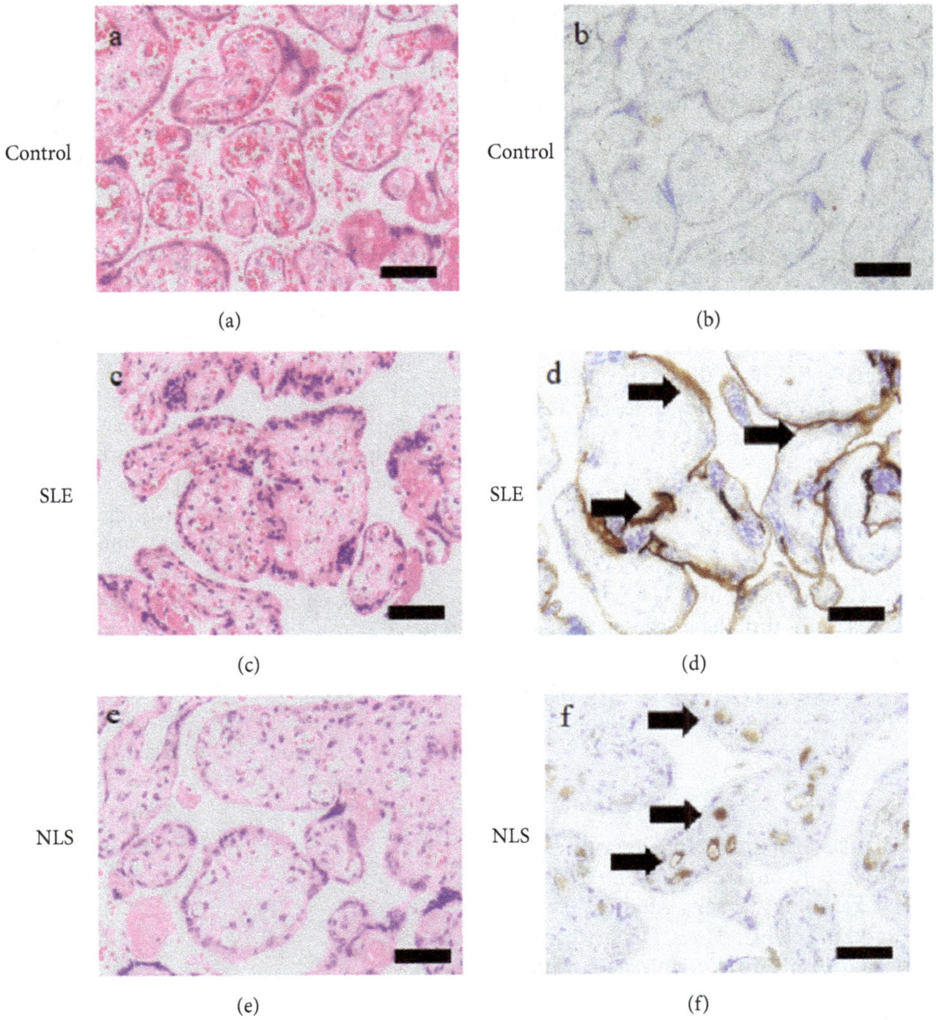

FIGURE 2: Histological findings from placentas obtained from the control pregnancy (28-year-old mother at 35 weeks of gestation, (a, b)), systemic lupus erythematous (SLE) pregnancy (40-year-old mother at 30 weeks of gestation, (c, d)), and neonatal lupus syndrome pregnancy (31-year-old mother at 35 weeks of gestation, (e, f)). (a, c, e) Representative images of tissue sections stained with hematoxylin and eosin (HE). (b, d, f) Representative anti-C4d immunostaining images (arrows). Scale bar = 50 μm.

Wisuthsarewong et al. [9] documented that 29.4% of NLS cases involved FGR. Our case also involved a neonate with FGR and a small placenta. In addition, histological findings revealed maternal vessel thrombosis. Maternal vasculopathy, including maternal vessel thrombosis, is associated with FGR. Several authors showed that maternal vasculopathy is related to maternal hypertension, but the association between maternal vasculopathy and collagen disease is unclear [10]. In our case, the mother had no history of hypertension; in addition, C4d deposits were not detected in the maternal vessels. Revaux et al. [11] reported that FGR and chronic intervillositis were associated with antiphospholipid syndrome and other autoimmune diseases; however, we could not detect chronic intervillositis or massive fibrin deposition. We considered that the small placenta and maternal vasculopathy were associated with FGR in this case.

NLS is a rare neonatal immune-mediated disease. Wisuthsarewong et al. [9] reported that the incidence of NLS is approximately 1 in 12,500 to 20,000 live births, and that it is slightly higher for girls and premature newborns. However, the true incidence of NLS has not been determined because of the high rate of underdiagnosed cases. Approximately 40-60% of mothers are asymptomatic when newborns are diagnosed with NLS [1, 2, 9]. Some mothers may have SLE, Sjögren syndrome, rheumatoid arthritis, or another undifferentiated autoimmune disease. Zuppa et al. [12] documented that the most frequent maternal autoimmune disease to accompany NLS was SLE (25/50); in their study, 15 mothers had primary Sjögren syndrome and 5 had SLE combined with Sjögren syndrome. In our case, the newborn's diagnosis was made based on neonatal skin findings and serum antibody levels of the newborn and the mother. The mother was suspected to have SLE 3 years before this pregnancy; after delivery, she was diagnosed with Sjögren syndrome.

The most common clinical manifestations of NLS are dermatologic, cardiac, hepatobiliary, and hematologic abnormalities [1, 2, 12]. Dermatologic lesions may be present at birth, but they often appear within the first few weeks of life.

Annular erythematous or polycystic plaque with or without scarring characterizes NLS and appears predominantly on the scalp, neck, or face. Periorbital erythema, referred to as "raccoon eye" or "owl eye," is a common characteristic. Our case also demonstrated characteristic dermatitis on the face, back, and upper and lower extremities, and the physicians suspected NLS with cutaneous lesions. The outcome of NLS is usually good when only skin lesions are present. Cardiac abnormalities, especially third-degree heart blockage, can be the most serious consequences of NLS. Li et al. [13] recently suggested that the frequency of congenital heart blockage was significantly lower for Asians than for Caucasians. Our case involved non-reassuring fetal status detected by the fetal heart monitor, but the newborn had no heart blockage. Her major symptoms were cutaneous lesions, and these have almost resolved.

4. Conclusion

We encountered a case of NLS and found C4d deposition in the placental capillaries and umbilical vessels. This is the first report of placental findings of NLS. These findings support the hypothesis that maternal antibodies affect the fetus through the placenta.

Acknowledgments

The authors thank Dr. Sachiko Minamiguchi, Department of Pathology, Faculty of Medicine, Kyoto University, Dr. Makoto Takeuchi, Department of Pathology, Osaka Medical Center and Research Institute, and Dr. Seichiro Hara, Department of Internal Medicine, Miyazaki Prefectural Nichinan Hospital, for their invaluable comments regarding this manuscript. We would also like to thank Editage (www.editage.jp) for English language editing. This study was supported by a grant-in-aid for clinical research from Miyazaki University Hospital.

References

[1] D. M. Friedman, A. Rupel, and J. P. Buyon, "Epidemiology, etiology, detection, and treatment of autoantibody-associated congenital heart block in neonatal lupus," *Current Rheumatology Reports*, vol. 9, no. 2, pp. 101–108, 2007.

[2] L. A. Lee, "The clinical spectrum of neonatal lupus," *Archives of Dermatological Research*, vol. 301, no. 1, pp. 107–110, 2009.

[3] V. Nickeleit, M. Zeiler, F. Gudat, G. Thiel, and M. J. Mihatsch, "Detection of the complement degradation product C4d in renal allografts: Diagnostic and therapeutic implications," *Journal of the American Society of Nephrology*, vol. 13, no. 1, pp. 242–251, 2002.

[4] S. Minamiguchi, Y. Mikami, N. Nakajima et al., "Complement split product C4d deposition in placenta in systemic lupus erythematosus and pregnancy-induced hypertension," *Pathology International*, vol. 63, no. 3, pp. 150–157, 2013.

[5] E. N. Kim, B. H. Yoon, J. Y. Lee et al., "Placental C4d deposition is a feature of defective placentation: observations in cases of preeclampsia and miscarriage," *Virchows Archiv*, vol. 466, no. 6, pp. 717–725, 2015.

[6] D. Cohen, R. B. Colvin, M. R. Daha et al., "Pros and cons for C4d as a biomarker," *Kidney International*, vol. 81, no. 7, pp. 628–639, 2012.

[7] M. G. Crespo-Leiro, A. Veiga-Barreiro, N. Domenech et al., "Humoral heart rejection (severe allograft dysfunction with no signs of cellular rejection or ischemia): incidence, management, and the value of C4d for diagnosis," *American Journal of Transplantation*, vol. 5, no. 10, pp. 2560–2564, 2005.

[8] C. M. Magro, A. Pope Harman, D. Klinger et al., "Use of C4d as a diagnostic adjunct in lung allograft biopsies," *American Journal of Transplantation*, vol. 3, no. 9, pp. 1143–1154, 2003.

[9] W. Wisuthsarewong, J. Soongswang, and R. Chantorn, "Neonatal lupus erythematosus: clinical character, investigation, and outcome," *Pediatric Dermatology*, vol. 28, no. 2, pp. 115–121, 2011.

[10] M. C. Audette, K. Levytska, S. J. Lye, N. Melamed, and J. C. Kingdom, "Parental ethnicity and placental maternal vascular malperfusion pathology in healthy nulliparous women," *Placenta*, vol. 66, pp. 40–46, 2018.

[11] A. Revaux, A. Mekinian, P. Nicaise et al., "Antiphospholipid syndrome and other autoimmune diseases associated with chronic intervillositis," *Archives of Gynecology and Obstetrics*, vol. 291, no. 6, pp. 1229–1236, 2015.

[12] A. A. Zuppa, R. Riccardi, S. Frezza et al., "Neonatal lupus: Follow-up in infants with anti -SSA/Ro antibodies and review of the literature," *Autoimmunity Reviews*, vol. 16, no. 4, pp. 427–432, 2017.

[13] Y. Li, Q. Wang, Y. Luo, and Y. Zhao, "Neonatal lupus erythematosus: a review of 123 cases in China," *International Journal of Rheumatic Diseases*, vol. 18, no. 7, pp. 761–767, 2015.

Management of Severe Epistaxis during Pregnancy: A Case Report and Review of the Literature

Maria Grazia Piccioni, Martina Derme, Laura Salerno, Elisa Morrocchi, Francesco Pecorini, Maria Grazia Porpora, and Roberto Brunelli

Department of Gynecological, Obstetrical and Urological Sciences, University of Rome "Sapienza", Viale del Policlinico, 155, 00161 Rome, Italy

Correspondence should be addressed to Laura Salerno; laurasalerno88@gmail.com

Academic Editor: Kyousuke Takeuchi

Background. Epistaxis is a common problem during pregnancy. Few cases of severe epistaxis, not associated with nasal lesions or clotting disorders, were described in the literature. We reported a case of severe epistaxis in a pregnant patient, exploring all the different possible management options. *Case.* A 33-year-old primigravida, who was 38 weeks pregnant, presented with spontaneous severe left-sided epistaxis. Her blood pressure was into normal ranges. Clotting disorders and nasal lesions were excluded. The patient clinical worsening, due to severe anemia, and the failure of conservative treatment have imposed an emergency caesarean section, with an immediate resolution of the nasal bleeding. *Conclusion.* Treatment of severe epistaxis must always consider conservative measures first-line with early recourse to otolaryngologist. In general, delivery of the fetus is considered curative.

1. Introduction

Epistaxis is a common problem during pregnancy, due to an increased nasal mucosa vascularity. The prevalence in pregnant women is 20.3% compared with 6.2% in nonpregnant ones [1]. Large volume epistaxis is rare for patients without preexisting risk factors or conditions, such as the use of anticoagulants or blood clotting disorders.

Few cases of severe epistaxis during pregnancy, not associated with nasal lesions or clotting disorders, were described in the literature, demonstrating a lack of familiarity regarding the appropriate management options in these clinical conditions.

We report a case of severe, prolonged epistaxis in a pregnant patient, during the third trimester, with no clear risk factors. We explored the different possible management options in this challenging case and we assume our experience may help in future similarly clinical situations.

2. Case Presentation

A 33-year-old primigravida, who was 38 weeks pregnant, presented with spontaneous severe left-sided epistaxis. Her first episode had started the previous week, with about seven-eight episodes a day. Her medical history was unremarkable. She had no personal or family history of bleeding tendencies, and she was not taking any regular medications. Her blood pressure was into normal ranges. She reported no previous episodes of epistaxis in her life. Routine blood tests were normal during the pregnancy.

We tried to control the bleeding first by administrating intravenous (IV) tranexamic acid, without resolution. So, we contacted the otolaryngologist, who performed an endoscopy, showing a left nasal floor bleeding varix. He decided for an anterior nasal packing: he inserted a tampon carefully along the floor of the left nostril, where it expanded on contact with blood. After the nasal tampon was been inserted, the otolaryngologist wetted it with a small amount of topical vasoconstrictor in order to hasten effectiveness. This procedure was repeated three times, inserting a total of six tampons (four in left nostril and two in the right one). Nevertheless, this conservative management of epistaxis failed. Within 4 hours of admission, patient haemoglobin had dropped from 12.5 to 7 mg/dl and she had a further bleed from the left nostril. The otolaryngologist did not consider a posterior nasal packing because the endoscopy showed an anterior

Table 1: Cases of severe epistaxis during pregnancy not associated with nasal lesion or clotting disorders.

Author/year	Number of patients	Management of epistaxis	Management of pregnancy
Green L K 1974 [2]	1	Local pressure; nasal packing	Emergency caesarean section
El Goulli M 1979 [3]	1	Nasal packing	Vaginal delivery
Howard DJ 1985 [4]	1	Nasal packing; bipolar diathermy; external carotid artery ligation; nasal balloon	Emergency caesarean section
Braithwaite J M [5]	1	Nasal packing; nasal balloon	Emergency caesarean section
Cooley 2002 [6]	1	Nasal packing; nasal balloon	Emergency caesarean section
Hardy 2008 [7]	1	Nasal packing; bipolar cautery; artery ligation	Vaginal delivery
Cornthwaite K 2013 [8]	1	Nasal packing; bipolar diathermy	Elective caesarean section
Crunkhorn RE 2014 [9]	1	Nasal packing; sphenopalatine artery (SPA) ligation; bipolar cautery; bipolar diathermy	Elective caesarean section
Our case 2018	1	IV* tranexamic acid nasal packing; bipolar cautery	Emergency caesarean section

Footnotes: * intravenous.

bleeding site. A new endoscopy to locate the exact site of bleeding for direct cauterization was not indicated in acute setting due to vascular congestion and mucosal oedema. Patient clotting studies were within the normal range. A blood transfusion was required, using two packed red blood cells (PRBCs). The patient also started antibiotic therapy with IV Cephazolin 2 g every 8 hours. Cardiotocography (CTG), biophysical profile, and fetal Doppler demonstrated fetal well-being.

During her second day of admission, repeated blood tests showed that her haemoglobin remained persistently low at 7.5 g/dl, despite the recent blood transfusion. The patient became tachycardic (rate 157 bpm), tachypnoeic (22 breaths per minute), and asthenic.

After accurate counselling with the patient and considering the failure of conservative treatment, we thereby decided for a surgical management of pregnancy. The patient delivered a healthy baby girl weighing 3.9 kg. The execution of caesarean section was followed by an immediate resolution of the nasal bleeding.

We discharged the patient from the hospital with nasal packing, in order to ensure the formation of an adequate clot. Five days later, the otolaryngologist performed an endoscopy to locate the exact site of bleeding for direct cauterization. The patient experienced no other episodes of epistaxis.

3. Discussion

Epistaxis in pregnancy is common but the vast majority of cases do not require medical attention. The prevalence of epistaxis in pregnant women is more than three times that in nonpregnant ones [1].

Several conditions predispose to epistaxis during pregnancy. In particular, the elevated oestrogen levels increase the vascularity of the nasal mucosa [10], which may potentiate and prolong the bleeding. Progesterone causes an increase in blood volume, which may exacerbate both vascular congestion and hence bleeding, and may mask blood loss in the event of severe epistaxis, due to apparently effective cardiovascular compensation [11]. Placental growth hormone has systemic effects, including vasodilation [11]. Indirect hormonal effects include vascular inflammatory and immunological changes that may predispose to nasal hypersensitivity and hence to problems such as nasal granuloma gravidarum [11]. In general, delivery or fetal death causes immediate cessation of the nasal bleeding, because some of the underlying factors, such as congestion and hyperemia, disappear.

Few cases of severe epistaxis during pregnancy were described in literature [2–8, 12] (Table 1). We excluded cases of epistaxis associated with nasal lesions, like granuloma gravidarum [9] and nasal polyp [13], or clotting disorders [14].

Treatment of severe epistaxis must always consider conservative measures first-line, like IV tranexamic acid administration, anterior packing and bipolar cautery. If conservative treatment fails, two radical treatments have to be considered: the one is surgical, in the form of vessel ligation, and the other is obstetrical and is termination of the pregnancy.

In our case, the patient clinical worsening and the failure of conservative treatment imposed an emergency caesarean section. The cervix was unfavorable for easy induction and a long induction of labor was considered contraindicated for this patient. Valsalva maneuvers could also aggravate the bleeding during labor, increasing the risk of fetal hypoxia. The decision to deliver was also influenced by the gestational age; in fact in the case of a preterm pregnancy, when maternal and fetal conditions are good, a conservative management is preferred, in order to avoid the possible risks associated with preterm birth.

Fetal anemia is a well-known cause of antenatal fetal distress. The case report by Braithwaite JM et al. [5] demonstrated that rapidly developing severe maternal anemia, due to recurrent blood loss of nonplacental origin, even in the absence of maternal hypotension, can cause fetal distress.

Severe epistaxis is potentially life-threatening to both mother and fetus.

This case highlights the importance of early recourse to ear, nose, and throat (ENT) referral, when epistaxis is unresponsive to simple measures. In general, when nasal lesions and clotting disorders cannot be identified, fetal delivery is considered curative, showing that hormonal changes during pregnancy may lead to significant alterations of nasal physiology, with oestrogen causing vascular congestion, mucosal oedema, and rhinitis, known as the "rhinitis of pregnancy". Moreover, pregnancy is associated with significant anatomic and physiologic remodeling of the cardiovascular system. Starting at 6-8 weeks of gestation and peaking at 32 weeks, maternal blood volume increases by 40–50% above nonpregnant volumes [15, 16]. Termination of pregnancy resolves hypervolemia and hormonal changes; in fact in all the cases reported in Table 1, we can observe a nasal bleeding resolution after delivery.

References

[1] M. Dugan-Kim, S. Connell, C. Stika, C. A. Wong, and D. R. Gossett, "Epistaxis of pregnancy and association with postpartum hemorrhage," *Obstetrics & Gynecology*, vol. 114, no. 6, pp. 1322–1325, 2009.

[2] L. K. Green, R. S. Green, and R. E. Harris, "Life-threatening epistaxis associated with pregnancy," *American Journal of Obstetrics & Gynecology*, vol. 120, no. 8, pp. 1113-1114, 1974.

[3] M. El Goulli and M. Chelli, "Severe epistaxis during pregnancy. A case history," *Journal de Gynécologie Obstétrique et Biologie de la Reproduction*, vol. 8, pp. 437–439, 1979.

[4] D. J. Howard, "Life-threatening epistaxis in pregnancy," *The Journal of Laryngology & Otology*, vol. 99, no. 1, pp. 95-96, 1985.

[5] J. M. Braithwaite and D. L. Economides, "Severe recurrent epistaxis causing antepartum fetal distress," *International Journal of Gynecology and Obstetrics*, vol. 50, no. 2, pp. 197-198, 1995.

[6] J. J. Hardy, C. M. Connolly, and C. J. Weir, "Epistaxis in pregnancy - not to be sniffed at!," *International Journal of Obstetric Anesthesia*, vol. 17, no. 1, pp. 94-95, 2008.

[7] K. Cornthwaite, K. Varadharajan, M. Oyarzabal, and H. Watson, "Management of prolonged epistaxis in pregnancy: Case report," *The Journal of Laryngology & Otology*, vol. 127, no. 8, pp. 811–813, 2013.

[8] R. E. M. Crunkhorn, A. Mitchell-Innes, and J. Muzaffar, "Torrential epistaxis in the third trimester: A management conundrum," *BMJ Case Reports*, vol. 2014, Article ID 203892, 2014.

[9] Y. Noorizan and H. Salina, "Nasal septal haemangioma in pregnancy," *Medical Journal of Malaysia*, vol. 65, no. 1, pp. 70-71, 2010.

[10] G. Goldstein and S. Govindaraj, "Rhinologic issues in pregnancy," *Allergy & Rhinology*, vol. 3, no. 1, pp. 13–15, 2012.

[11] S. E. Sobol, S. Frenkiel, D. Nachtigal, D. Wiener, and C. Teblum, "Clinical manifestations of sinonasal pathology during pregnancy," *Journal of Otolaryngology*, vol. 30, no. 1, pp. 24–28, 2001.

[12] S. M. Cooley, M. Geary, M. P. O'Connell, and D. P. Keane, "Hypovolaemic shock secondary to epistaxis in pregnancy," *Journal of Obstetrics & Gynaecology*, vol. 22, no. 2, pp. 229-230, 2002.

[13] P. M. J. Scott and A. Van Hasselt, "Case report of a bleeding nasal polyp during pregnancy," *Ear, Nose & Throat Journal*, vol. 78, no. 8, p. 592, 1999.

[14] G. Aynağolu, G. D. Durdağ, B. Özmen, and F. Söylemez, "Successful treatment of hereditary factor VII deficiency presented for the first time with epistaxis in pregnancy: A case report," *The Journal of Maternal-Fetal and Neonatal Medicine*, vol. 23, no. 9, pp. 1053–1055, 2010.

[15] F. E. Hytten and D. B. Paintin, "Increase in plasma volume during normal pregnancy," *Obstetrical & Gynecological Survey*, vol. 70, pp. 602–607, 1963.

[16] M. M. Costantine, "Physiologic and pharmacokinetic changes in pregnancy," *Frontiers in Pharmacology*, vol. 5, no. 65, 2014.

46

A Clinical Study on Initial Experience of COVID-19 ARDS in Obstetric Patients at a Tertiary Care Centre in India

Sheeba Marwah,[1,2] Reenu Kanwar,[1,2] Shahida Naghma,[1,2] Anjali Dabral,[1,2] and Nitesh Gupta[2,3]

[1]Department of Obstetrics and Gynaecology, New Delhi 110029, India
[2]VMMC and Safdarjung Hospital, New Delhi 110029, India
[3]Department of Pulmonary, Critical and Sleep Medicine, New Delhi 110029, India

Correspondence should be addressed to Anjali Dabral; dranjalidabralacademic@gmail.com

Academic Editor: Seung-Yup Ku

Coronavirus disease 2019 (COVID-19) is caused by a novel coronavirus (severe acute respiratory syndrome coronavirus 2 (SARS-CoV-2)) which causes severe viral pneumonia rapidly leading to acute respiratory distress syndrome (ARDS). Pregnant women are considered more vulnerable to severe viral respiratory infections owing to the physiological changes in pregnancy. In COVID-19, patient can present with a variety of symptoms of which dyspnoea is one that is also commonly seen in the late stages of pregnancy. The clinical presentation as well as response to therapy is highly variable, and since no conclusive proven treatment is available yet, prevention and symptomatic treatment remains the mainstay of management. Thus, we report a case series of four SARS-CoV-2-positive obstetric patients who presented with severe ARDS in a tertiary care hospital, posing diagnostic and therapeutic challenges to the clinician, and were managed with a holistic multidisciplinary stepwise approach. Through this, an effort has been made to sensitize the attending obstetrician on diverse presentation of COVID-19 disease and to emphasize the importance of prevention, early pick up, and timely optimal management of pneumonia in pregnant females with COVID-19. The clinical presentation of respiratory illness due to SARS-CoV-2 in pregnancy can be mistaken for exaggerated physiological changes of pregnancy leading to delay in seeking medical care. During the current pandemic, high suspicion for COVID-19 should be kept. If found symptomatic, immediate care should be sought in a designated facility and managed accordingly preferably with a multidisciplinary approach.

1. Introduction

The present COVID-19 pandemic with a worldwide spread is caused by SARS-CoV-2. Coronavirus disease is believed to be a zoonotic disease, with the intermediate host being unclear [1]. It is commonly transmitted through air, respiratory droplets, contact, and even fecal-oral route [2]. Coronavirus disease can present with fever, cough, and dyspnoea often followed by pneumonia. The World Health Organization (WHO) has termed the pneumonia caused by SARS-CoV-2 as the coronavirus disease 2019 (COVID-19) [3, 4].

About 80% of COVID-positive patients are classified as mild and the remaining 20% as severe or critical [5, 6] which are associated with complications like ARDS (acute respiratory distress syndrome), disseminated intravascular coagulopathy, renal failure, secondary bacterial pneumonia sepsis, shock with organ failure, and respiratory failure. Pregnant women are considered more vulnerable to severe viral respiratory infections. Till date, no treatment has been proven to be curative for the SARS-CoV-2 virus; hence, supportive treatment with supplemental oxygen therapy (if required) is the key for management.

The review of literature till date illustrates no additional risk in the morbidity and mortality associated with COVID-19 in pregnant women, but owing to the physiological changes in pregnancy like diaphragm elevation, increased oxygen consumption, and oedema of respiratory tract mucosa; they become intolerant to hypoxia [7–10]. In addition, hypercoagulable state in pregnancy increases the risk of pulmonary microvascular thrombosis. Due to all these factors, any superimposed insult by the virus may contribute to exacerbations of respiratory diseases in the antenatal and postpartum period. Because of similarity in exaggerated physiological symptoms in normal pregnancy and in any respiratory illness, there might be a possible delay in seeking medical care by patients during pregnancy. This topped with variable presentation of COVID-19 pneumonia, which can easily be misleading to the attending clinician. Thus, an attempt is made to describe a case series of four obstetric patients admitted in a tertiary hospital, emphasizing the importance of prevention, early diagnosis, and management of COVID pneumonia in these cases.

2. Case Presentation

2.1. Case 1. A 26-year-old female P1L1 (para 1, living 1) with no previous comorbidities had full-term normal vaginal delivery. Her antenatal period was thoroughly supervised and uneventful. She was completely asymptomatic till day 5 of postpartum period, when she presented with shortness of breath with dry cough for 2 days. She was referred to our tertiary care hospital for further management in view of clinically deteriorating symptoms. At the time of presentation in emergency room (ER), she had fair general condition: pulse—120/min, BP (blood pressure)—104/70 mmHg, RR (respiratory rate)—36/min, SPO_2 (oxygen saturation)—64% on room air, cardiovascular system—normal, chest ex—B/L (bilateral) crepitations present, B/L decreased breath sounds, P/A (per-abdomen)—uterus 16 weeks, well contracted, nontender, P/V (per vaginum)—episiotomy healthy, lochia healthy. On reviewing her records, chest X-ray (done 24 hrs back) showed patchy peripheral extensive consolidation along with ground-glass opacities in B/L lung fields predominantly in mid and lower zones suggestive of atypical pneumonia. ECG (echocardiograph) showed sinus tachycardia. After initial management and evaluation, she was admitted in SARI (severe acute respiratory distress isolation) ward in collaboration with Medicine Department. All routine investigations, cultures, and ABG (arterial blood gas analysis) were sent. COVID-19 testing was done using nasopharyngeal swab. She was tested positive for SARS-CoV-2 and was shifted to designated COVID-19 ICU (intensive care unit). Patient was put on NRBM (nonrebreathing mask) at 15 lt/min followed by NIV (noninvasive ventilation). Because of inability to maintain oxygen saturation, patient required intubation and was put on mechanical ventilation for a day. She was provided with supportive care guided by Government of India (GOI) guidelines, including the antiviral drug (remdesivir) and higher intravenous antibiotics with steroid therapy for 10 days. She was extubated on the very next day and was put on NIV again. Her blood reports were within normal range except indicative of infection: haemoglobin—12.2 gm/dl, TLC (total leucocyte count)—16,300, platelets—1,13,000, INR (international normalized ratio)—1.18, LFT/KFT (liver function tests/kidney function tests)—normal. Ultrasound chest was done on day 10 suggestive of B/L consolidation in left to right and no evidence of any effusion. During her hospital stay, she complained of pain left-sided abdomen. She was evaluated in conjunction with gastroenterologist. An ultrasound of the whole abdomen was done and she was diagnosed to have portal cavernoma, which did not require any active intervention. In view of persistent tachycardia, cardiology consultation was done. Her 2D echo (2-dimensional echocardiogram) revealed ejection fraction—55%, no clots, no RWMA (regional wall motion abnormalities). She was subjected to serial chest radiographs, as advised by pulmonologist, which showed a gradual resolution in sizes of patches and opacity as shown in Figures 1(a)–1(d).

There was no history of any contact with the COVID-19-positive patient; her newborn baby was also tested positive for SARS-CoV-2 and required admission in nursery but was discharged after 7 days. Her remaining contact tracing was negative. After almost 7 weeks of hospital stay, she was tested negative for COVID-19 disease in 2 consecutive reports. Due to the massive spread of infection to lower respiratory tract, the patient was required with NRBM for maintaining saturation for almost 2 months but severity of symptoms decreased significantly. She gradually started maintaining oxygen saturation on room air. At the time of writing this paper, the patient has been discharged back home in good health to join her family.

2.2. Case 2. A 34-year-old woman G2P1L1 (gravida 2, para 1, living 1) at 39 weeks of POG with previous LSCS was presented in the Gynaecology Casualty with complaints of fever, cough, and breathlessness for 5 days. She had an uneventful antenatal period with no previous respiratory/-cardiac disease or any history of high BP records. At the time of presentation, her general condition was dyspnoeic: pulse—130/min, BP—160/112 mmHg, urine albumin—+3, temperature—98.3°F, RR—24/min, SPO_2—94% (room air), CVS—normal, chest examination—B/L crepitations present, B/L decreased breath sounds, on P/A examination—36 wks, cephalic, foetal heart sound (FHS) absent, uterus relaxed, no scar tenderness, nontender, P/V—1 cm dilated, uneffaced, membrane present, vertex—3, pelvis adequate.

In view of high BP with urine albumin +3 and crepitations in B/L chest, diagnosis of severe preeclampsia with pulmonary edema with differential of COVID-19 was made. She was put on oxygen mask with reservoir, injectable diuretics were given, and urgent ultrasound was done in ER which revealed intrauterine death. After initial stabilization in causality, patient was admitted in SARI Ward. She was put on NIV as she was not maintaining saturation (<90%) (haemoglobin—11.3 gm/dl, TLC—9300, platelets—1.75 lakhs/mm^3, INR—1.02, KFT/serum electrolytes—normal, LFT—1/243/256/542). Chest X-ray was done which showed inhomogeneous airspace in peripheral distribution with B/L blunting of costophrenic angles likely due to pleural effusion. COVID-19 testing was done with nasopharyngeal swab on the day of admission which came negative. Patient went in spontaneous labor and was shifted to the labor room for monitoring of progress of labor where she required with NRBM to maintain oxygen saturation. She was started on antibiotics and antiviral drugs. Because of the persistent high blood pressure, cardiology opinion was sought. 2D echo was done which was essentially normal. As there was strong clinical suspicion of COVID-19 pneumonia, repeat testing was done after 2 days and patient was diagnosed to

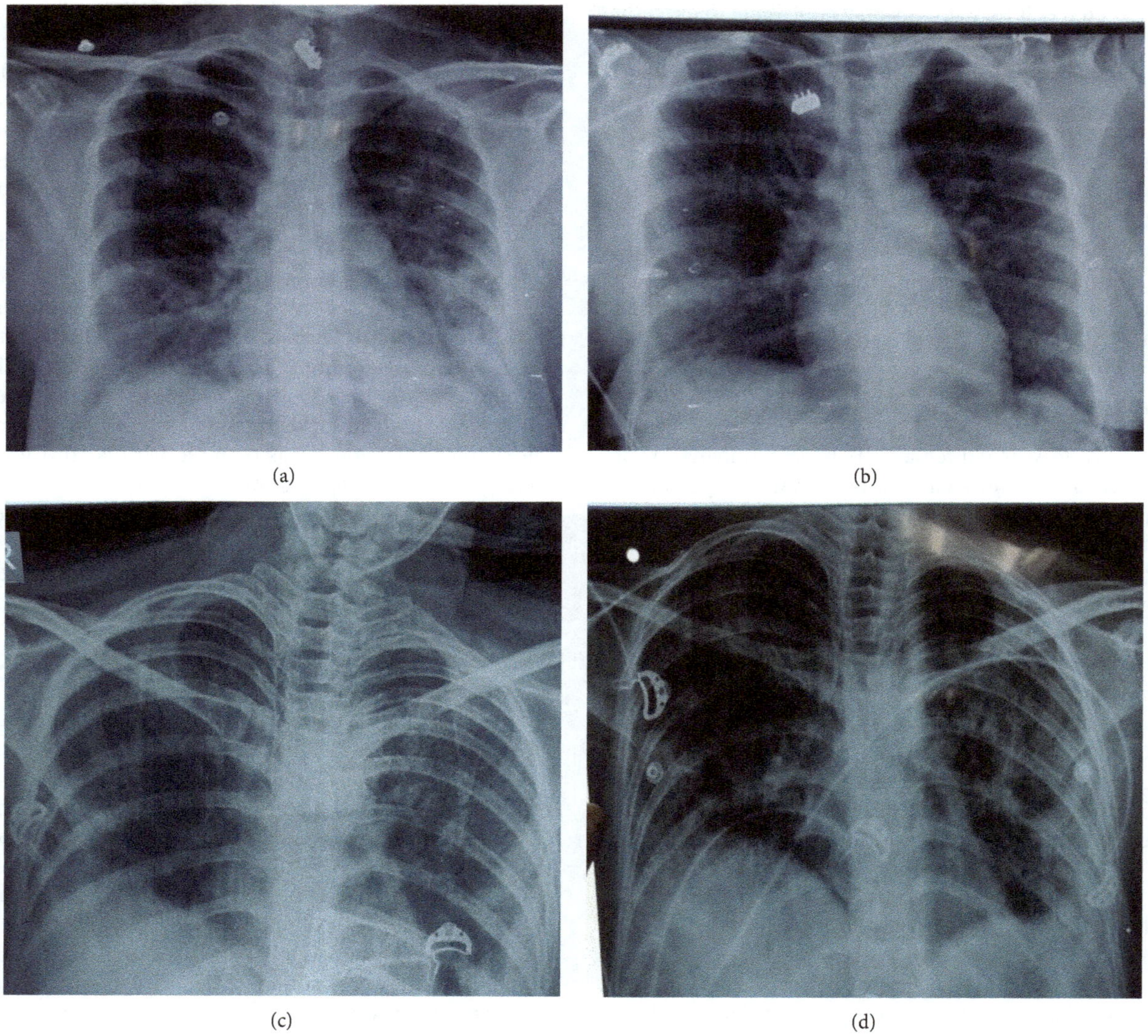

FIGURE 1: Radiological findings: (a) postnatal day 7, (b) postnatal day 11, (c) postnatal day 30, and (d) postnatal day 36.

be SARS-CoV-2 positive. Patient was immediately shifted to a COVID-19-designated ICU. She went in spontaneous labor and delivered a fresh still born baby girl of 2.45 kg. There was no intrapartum complications. Postnatally, further serial chest X-rays showed radiological improvement in the form of decrease in pleural effusion and clearing of costophrenic angles. After delivery, she required high flow oxygen for almost a week following which she was gradually shifted to oxygen mask and started maintaining oxygen on a room air. After being asymptomatic for a week, patient was discharged for further home isolation as per GOI guidelines with an advice to follow up after 2 weeks or SOS.

2.3. Case 3. A 30-year-old female G2P1L1 at 37 weeks and 2 days of gestation with gestational hypertension was presented in the Gynaecology Casualty of our hospital with complaints of breathlessness for 2 days. Patient was referred from a government hospital in view of breathlessness with pulmonary edema. Her antenatal period was uneventful. At the time of presentation, patient was visibly dyspnoeic: pulse—118/min, BP—170/122 mmHg, urine albumin—+3, temperature—afebrile, RR—28/min, SPO_2—96% (room air), CVS—normal, chest examination—B/L crepitations present, B/L decreased breath sounds, on P/A examination—34 weeks, cephalic, FHS present and regular, uterus relaxed, P/V—Os closed, uneffaced, pelvis adequate. Diagnosis of severe preeclampsia with pulmonary edema was made, and patient was initiated on diuretic while being on high flow oxygen. She was prepared for emergency LSCS (lower segment caesarean section) under a high-risk consent. COVID-19 testing was done preoperatively. Emergency LSCS was done under general anaesthesia. A baby boy of 1.9 kg was delivered and was shifted to NICU (neonatal intensive care unit) in view of low respiratory efforts and low birth weight. Baby was tested negative for COVID-19 disease. An attempt to extubate the patient was made postsurgery but could not be done in view of poor chest condition. She was shifted to ICU in immediate postoperative period. Injectable antibiotics was given along with diuretics. Her COVID-19 test came back positive. She was shifted to COVID-19 ICU where the patient was given supportive care in the form of mechanical ventilation, antibiotics, and obstetrics postop care. Her baby was also tested positive and was managed in NICU. She was extubated on the next day and was put on NIV. After 3 days, she was able to maintain oxygen saturation without support. She was later shifted to the Gynaecology COVID-19 ward and discharged from there after 10 days with a baby boy.

2.4. Case 4. A 26-year-old female G2P1L0 (gravida 2, para 1, living 0) at 37 weeks and 5 days of POG with hypothyroidism was presented in the Gynaecology Casualty with complaints of leaking per vaginum for 12 hrs. There were no complaints of fever, cough, and breathlessness. At the time of presentation, her general condition was fair: pulse—86/min, BP—112/76 mmHg, temp—97.6°F, RR—24/min, SPO_2—94% (room air), CVS—S1S2+, chest ex—B/L clear, on P/A ex—34 wks, cephalic, FHS present, and regular (140/min), uterus contraction present, P/V—2 cm dilated, 50% effaced, membrane absent, vertex—2, pelvis adequate.

She was admitted in the labor room where she progressed gradually and spontaneously and had full-term normal vaginal delivery of a baby boy of 2.4 kg. The baby and mother were doing absolutely fine until postnatal day 2, when she started having difficulty in breathing and a cough (on examination, pulse—100/min, BP—132/90 mmHg, SPO_2—94%, temp—100.8°F, heart—normal, no murmur, chest ex—B/L crepitations present). She was managed immediately with oxygen support, diuretics, and analgesics. A vital monitor was attached. Her COVID-19 testing was done, and meanwhile, the patient was kept in isolation. Cardiology referral was done. ECG was found to be normal, and pro-BNP (brain natriuretic peptide) came out negative. Her lab reports were as follows: Hb—13.5 gm/dl, TLC—11,500, PT—1,70,000. Her chest X-ray showed B/L consolidation predominantly in lower zones with no evidence of pleural effusion. She came out COVID-19 positive and was shifted to a designated COVID-19 ICU as she was not maintaining oxygen saturation with an oxygen mask at 10 lt/min. In ICU, she was put on NRBM for 2 days along with multivitamins and zinc supplements. Taking antibiotics was continued for 5 days. After 5 days of diagnosis, she started maintaining oxygen saturation on room air with radiological improvement in serial X-rays. Patient was moved back to the COVID-19-designated ward. Her baby tested negative for COVID-19. At the time of writing this paper, patient is still admitted in the hospital with no symptoms. She is planned to be discharged after testing negative.

3. Discussion

The ongoing COVID-19 pandemic is a global public health emergency, the course and outcome of the disease being highly unpredictable. Illness caused by SARS-CoV-2 ranges from asymptomatic viraemia to symptomatic disease similar to influenza like illness in various stages and can even be fatal. Also, the morbidity associated with physiology of pregnancy overlapping with respiratory illness leads to deferment in seeking timely help. Therefore, early diagnosis and critical management of these women becomes an important confounding factor for associated comorbidity in such patients. Over the past few months, lots of insights have been gained on COVID-19, but robust evidence on respiratory symptoms of pregnant women with SARS-COV-2 are unavailable; hence, we present a narrative case series of 4 young females affected with SARS-CoV-2 during pregnancy. A comparative evaluation of present series with the limited body of literature available in current times has been discussed (Table 1).

Recent studies have revealed negligible difference in presentation of COVID-19 infection in pregnant and nonpregnant women. However, associated comorbidities especially hypertensive disorders of pregnancy can worsen the stages of COVID-19 and thus their outcome. This is consistent with the study by Chen and colleagues, wherein the clinical characteristics reported in pregnant women with confirmed COVID-19 infection were similar to those reported for nonpregnant adults with confirmed COVID-19 infection in the general population and were indicative of a relatively optimistic clinical course and outcomes for COVID-19 infection [7, 10].

However, contact with a positive patient is a known risk factor for acquiring SARS-CoV-2 virus but it was absent in all the cases in the current study. Similarly, the observations reported by Sahin et al. wherein they found that 75% of the patients had negative history of close contact. This reiterates the importance of high clinical suspicion of COVID-19 in the presence of clinical findings even without significant history of exposure [11].

The presenting symptoms in the patients under current study included fever, cough, cold, chest pain, shortness of breath, and myalgia which were consistent to the findings of previous researchers [11, 12].

Even though in-house HRCT for SARS-CoV-2-positive patients was not available, all four women in the current series underwent chest X-rays which revealed peripheral patchy infiltrates in B/L lungs. This finding was peculiarly parallel to the most frequent CT finding reported by most of the investigators in COVID-19 pneumonia in pregnancy [5, 12]. This highlights the importance of adopting a step-by-step approach to the management of dyspnoea in pregnancy including all preliminary investigations like chest radiographs even in modern times.

Inflammatory markers (serum ferritin, interleukin 6, C-reactive protein, and serum LDH) were increased in all 4 women. This is in synchrony with several other studies and adding to the evidence in the role of anti-inflammatory agents in COVID-19 disease, thus emphasizing the importance of proinflammatory cytokines in disease progression [13].

Amongst the four patients reported in our series, two presented with findings consistent with COVID-19 pneumonia. While the other two of them presented with acute respiratory distress syndrome owing to pulmonary edema. The largest case narrative on COVID-19 pneumonia in pregnancy, conducted in Spain, showed that pregnant females have a 61.5% chance of developing pneumonia as compared to the general population between age groups 30-40 years [14]. Since the advent of novel SARS-CoV-2, only few isolated cases of COVID-19 pneumonia in pregnancy have been reported. It is associated with varied complications including acute respiratory distress syndrome, disseminated intravascular coagulopathy, renal failure, secondary bacterial pneumonia sepsis, shock with organ failure, respiratory

Table 1

S no	Studies	Study population	Type of study	Study centre	Observations
1.	Chen et al.	118 pregnant women	Epidemiological review	China	(i) 8%—severe disease (ii) 0.008%—required NIV (iii) Mortality—nil
2.	San-Juan et al.	52 pregnant women with COVID-19	Single-centred cohort study	Spain	(i) Pneumonia—61.5% (>50% required supplemental oxygen) (ii) Most common radiological findings were bilateral ground-glass opacities (46.8%) followed by bilateral or unilateral alveolar infiltrates (40.6%) (iii) ARDS—25% (iv) IMV—6.2%
3.	Knight et al.	427 pregnant women with COVID-19	Prospective population-based cohort study	All obstetric unit in UK	(i) Needed critical care—10% (ii) ECMO—1% (iii) Pneumonia on imaging—24%
4.	Kayem et al.	617 pregnant women with COVID-19	Case series	France	(i) Typical chest CT features of pneumonia—8.3% (ii) Nasal oxygen therapy—13.5% (iii) NIV—1.6% (iv) Invasive mechanical ventilation—4.7% (v) ECMO—1% (vi) Association with hypertensive disorders—3.4%
5.	Present case series	4 pregnant women with COVID-19-related ARDS	Case series	India	(i) Typical chest radiograph features of pneumonia—25% (ii) NIV—25% (iii) NRBM—25% (iv) Invasive ventilation—50% (v) Association with hypertensive disorders—50%

failure requiring mechanical ventilation, or refractory hypoxemia requiring extracorporal membrane oxygenation. However, such serious complications could be averted successfully in our patients due to vigilant monitoring and timely intervention due to high index of suspicion.

All of the four patients in the series were successfully discharged; this was in congruence with a systematic view of 41 pregnancies affected by COVID-19 and another report of 108 pregnancies, which also reported no maternal deaths [15, 16]. However, a different observation was made by an Iranian case series wherein they reported 7 maternal deaths in nine pregnant women with critical COVID-19 [17].

Out of 4 cases included in the current study, 3 had live births; whereas, one was a diagnosed intrauterine death. Out of these, only one baby (Case 1) was tested positive who was also discharged after 7 days in a healthy condition. However, this could be a horizontal spread and so vertical transmission could not be documented in this particular case due to the absence of breast milk, histopathological examination of placenta, cord blood, and amniotic fluid. The largest systemic review and meta-analysis studying the vertical transmission in coronavirus positive cases included 39 studies (1316 pregnant women) and also concluded no transmission of COVID-19 from the mother to the foetus in utero till date [18].

There is no evidence-based treatment for COVID-19-associated pneumonia yet, and the treatment mainly focuses on supportive therapy, improving immunity and supplemental oxygen therapy. All four patients included in the study were given steroid since day 1 of admission as per protocol and government of India guidelines and they responded well to the therapy. This is alike the inference of RECOVERY trial which depicted that steroids significantly decrease the 28-day mortality for individuals with COVID-19-positive patients requiring oxygen (age-adjusted rate ratio 0.83; 95% CI 0.75–0.93; $P < 0.001$) [19].

There is limited data available on the use and safety of remdesivir (an antiviral nucleotide prodrug that effectively inhibits replication of SARS-CoV-2 in vitro) in pregnancy. Although recent case reports documented no side effects of remdesivir in pregnant women, it cannot be concluded to be safe in pregnancy since all these women had administered the drug in the 2nd/3rd trimester only [20–22]. Therefore, none of the women were given remdesivir as part of therapy in the current study in antenatal period. In another case series by Burwick et al., of 86 women (67 were pregnant, 19 have immediate postpartum), remdesivir was administered on a compassionate basis for severe COVID-19 infection and resulted in high clinical recovery, though with increased rate of preterm delivery [23].

Amoxicillin and azithromycin are classified as class B by FDA and commonly used in pregnancy and breastfeeding [24, 25]. All of the cases in current study with ARDS were given azithromycin as per institutional protocol. Although antibacterial therapy should be started, only if a bacterial infection is suspected, but the initiation was justifiable in our patients as prophylaxis against community-acquired pneumonia in all women with COVID-19 disease.

Symptomatic pregnant women should seek timely medical consultation and help, and women with clinical suspicion of infection should be isolated and investigated. Women diagnosed with infection should be promptly admitted to a negative pressure isolation ward, preferably in a designated hospital with adequate facilities and multidisciplinary expertise to manage critically ill obstetric patients. Adequate rest, hydration, nutritional support, and water and electrolyte balance should be ensured. It is essential to monitor vital signs and oxygen saturation closely. Depending on the severity of the disease, supplemental oxygen inhalation (60%-100% concentration at a rate of 40 l/min) should be given via high flow nasal cannula depending on the severity of hypoxemia. Intubation and mechanical ventilation or even extracorporal membrane oxygenation (ECMO) may be required to maintain oxygenation as was seen in two of our cases (cases 1 and 3).

4. Conclusion

COVID-19 is a global health threat because of its varied presentation and unpredictable behaviour. The outcome is multifactorial; hence, delay in seeking medical care can have adverse implications. Active infection in pregnancy may present with severe respiratory illness in antenatal and postnatal females owing to the physiological changes in the immune and respiratory system. Dyspnoea in pregnancy, often missed, is a grave complication of COVID-19 infection in pregnancy, which if picked up in time can result in optimal maternal and foetal outcome by avoiding serious complications. Diverse presentations and the need to suspect COVID-19 infection earlier in such patients should be emphasised to gynaecologists. Pregnant women being high risk should refrain from unnecessary travel, avoid crowded places, and more importantly, practice and maintain good personal and social hygiene. They should check their temperature regularly and immediately inform their doctor if they experience shortness of breath, cough, or fever. If found symptomatic, immediate care should be sought in designated facility with multidisciplinary approach. To date, research studies conducted in pregnant women with COVID-19 have showed only few maternal and neonatal complications [26], but more concrete evidence and further studies are required to gain insight on its behaviour in pregnancy as these studies included a small number of women over a short period of time.

Consent

All subjects gave their informed consent to participate. No written consent for publication has been obtained from the patients as there is no patient identifiable data included in this case series.

Authors' Contributions

All authors contributed equally to this work.

Acknowledgments

The authors are extremely grateful to all the patients for participating in the study and also extend thanks to participants including doctors, nursing staff, and researchers from the Department of Obstetrics and Gynaecology, Department of Radiology, and Department of Pulmonary Medicine in Safdarjung Hospital.

References

[1] P. Zhou, X. L. Yang, X. G. Wang et al., "A pneumonia outbreak associated with a new coronavirus of probable bat origin," *Nature*, vol. 579, no. 7798, pp. 270–273, 2020.

[2] C. W. Lu, X. F. Liu, and Z. F. Jia, "2019-nCoV transmission through the ocular surface must not be ignored," *The Lancet*, vol. 395, no. 10224, article e39, 2020.

[3] A. E. Gorbalenya, S. C. Baker, R. S. Baric et al., "Severe acute respiratory syndrome-related coronavirus: the species and its viruses – a statement of the coronavirus study group," 2020.

[4] World Health Organization, *Director-general's remarks at the media briefing on 2019-nCoV on 11 February 2020*, WHO, 2020.

[5] C. Huang, Y. Wang, X. Li et al., "Clinical features of patients infected with 2019 novel coronavirus in Wuhan, China," *The Lancet*, vol. 395, no. 10223, pp. 497–506, 2020.

[6] Z. Wu and J. M. McGoogan, "Characteristics of and important lessons from the coronavirus disease (COVID-19) outbreak in China: summary of a report of 72314 cases from the Chinese Centre for Disease Control and Prevention," *JAMA*, vol. 323, pp. 1239–1242, 2020.

[7] J. Yan, J. Guo, and H. Yang, "Coronavirus disease 2019 in pregnant women: a report based on 116 cases," *American Journal of Obstetrics and Gynecology*, vol. 223, no. 1, pp. 111.e1–111.e14, 2020.

[8] W. H. Goodnight and D. E. Soper, "Pneumonia in pregnancy," *Critical Care Medicine*, vol. 33, pp. 390–397, 2005.

[9] M. P. O'Day, "Cardio-respiratory physiological adaptation of pregnancy," *Seminars in Perinatology*, vol. 21, no. 4, pp. 268–275, 1997.

[10] L. Chen, Q. Li, D. Zheng et al., "Clinical characteristics of pregnant women with COVID-19 in Wuhan, China," *The New England Journal of Medicine*, vol. 382, article e100, 2020.

[11] D. Sahin, A. Tanacan, S. A. Erol et al., "Updated experience of a tertiary pandemic center on 533 pregnant women with COVID-19 infection: a prospective cohort study from Turkey," *International Journal of Gynecology and Obstetrics*, vol. 151, pp. 328–334, 2021.

[12] S. Wan, Y. Xiang, W. Fang et al., "Clinical features and treatment of COVID-19 patients in Northeast Chongqing," *Journal of Medical Virology*, vol. 92, no. 7, pp. 797–806, 2020.

[13] F. Zeng, Y. Huang, Y. Guo et al., "Association of inflammatory markers with the severity of COVID-19: a meta-analysis," *International Journal of Infectious Diseases*, vol. 96, pp. 467–474, 2020.

[14] R. San-Juan, M. Fernández-Ruiz, F. López-Medrano et al., "Incidence and clinical profile of COVID-19 pneumonia in pregnant women: a single centre cohort study from Spain," *EClinicalMedicine*, vol. 23, article 100407, 2020.

[15] D. Di Mascio and F. D'Antonio, "Outcome of coronavirus spectrum infections (SARS, MERS, COVID-19) during pregnancy: a systemic review and meta analysis," *American Journal of Obstetrics & Gynecology MFM*, vol. 2, no. 2, article 100107, 2020.

[16] M. Zaigham and O. Andersson, "Maternal and perinatal outcomes with COVID-19: a systematic review of 108 pregnan-

cies," *Acta Obstetricia et Gynecologica Scandinavica*, vol. 99, no. 7, pp. 823–829, 2020.

[17] S. Hantoushzadeh, A. A. Shamshirsaz, A. Aleyasin et al., "Maternal death due to COVID-19," *American Journal of Obstetrics and Gynecology*, vol. 223, no. 1, pp. 109.e1–109.e16, 2020.

[18] K. Diriba, E. Awulachew, and E. Getu, "The effect of coronavirus infection (SARS-CoV-2, MERS-CoV, and SARS-CoV) during pregnancy and the possibility of vertical maternal–fetal transmission: a systematic review and meta-analysis," *European Journal of Medical Research*, vol. 25, no. 1, article 39, 2020.

[19] University of Oxford, *RECOVERY; Randomised evaluation of COVID-19 therapy*.

[20] G. A. Maldarelli, M. Savage, S. Mazur, C. Oxford-Horrey, M. Salvatore, and K. M. Marks, "Remdesivir treatment for severe COVID-19 in third-trimester pregnancy: case report and management discussion," *Open Forum Infectious Diseases*, vol. 7, no. 9, 2020.

[21] M. Naqvi, P. Zakowski, L. Glucksman, S. Smithson, and R. M. Burwick, "Tocilizumab and remdesivir in a pregnant patient with coronavirus disease 2019 (COVID-19)," *Obstetrics & Gynecology*, vol. 136, no. 5, pp. 1025–1029, 2020.

[22] J. Anderson, J. Schauer, S. Bryant, and C. R. Graves, "The use of convalescent plasma therapy and remdesivir in the successful management of a critically ill obstetric patient with novel coronavirus 2019 infection: a case report," *Case Reports in Women's Health.*, vol. 27, 2020.

[23] R. M. Burwick, S. Yawetz, K. E. Stephenson et al., "Compassionate use of remdesivir in pregnant women with severe coronavirus disease 2019," *Clinical Infectious Diseases*, 2020.

[24] U.S Food and Drug Administration, *Amoxicillin drug approval package*, pharmacology review, FDA, Silver Spring (MD), 2000.

[25] U.S Food and Drug Administration, "Azithromycin drug approval package," FDA, Silver Spring (MD), 2006.

[26] Centers for disease control and prevention, *Coronavirus disease 2019 (COVID-19) situation summary*.

Pregnancy in a Woman with Latent Myeloproliferative Neoplasm Induced Chronic Portal Vein Thrombosis, Portal Cavernoma, and Gastric Varices

Andréanne Durivage, Geneviève Le Templier, Annabelle Cumyn, and Nadine Sauvé

Department of General Internal Medicine, Faculty of Medicine, University of Sherbrooke, Quebec, Canada

Correspondence should be addressed to Andréanne Durivage; andreanne.durivage@usherbrooke.ca

Academic Editor: Edi Vaisbuch

Extra-hepatic portal vein thrombosis (EHPVO) represents the obstruction of the portal vein outside the liver and is not related to chronic liver disease or neoplasia. In chronic EHPVO, collateral veins and portal hypertension develop, resulting in splenomegaly and variceal formation. Myeloproliferative neoplasms (MPN) are the most frequent acquired etiology of EHPVO. These conditions put pregnant women at increased risk of vascular complications, including venous thrombosis, occlusion of the placental circulation, and variceal bleeding. In this report, we present a 36-year-old pregnant woman with chronic, anticoagulated EHPVO secondary to latent MPN who developed severe intrauterine growth restriction and had cesarean section at 32+1 weeks for increased umbilical doppler resistance and breech presentation. The article will emphasize outcome and management of pregnancies complicated by chronic EHPVO, portal hypertension, and MPN.

1. Introduction

Extra-hepatic portal vein thrombosis (EHPVO), also named noncirrhotic portal vein thrombosis (PVT), represents obstruction of the extra-hepatic portal vein unrelated to chronic liver disease or neoplasia [1]. Portal venous obstruction is caused by both thrombotic (acquired or hereditary) and nonthrombotic causes. The acquired conditions include abdominal inflammation, infections, surgery, obesity, oral contraceptive intake, pregnancy, postpartum period, and myeloproliferative neoplasms (MPN), which is the most frequent [1, 2]. *Valla et al* reported an incidence of 58% of latent MPN in western patients with EHPVO of unknown etiology. Among those patients, 57% developed an overt MPN during followup [3]. On the other hand, very few PVT are diagnosed throughout pregnancy or postpartum, representing less than 4% of PVT cases in the latest series [4].

In the absence of recanalization, a network of collateral veins develops as a compensatory mechanism of venous rescue to bypass the obstruction [2, 5]. These porto-portal collaterals are given the name "portal cavernoma" [6]. They begin to form rapidly in the first 6 to 20 days following acute thrombosis and are complete 3 to 5 weeks thereafter [2]. Thus, the presence of collateral veins on imaging and signs of portal hypertension, such as splenomegaly and varices, confirm the diagnosis of chronic EHPVO [7]. Hypersplenism and variceal bleeding are frequent manifestations of chronic PVT [6]. Splenomegaly, ranging from moderate to massive, is always present and can be a presenting feature [1]. Furthermore, 30-40% of patients with chronic PVT develop gastric varices secondarily to portal hypertension [6]. There is a constant risk of gastrointestinal bleeding associated with portal cavernoma, sometimes fatal [5].

Women of childbearing age represent nearly 25% of patients with noncirrhotic PVT [5, 6]. Because liver function is usually maintained, their fertility is considered normal [4, 6]. It is well established that pregnancy is associated with an increased risk of thrombosis, a risk that is roughly six times higher than in nonpregnant women [8]. MPN also amplifies thrombotic risk, making pregnant woman with this condition at higher risk of vascular complications including venous thromboembolism and occlusion of the placental circulation

[8]. With that in mind, we present a 36-year-old woman with chronically anticoagulated PVT secondary to latent myeloproliferative neoplasm who was referred to our clinic for preconception counselling. The report will emphasize on outcome and management of pregnancies complicated by chronic PVT, portal hypertension, and MPN.

2. Case Report

A 36-year-old gravida 1 para 0 presented to the obstetric medicine clinic for preconception counselling. Her medical history was notable for chronic thrombosis of the extra-hepatic portal, splenic, and mesenteric veins since 2011. She had developed cavernous transformation in her portal vein, portal hypertension, splenomegaly, and secondary grade 1-2 gastric varices. A few years after the thrombosis was discovered, a diagnosis of latent myeloproliferative neoplasm was made on the basis of a positive Jak-2 mutation (V617F, 1.65% mutational allele burden) and increased cellularity on the bone marrow biopsy. Until now, she has never developed polycythemia, thrombocytosis, or leukocytosis (last hemoglobin level 135 g/L, platelet count 349×10^9/L, and leukocytes count 8.8×10^9/L). The patient was also known for essential hypertension, hypothyroidism, migraine, and obesity. Her first pregnancy (2011), while on depo-provera and warfarin, was interrupted voluntarily. In 2012, she had bilateral salpingectomy with unilateral left ovariectomy for possible endometriosis.

On medication review, she had taken warfarin after the thrombosis diagnosis until it was replaced by dalteparin (18 000 units once a day, subcutaneous injection) because of difficulty to reach and maintain the target international normalized ratio (INR) despite doses greater than 20 mg daily. The patient decided to stop dalteparin nine months after the initial thrombosis. It was not replaced by another anticoagulant because of the risk of variceal bleeding. However, aspirin 80 mg once daily was prescribed to address established platelets, leukocytes, and endothelium interaction in the pathogenesis of vascular occlusion in MPN [8, 9]. Aspirin was replaced by clopidogrel 75 mg once daily after she developed an allergic reaction. Rivaroxaban 20 mg once daily was finally added to her medication when splenic infarctions were discovered at the time of an episode of abdominal pain. At her preconception visit, she was taking rivaroxaban 20 mg once daily and clopidogrel 75 mg once daily.

After a frank and open counselling about the risks associated with a pregnancy, namely, thrombosis (especially considering the *in vitro* fertilization and MPN) and variceal bleeding, she decided to begin the process of *in vitro* fertilization. Rivaroxaban was replaced by once a day subcutaneous therapeutic dose of dalteparin (18 000 units) and clopidogrel was stopped. She was already taking nadolol 20 mg once daily for her gastric varices.

At her 5th week of pregnancy, she had vaginal bleeding, but after a few days of bed rest, it did not recur. Her ultrasound at gestational week 22 showed fetal growth at the 10th percentile. She was hospitalized for 48h at 26 weeks of pregnancy for severe intrauterine growth restriction (IUGR) secondary to placental insufficiency. Nadolol may have also contributed to the IUGR [10]. There was no preeclampsia so she was discharged from the hospital. She finally had a cesarean section at 32+1 weeks for severe IUGR and increased umbilical doppler resistance. This delivery route was chosen because of breech presentation.

At her 3 weeks postpartum followup, she confirmed her decision not to pursue breastfeeding. After a long discussion, it was then decided to stop dalteparin and start apixaban 2.5 mg twice daily, a reduced dose to minimize the risk of variceal bleeding while preventing another thrombosis.

3. Discussion

Outcomes of such cases are uncommon in the medical literature. In the last decade, a total of 83 pregnancies in 43 patients with PVT and portal hypertension were reported in 3 studies [5, 7, 11]. Firstly in 2008, a research reported 12 pregnancies in 5 patients with noncirrhotic portal hypertension [11]. Only one woman had hematemesis at 8 weeks of gestation and was successfully managed with blood transfusion and endoscopic sclerotherapy. In this series, the incidence of small for gestational age babies was increased (44%) [11]. The second study in 2011 reported 26 pregnancies in 14 women with EHPVO [7]. None had variceal bleeding during pregnancy. Anemia and thrombocytopenia were the most common complications caused by hypersplenism. Authors concluded that outcomes are expected to be good if the disease is diagnosed and adequately treated before conception [7]. Finally, in 2012, *Hoekstra et al.* reported 45 pregnancies in 24 patients with PVT [5]. Three patients had esophageal varices bleeding during pregnancy, all without adequate prophylaxis. Postpartum bleeding occurred in 4 women, with only one being anticoagulated at that time. No difference was appreciated in bleeding rate whether patients were anticoagulated or not. There was an association between higher platelet count at diagnosis of PVT and unfavorable outcome during pregnancy. HELLP (hemolysis, elevated liver enzymes, low platelet count) syndrome complicated 2 pregnancies, both presenting infarcts on placental inspection. One of these women had underlying MPN, suggesting this prothrombotic disorder may cause unfavorable pregnancy outcome by occluding placental vessels [5].

Direct oral anticoagulants (DOAC) are sometimes used "off-label" for the treatment of PVT [12]. These medications offer some advantages over vitamin K antagonists, specifically the stable dose without the necessity for laboratory monitoring [13]. Despite the paucity of data on the use of DOACs in the treatment of venous thrombosis in atypical locations, their use is expanding in splanchnic venous thrombosis (SVT) [12, 13]. *De Gottardi et al.* presented the largest series on DOACs in patients with SVT. In this retrospective study, among the 58 patients without cirrhosis, 38 (65%) were anticoagulated for PVT. Adverse events happened in five patients (8,6%), 2 thrombotic and 3 hemorrhagic complications, leading to the change of anticoagulant in 4 cases [12].

Even if DOACs seem to be safe and effective in SVT, further data are needed [12, 13].

What about the risk of variceal bleeding in pregnancy? There are two perspectives on the matter. Firstly, some authors think that variceal bleeding increases with pregnancy [1, 6, 10, 14]. Even in women with no prior history of variceal bleeding, the gravid state can sometimes trigger a first episode [1]. This feared complication can happen at all stages of pregnancy but is more frequent in second and third trimesters and during the second stage of labor [10]. The increased risk of bleeding comes from the physiological hemodynamic changes of pregnancy, which bring a hyperdynamic and hypervolemic state and thus increase the inflow to the collaterals [6, 10, 14]. Conversely, *Sumana et al* and *Kochhar et al* hypothesize that even if cardiac output and blood volume increase during pregnancy, the splanchnic blood flow and the portal pressure remained stable because the majority of the additional blood circulates through the uterine arteries to the fetus [11, 15]. Indeed, variceal bleeding during pregnancy is probably less frequent than initially thought [11].

When the woman has a history of variceal bleeding, it is important to treat the varices before conception, either with endoscopic variceal ligation or sclerotherapy, since the incidence of upper gastrointestinal bleeding decreases with prepregancy eradication of varices [1, 6, 7, 11, 16]. Even in the absence of prior variceal bleeding, primary prophylaxis should be given to pregnant woman at risk [6, 10]. There is not enough data to decide whether beta-blockers or endoscopic therapy should be favored [1, 17]. Nonselective beta-blockers are considered safe in pregnancy, though nadolol and propranolol may induce growth retardation, fetal bradycardia, and neonatal hypoglycemia [10].

Lastly, delivery route should be chosen according to standard indications [1, 11]. Vaginal delivery is preferred with adequate analgesia and assisted second stage of labor to limit straining effort [4, 6, 10, 11]. Cesarean section should be reserved for usual obstetric reasons [1, 11]. Risks specific to caesarean delivery must be considered in women with portal hypertension, including surgical bleeding from thrombocytopenia or direct injury to abdominal wall varices and postoperative ascitic decompensation [4, 6]. Moreover, caesarean operation augments the chance of postpartum venous thromboembolism, a risk that is already high in women with PVT [4].

4. Conclusion

Although there will always be a risk of variceal bleeding during pregnancy in woman with PVT and portal hypertension, outcome is generally good in the presence of preconception evaluation and primary or secondary prophylaxis for varices with beta-blockers and endoscopic therapy. Available data permit us to propose that pregnancy is not contraindicated in these patients when the disease is treated and stable. Anticoagulation should be continued to prevent new thrombosis. Pregnant women at risk should be followed in a center where expertise and multidisciplinary team are available.

References

[1] S. K. Sarin, J. D. Sollano, Y. K. Chawla et al., "Consensus on extra-hepatic portal vein obstruction," *Liver International*, vol. 26, no. 5, pp. 512–519, 2006.

[2] F. Savoia, C. Ferrara, A. Sansone, G. Bifulco, C. Nappi, and C. Di Carlo, "Portal cavernoma during pregnancy," *Case Reports in Obstetrics and Gynecology*, vol. 2013, Article ID 396083, 4 pages, 2013.

[3] D. Valla, N. Casadevall, M. G. Huisse et al., "Etiology of portal vein thrombosis in adults. a prospective evaluation of primary myeloproliferative disorders," *Gastroenterology*, vol. 94, no. 4, pp. 1063–1069, 1988.

[4] J. Bissonnette, F. Durand, E. de Raucourt et al., "Pregnancy and vascular liver disease," *Journal of Clinical and Experimental Hepatology*, vol. 5, no. 1, pp. 41–50, 2015.

[5] J. Hoekstra, S. Seijo, P. E. Rautou et al., "Pregnancy in women with portal vein thrombosis: results of a multicentric European study on maternal and fetal management and outcome," *Journal of Hepatology*, vol. 57, no. 6, pp. 1214–1219, 2012.

[6] I. Üstüner, R. A. Akdoğan, E. S. G. Güven et al., "Pregnancy in the setting of asymptomatic non-cirrhotic chronic portal vein thrombosis complicated by pre-eclampsia," *Case Reports in Obstetrics and Gynecology*, vol. 2013, Article ID 984271, 4 pages, 2013.

[7] N. Aggarwal, S. Chopra, A. Raveendran, V. Suri, R. K. Dhiman, and Y. K. Chawla, "Extra hepatic portal vein obstruction and pregnancy outcome: largest reported experience," *Journal of Obstetrics and Gynaecology Research*, vol. 37, no. 6, pp. 575–580, 2011.

[8] T. Barbui and G. Finazzi, "Myeloproliferative disease in pregnancy and other management issues," *Hematology ASH Education Program*, vol. 2006, no. 1, pp. 246–252, 2006.

[9] A. Falanga, M. Marchetti, A. Vignoli, D. Balducci, and T. Barbui, "Leukocyte-platelet interaction in patients with essential thrombocythemia and polycythemia vera," *Experimental Hematology*, vol. 33, no. 5, pp. 523–530, 2005.

[10] N. Aggarwal, N. Negi, A. Aggarwal, V. Bodh, and R. K. Dhiman, "Pregnancy with Portal Hypertension," *Journal of Clinical and Experimental Hepatology*, vol. 4, no. 2, pp. 163–171, 2014.

[11] G. Sumana, V. Dadhwal, D. Deka, and S. Mittal, "Non-cirrhotic portal hypertension and pregnancy outcome," *Journal of Obstetrics and Gynaecology Research*, vol. 34, no. 5, pp. 801–804, 2008.

[12] A. De Gottardi, J. Trebicka, C. Klinger et al., "Antithrombotic treatment with direct-acting oral anticoagulants in patients with splanchnic vein thrombosis and cirrhosis," *Liver International*, vol. 37, no. 5, pp. 694–699, 2017.

[13] G. Finazzi, V. De Stefano, and T. Barbui, "Splanchnic vein thrombosis in myeloproliferative neoplasms: treatment algorithm 2018," *Blood Cancer Journal*, vol. 8, no. 7, p. 64, 2018.

[14] D. M. Paternoster, A. R. Floreani, A. Paggioro, and E. Laureti, "Portal hypertension in a pregnant woman," *Minerva Ginecologica*, vol. 48, no. 6, pp. 243–245, 1996.

[15] R. Kochhar, "Pregnancy and its outcome in patients with noncirrhotic portal hypertension," *Digestive Diseases and Sciences*, vol. 44, no. 7, pp. 1356–1361, 1999.

[16] P. Dasari and S. Balusamy, "Portal vein thrombosis during pregnancy," *BMJ Case Reports*, 2013.

[17] R. de Franchis, "Revising consensus in portal hypertension: report of the Baveno V consensus workshop on methodology of diagnosis and therapy in portal hypertension," *Journal of Hepatology*, vol. 53, no. 4, pp. 762–768, 2010.

48

Successful Management of the Fetal Severe Anemia Associated with Jra Alloimmunization by Intrauterine Transfusion of Jr(a+) Red Blood Cells

Masatake Toshimitsu,[1] Shinichi Nagaoka,[1] Shuusaku Kobori,[1] Yuichiro Takahashi,[2] and Jun Murotsuki[1]

[1]*Department of Maternal and Fetal Medicine, Miyagi Children's Hospital, Miyagi 989-3126, Japan*
[2]*Department of Fetal and Maternal Medicine, Nagara Medical Center, Gifu, Japan*

Correspondence should be addressed to Jun Murotsuki; murotsuki@miyagi-children.or.jp

Academic Editor: Yoshio Yoshida

Objective. We present a case of fetal severe anemia associated with Jra alloimmunization, which was managed using Doppler measurement of the peak systolic velocity of the fetal middle cerebral artery (MCA-PSV) and intrauterine transfusion (IUT) of Jr(a+) red blood cells (RBCs). We also review the previous case reports on fetal or neonatal anemia associated with Jra alloimmunization. *Case Report.* A woman with Jra alloimmunization was referred to our department at 29 weeks of gestation. As fetal MCA-PSV exceeded 1.55 multiples of the median, fetal blood sampling was performed and demonstrated severe anemia. During the course, a total of two IUTs were performed using Jr(a+) RBCs. The neonate was delivered by repeated cesarean section at 35 weeks of gestation and showed no apparent signs of hemolysis. *Conclusion.* Based on the literature review, fetal anemia associated with Jra alloimmunization becomes severe during mid-gestation and may not develop during late gestation. The severity of fetal anemia is predicted by MCA-PSV Doppler assessment rather than the maternal anti-Jra titers. Timely IUT of Jr(a+) RBCs can help to prolong the pregnancy to term in emergency situations wherein compatible blood of Jr(a-) RBCs is not available soon.

1. Introduction

Fetal anemia can cause fetal high-output cardiac failure, fetal hydrops, iatrogenic preterm delivery, and fetal demise [1]. Therefore, fetal anemia is still an important cause of fetal and neonatal mortality and morbidity in modern obstetric practice.

The Jra antigen, which is a high-incidence red blood cell (RBC) antigen, is known to be involved in hemolytic anemia of the fetus and newborn [2, 3]. The expression of Jra antigen is regulated by the *ATP-binding cassette G2* (*ABCG2*) gene on chromosome 4q22.1 and Jra antigen is located on ABCG2 transporter, which is highly expressed on cells of the erythroid lineage [3, 4]. The Jr(a-) phenotype results from the inheritance of ABCG2 null alleles caused by frameshift or nonsense mutations such as c.1515delC (p.Ala505fs), c.376C>T (p.Gln126Ter), c.421C>A (p.Gln14Lys), and c.1723C>T (p.Arg575Ter), particularly in Japanese individuals [3, 5, 6]. Furthermore, the variation in the Jra antigen density on RBCs among Jr(a+) individuals with genetic mutations at 376 and 421 has also been reported [7].

Although anti-Jra can be produced in Jr(a-) women due to pregnancy or incompatible Jr(a+) RBC transfusion and cross the placenta, the effect of anti-Jra on fetal anemia remains unclear [4, 7–11]. For example, the fetal anemia associated with anti-Jra positivity is reported to be mild [8, 9]. In contrast, several reports have shown an association between Jra alloimmunization and fetal or neonatal severe anemia requiring intervention [4, 10, 11]. In addition, in one case, neonatal death occurred due to Jra alloimmunization [10].

We report a case of fetal severe anemia associated with Jra alloimmunization that was successfully managed by close fetal monitoring and intrauterine transfusion (IUT) of Jr(a+)

Table 1: The fetal blood analysis.

GA Weeks + days	Pre-IUT Hb(g/dL)/ Hct(%)	Post-IUT Hb(g/dL)/ Hct(%)	Volume of IUT (ml)	T-bil (mg/dL)	DAT
30+0 (first IUT)	3.5/ 9.9	7.2/ 22.1	70	N/A	N/A
31+2 (second IUT)	6.1/ 18.6	9.5/ 29.1	35	N/A	N/A
35+1 (at birth)	9.2/ 28.4		-	1.7	+

GA: gestational age; Hb: hemoglobin; Hct: hematocrit; IUT: intrauterine transfusion; T-bil: total bilirubin; DAT: direct antiglobulin test; N/A: not available.

RBCs. We also analyzed the clinical characteristics and perinatal outcome of fetal anemia due to Jra alloimmunization. Cases were obtained by searching PubMed or Medical Online for the terms "Jr(a)", "hemolytic disease", "fetus", and "anemia". All reports and publications in English or Japanese from 2006 to 2016 were reviewed. Cases at Nagara Medical Center, a tertiary center in Japan, were also included.

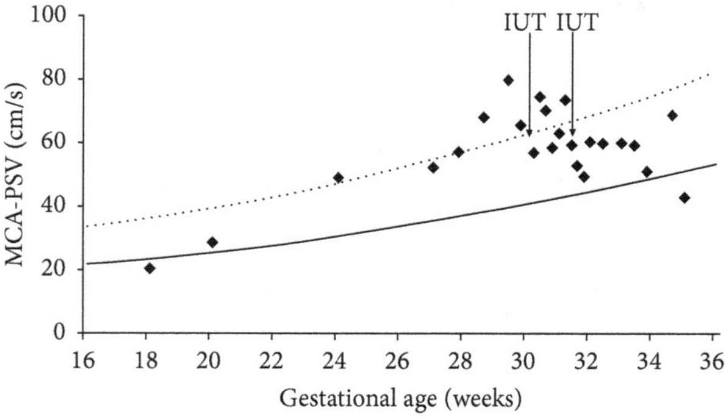

Figure 1: *The peak systolic flow velocity of the fetal middle cerebral artery during pregnancy.* (—) The median MCA-PSV level in normal pregnancies; (··) 1.55 MoM; (◆) our case. MCA-PSV: the peak systolic flow velocity of the fetal middle cerebral artery; MoM: multiple of the median.

2. Clinical Case

The patient was a 34-year-old Japanese woman (gravida 5 para 2, including 2 miscarriages) with blood group O type RhD (+). She was referred to our department in the 29th week of her fifth pregnancy for perinatal management. She had no relevant medical history and had never received a blood transfusion. Screening performed when she was pregnant with her first child revealed Jr(a-) and anti-Jra with a titer of 1:512. Her Jr(a-) genotype was c.376T/T and c.421C/C. Her partner was Jr(a+) with c.376C/C and c.421C/A. Her first child of 2590 g was delivered at 36 weeks of gestation by cesarean section (CS) at a different hospital due to breech presentation and did not have any other episodes of anemia or jaundice. When pregnant with her second child, the titer of anti-Jra changed from 1:128 to 1:256. Her second child was delivered at 37 weeks and 6 days of gestation by planned repeat CS at a different hospital due to previous CS. Her second child of 2808 g was diagnosed with anemia (Hb 8.4 g/dL) based on a positive direct antiglobulin test (DAT), but did not display jaundice. The second child was diagnosed as being heterozygous for c.376C/T with c.421C/C and exhibited the Jr(a+) phenotype.

Her current pregnancy was a naturally conceived and normal singleton pregnancy. The titer of anti-Jra at 20 weeks of gestation was 1:256. No other antibodies against blood group antigens were identified. The fetus was monitored by ultrasound scans and Doppler measurements of the peak systolic flow velocity of the fetal middle cerebral artery (MCA-PSV). Although the titer of anti-Jra did not change (1:256), the MCA-PSV level began to increase at 24 weeks and exceeded 1.55 multiples of the median (MoM) at 28 weeks (Figure 1). She was referred to our department at 29 weeks and 6 days due to suspected fetal anemia. Our ultrasound examination showed that the estimated fetal body weight corresponded to the Japanese standard for the gestational age and that there were no fetal or placental structural abnormalities. The MCA-PSV level (65.6 cm/s) was >1.55 MoM (Figure 1). The fetal cardiothoracic area ratio (CTAR) was 42.0% without any signs of hydrops, such as ascites or skin edema. The next day, percutaneous umbilical cord blood sampling (PUBS) was carried out and revealed fetal severe anemia (Hb 3.5 g/dL, Hct 9.9%) (Table 1). An immediate IUT via the umbilical cord was performed with group O RhD (-), Jr(a+) concentrated RBC units. After the first IUT, the Hb and Hct levels increased to 7.2 g/dL and 22.1%, respectively (Table 1). On the sixth day after the first IUT (30 weeks and 6 days), the titer of anti-Jra increased from 1:256 to 1:512. The IgG subclass was found to be IgG1 and IgG3. On the seventh day after the first IUT, the MCA-PSV level was >1.55 MoM, suggesting the exacerbation of fetal anemia (Figure 1). Thus, a second PUBS and a second IUT was performed with group O RhD (-), Jr(a+) concentrated RBC units on the ninth day after the first IUT. The fetal Hb and Hct levels before the second IUT were 6.1 g/dL and 18.6%, respectively (Table 1), while those after the second IUT were 9.5 g/dL and 29.1%, respectively (Table 1). After the second IUT, an ultrasound examination showed that the MCA-PSV level remained within the normal range and that the CTAR level had normalized to 31.6% (Figure 1). She returned to her referring hospital, where she was managed from 32 weeks of gestation. At 34 weeks of gestation, the fetal MCA-PSV and CTAR levels increased to <1.5 MoM and 39%, respectively (Figure 1). The exacerbation of fetal anemia was suspected; thus, a repeat CS was performed at 35 weeks and 1 day of gestation due to previous CS at the referring hospital. The neonate of 2114 g had anemia (Hb 9.2 g/dL, Hct 28.4%) with a positive DAT, without jaundice (total bilirubin 1.7 mg/dL) (Table 1). On the second day after birth, the neonatal anemia worsened (8.0 g/dL) and a blood transfusion was performed.

Neither neonatal anemia nor jaundice developed after the single blood transfusion. The neonate was discharged from the hospital without phototherapy.

To investigate the phenotype and the Jra antigen density of the neonate, an analysis of the *ABCG2* gene was performed at Japanese Red Cross Tohoku Block Center. Genomic DNA was extracted from the peripheral blood and PCR-SSP was used to examine the genetic base substitutions at positions 376, 421, 1515, and 1723, which are most common in Japanese Jr(a-) individuals [7]. The neonate's phenotype was classified as Jr(a+); the neonate was heterozygous for c.376C/T with no mutation at position 421 (c.421C/C), which was the same genotype of the second child.

3. Discussion

We presented a case of fetal severe anemia associated with Jra alloimmunization in which the pregnancy was successfully prolonged by Doppler measurements of the MCA-PSV and timely IUT. This is also the first case report describing the performance of IUT using Jr(a+) concentrated RBC units. In the present case, fetal anemia did not develop after the IUT of Jr(a+) RBCs and the neonate's blood exam did not show any evidence of hemolysis.

Several clinical investigations and experimental studies have been performed to elucidate the precise pathogenesis of fetal anemia associated with Jra alloimmunization [4, 7, 9–17]. There are ten reports, including our own, describing fetal or neonatal anemia in association with Jra alloimmunization (Table 2). A review of the literature revealed several features of the clinical course of fetal anemia with Jra alloimmunization (Table 2). First, the cases that required IUT suggested that the fetal anemia becomes severe during mid-gestation; however, it is unclear when anemia occurs. Furthermore, the fetal anemia was not exacerbated during late gestation. In the present case, fetal anemia did not develop after the second IUT of Jr(a+) RBCs (Table 1). Although the exact mechanisms underlying the development of fetal severe anemia during mid-gestation and the transfusion effect of IUT of Jr(a+) RBCs are unknown, they may be related to the change of ABCG2 expression in erythroid lineage cells with advancing gestational ages [4]. A high expression of ABCG2 on erythroid progenitor cells during mid-gestation may lead to a high affinity for anti-Jra, resulting in development of fetal anemia during mid-gestation [4]. In contrast, a low expression of ABCG2 on RBCs after late gestation may contribute to prevention of the exacerbation of fetal anemia and preservation of efficacy of incompatible transfusion using adult Jr(a+) RBCs [4]. Thus, a single IUT may be sufficient to allow the pregnancy to progress until term without repeated IUTs. However, cases treated with IUT may still require neonatal blood transfusion. Second, the severity of fetal anemia is not directly correlated with the titer of anti-Jra, suggesting that the measurement of the maternal antibody titers alone is not a reliable method for predicting fetal anemia. Future studies with larger sample size focused on the value of the first titer or repeated titer determination in the management of Jra alloimmunization requiring frequent monitoring to detect fetal anemia are helpful to identify the fetus with need for IUT. In the present case, PUBS was indicated based on the measurement of the fetal MCA-PSV. In the majority of cases that were treated with IUT, the timing of the first PUBS was based on the assessment of the fetal MCA-PSV. Although there are no clear data regarding the optimal intervals between repeated Doppler measurements of the fetal MCA-PSV, measurement of the MCA-PSV may be useful in the management of Jra alloimmunization. Third, anti-Jra-mediated fetal anemia was characterized by anemia without developing hyperbilirubinemia at PUBS and at birth. However, there are several limitations. First, the unconjugated fetal bilirubin crosses the placenta. In the present case, we did not evaluate the level of total bilirubin in PUBS at 30 weeks of gestation due to the limited blood sample volume (Table 1). Second, the fetal anemia was not exacerbated after late gestation based on the literature review, including this one (Table 2). Therefore, we cannot assess the contribution of hemolysis to fetal anemia based on the bilirubin levels.

In this review, the majority of clinical data analyzed are derived from Japanese women (9 women were Japanese and 1 was Caucasian of Gypsy Spanish origin [10]), so it is necessary to be cautious about applying our results to other racial groups.

Experimental studies have demonstrated that the ABCG2 is expressed on not only cells of the erythroid lineage but also the placenta and that it is a plasma membrane protein extruding endogenous and exogenous substrates, such as xenobiotics, heme, porphyrin, and uric acid [15–17]. The maintenance of cellular porphyrin and heme homeostasis, which constitute an essential component of hemoglobin, by ABCG2 is thought to perform a vital physiological function in erythropoiesis [17]. Taken together, these clinical and experimental findings suggest that anti-Jra antibodies may directly affect the function of ABCG2 and may cause fetal anemia due to ineffective erythropoiesis.

One of the important findings in our case was that pregnancy could be prolonged by incompatible IUT with Jr(a+) RBC units. In the present case, we were not able to obtain Jr(a-) RBC units because of the low incidence of Jr(a-). As a result, a total of 105 ml of Jr(a+) RBCs were transfused and fetal anemia did not develop after the second IUT. The sufficient efficacy of incompatible transfusion using adult Jr(a+) RBCs may be partly due to a low expression of ABCG2 on adult RBCs compared with fetus [4]. In the setting of incompatible transfusions in adults, whereas most reported cases showed a mild and delayed hemolytic transfusion reaction, an acute hemolytic transfusion reaction also has been reported, suggesting that anti-Jra is a possible cause of transfusion-related hemolysis [18–20]. Therefore, IUT of Jr(a+) RBCs may be considered, especially in emergency situations wherein compatible blood of Jr(a-) RBCs is not available soon [20].

Another important finding in our case was the different outcomes between the second child who did not require IUT and the present child who required IUT. Since the severity of fetal anemia may be independent of the maternal anti-Jra, we hypothesized that the Jra antigen density on fetal RBCs contributes to the severity of anemia. In contrast to

Table 2: Theclinical details and outcomes of the reported cases of Jra alloimmunization, including the present case.

Case	GA at first PUBS or IUT (weeks)	MCA-PSV at first PUBS (MoM)	Hb (g/dL)/Hct (%)/T-bil (mg/dL) at first PUBS	Number of IUTs	Type of blood transfusion	GA at birth (weeks)	Interval between the last IUT and birth (weeks)	Hydrops fetalis	Hb (g/dL)/Hct (%)/T-bil (mg/dL) at birth	Maximum anti-Jra titer	Neonatal transfusion	Neonatal outcome
Cases with IUT (n = 6)												
Present case	30	>1.55	3.5/ 9.9/ N/A	2	Jr(a+)	35	5	-	9.2/ 28.4/ 1.7	512	+	Alive
Case 2 (unrelated)	29	>1.55	5.3/ 15.7/ 1.4	1	Jr(a-)	37	8	-	9.4/ 29.0/ 1.1	256	-	Alive
Ishihara et al. [11]	30	>1.55	3.5/ 7.9/ 1.0	4	Jr(a-)	35	1	+	7.2/ N/A/ 1.0	512	+	Alive
Fujita et al. [4]	30	>1.5	8.5/ 26.8/ N/A	1	Jr(a-)	37	7	-	11.8/ 35.4/ 2.0	512	-	Alive
Aikou et al. [12]	30	>1.5	5.4/ 15.7/ 2.3	1	Jr(a-)	38	8	-	10.8/ 31.8/ 2.1	32	-	Alive
Yahara et al. [13]	27	N/A	3.4/ 11.4/ 1.9	2	Jr(a-)	37	6	+	12.2/ 37.0/ 1.0	16	-	Alive
Cases without IUT (n = 4)												
Sasamoto et al. [14]	-	-	-	0	-	33	-	-	8.2/ 25.4/ 0.9	1024	-	Alive
Peyrard et al. [10]	-	-	-	0	-	36	-	+	6.4/ N/A/ 2.5	1024	+	Neonatal death
Endo et al. [7]	-	-	-	0	-	37	-	-	8.4/ 25.8/ 1.9	256	-	Alive
Masumoto et al. [9]	-	-	-	0	-	37	-	-	11.5/ N/A/ N/A	64	-	Alive

GA: gestational age; Hb: hemoglobin; Hct: hematocrit; PUBS: percutaneous umbilical cord blood sampling; IUT: intrauterine transfusion; T-bil: total bilirubin; N/A: not available. Case 2 is unrelated to ours. The clinical data of case 2 was provided by the Department of Fetal-Maternal Medicine, Nagara Medical Center.

our hypothesis, the Jr(a+) genotype was the same in both children, suggesting that their Jra antigen density was similar and implicating the impact of ABCG2 on erythropoiesis and compensatory mechanisms when ABCG2 is inhibited by anti-Jra. There are several possibilities that could explain the intrafamilial phenotypic variability in the perinatal outcomes. One possibility is that increasing sensitization due to a previous Jra positive child may be involved in the development of fetal severe anemia. It is known that the degree of fetal anemia due to red cell alloimmunization depends on the number of affected pregnancies. Another possibility is anti-Jra titer variability. Intra- and interlaboratory variability in the titer measurement constitute a major point of concern. In addition, antibody titration, a semiquantitative method to detect the reactivity, may not reflect true biological activity in the Jra alloimmunization. Although our main goal in the management of pregnancies complicated by Jra alloimmunization is to detect fetuses that are at higher risk of developing severe anemia in order to prevent fetal hydrops [21], the clinical course of fetal anemia may be affected by various factors, such as the Jra antigen density of cells of the erythroid lineage and placenta, the maternal antibody titer, and the numbers of affected pregnancies. It is important to recognize that fetal severe anemia can occur, even if a previous child did not develop anemia.

In conclusion, it is necessary to recognize Jra alloimmunization as a possible cause of fetal severe anemia, and that this may occur through ineffective erythropoiesis and hemolysis. We think that careful obstetric management is needed, including routine Doppler measurements of the fetal MCA-PSV to detect anemia, the sampling of fetal blood by PUBS when fetal anemia is detected, and when necessary timely IUT to improve the neonatal outcomes by preventing fetal hydrops and fetal anemia-associated prematurity.

Acknowledgments

We would like to thank Takahiro Koshino, Yamagata Prefectural Central Hospital, and Shoichi Ito, Japanese Red Cross Tohoku Block Center, who participated in this survey.

References

[1] N. Abbasi, J. Johnson, and G. Ryan, "Fetal anemia," *Ultrasound in Obstetrics & Gynecology*, vol. 50, no. 2, pp. 145–153, 2017.

[2] K. J. Moise, "Fetal anemia due to non-Rhesus-D red-cell alloimmunization," *Seminars in Fetal and Neonatal Medicine*, vol. 13, no. 4, pp. 207–214, 2008.

[3] L. Castilho and M. E. Reid, "A review of the JR blood group system," *Immunohematology*, vol. 29, no. 2, pp. 63–68, 2013.

[4] S. Fujita, H. Kashiwagi, T. Tomimatsu et al., "Expression levels of ABCG2 on cord red blood cells and study of fetal anemia associated with anti-Jra," *Transfusion*, vol. 56, no. 5, pp. 1171–1181, 2016.

[5] M. Tanaka, I. Kamada, J. Takahashi, K. Kimura, H. Matsukura, and Y. Tani, "Defining the Jr(a-) phenotype in the Japanese population," *Transfusion*, vol. 54, no. 2, pp. 412–417, 2014.

[6] K. Hue-Roye, T. Zelinski, A. Cobaugh et al., "The JR blood group system: Identification of alleles that alter expression," *Transfusion*, vol. 53, no. 11, pp. 2710–2714, 2013.

[7] Y. Endo, S. Ito, and Y. Ogiyama, "Suspected anemia caused by maternal anti-Jra antibodies: a case report," *Biomarker Research*, vol. 3, no. 23, 2015.

[8] P. Toy, M. Reid, T. Lewis, S. Ellisor, and D. R. Avoy, "Does anti-jr cause hemolytic disease of the newborn?" *Vox Sanguinis*, vol. 41, no. 1, pp. 40–44, 1981.

[9] A. Masumoto, H. Masuyama, Y. Sumida, T. Segawa, and Y. Hiramatsu, "Successful management of anti-Jra alloimmunization in pregnancy: A case report," *Gynecologic and Obstetric Investigation*, vol. 69, no. 2, pp. 81–83, 2010.

[10] T. Peyrard, B.-N. Pham, L. Arnaud et al., "Fatal hemolytic disease of the fetus and newborn associated with anti-Jra," *Transfusion*, vol. 48, no. 9, pp. 1906–1911, 2008.

[11] Y. Ishihara, S. Miyata, Y. Chiba, and T. Kawai, "Successful treatment of extremely severe fetal anemia due to anti-Jr a alloimmunization," *Fetal Diagnosis and Therapy*, vol. 21, no. 3, pp. 269–271, 2006.

[12] K. Aikou, A. Kuramoto, H. Matsuura et al., "Intrauterine fetal blood transfusion for severe fetal anemia with anti-Jra:acase report," *The Journal of Fukuoka College of Obstetricians and Gynecologists*, vol. 37, pp. 8–11, 2013 (Japanese).

[13] K. Yahara, T. Inaoka, and H. Yasui, "A case of pregnant woman with anti-Jra which required intrauterine transfusion," *Japanese Journal of Transfusion and Cell Therapy*, vol. 57, no. 344, 2011 (Japanese).

[14] N. Sasamoto, T. Tomimatsu, K. Nagamine et al., "Fetal and neonatal anemia associated with anti-Jr a: A case report showing a poorly hemolytic mechanism," *Journal of Obstetrics and Gynaecology Research*, vol. 37, no. 8, pp. 1132–1136, 2011.

[15] Q. Mao, "BCRP/ABCG2 in the placenta: Expression, function and regulation," *Pharmaceutical Research*, vol. 25, no. 6, pp. 1244–1255, 2008.

[16] D. Yeboah, M. Sun, J. Kingdom et al., "Expression of breast cancer resistance protein (BCRP/ABCG2) in human placenta throughout gestation and at term before and after labor," *Canadian Journal of Physiology and Pharmacology*, vol. 84, no. 12, pp. 1251–1258, 2006.

[17] G. O. Latunde-Dada, A. H. Laftah, P. Masaratana, A. T. McKie, and R. J. Simpson, "Expression of ABCG2 (BCRP) in mouse models with enhanced erythropoiesis," *Frontiers in Pharmacology*, vol. 5, no. 135, 2014.

[18] M. Y. Kwon, L. Su, P. A. Arndt, G. Garratty, and D. P. Blackall, "Clinical significance of anti-Jra: Report of two cases and review of the literature," *Transfusion*, vol. 44, no. 2, pp. 197–201, 2004.

[19] S. Yuan, R. Armour, A. Reid et al., "Case report: massive postpartum transfusion of Jr(a+) red cells in the presence of anti-Jra," *Immunohematology*, vol. 21, no. 3, pp. 97–101, 2005.

[20] J. Poole and G. Daniels, "Blood group antibodies and their significance in transfusion medicine," *Transfusion Medicine Reviews*, vol. 21, no. 1, pp. 58–71, 2007.

[21] I. T. Lindenburg, V. E. Smits-Wintjens, J. M. Van Klink et al., "Long-term neurodevelopmental outcome after intrauterine transfusion for hemolytic disease of the fetus/newborn: The LOTUS study," *American Journal of Obstetrics & Gynecology*, vol. 206,no. 141, pp. e1–e8, 2012.

A Case of Monochorionic-Triamniotic Triplet Pregnancy with TRAP Sequence Successfully Treated with Radiofrequency Ablation with a Parallel Circuit Consisting of Anastomosed Blood Vessels between the Direct Pump Fetus and the Indirect Pump Fetus

Shusaku Kobori, Masatake Toshimitsu, Shinichi Nagaoka, and Jun Murotsuki

Department of Maternal and Fetal Medicine, Miyagi Children's Hospital, Sendai, Miyagi 989-3126, Japan

Correspondence should be addressed to Jun Murotsuki; murotsuki@miyagi-children.or.jp

Academic Editor: Edi Vaisbuch

Monochorionic-triamniotic triplet pregnancy with twin reversed arterial perfusion (TRAP) sequence is one of the rare complications of multiple pregnancy and has been reported by only a few. Here, we report a case of monochorionic-triamniotic triplet pregnancy with TRAP sequence successfully treated with radiofrequency ablation, which did not develop polyhydramnios and heart failure although the estimated weight of the acardiac fetus increased twice as much as that of the direct pump fetus. Interestingly, the anastomosed blood vessels between the direct and indirect pump fetuses comprised a parallel circuit, which provided blood flow to the acardiac fetus. We hypothesized that the burden on the pump fetus in monochorionic pregnancy with TRAP sequence would be different between triplet and twin pregnancies.

1. Introduction

Twin reversed arterial perfusion (TRAP) sequence is one of the rare complications of multiple pregnancy. It occurs for approximately 1% of monochorionic pregnancies [1]. Monochorionic triplet pregnancies occur at a rate of 1 in 45000 deliveries [2]. However, with progress of assisted reproductive technologies, the rate of multiple pregnancies (triplets and above) has dramatically risen over the last 20 years. Accordingly, the rate of monochorionic triplet pregnancy with TRAP sequence seems to have increased during the same period. In monochorionic twin pregnancy with TRAP sequence, there are several vascular anastomoses between an acardiac fetus and the other fetuses. In monochorionic triplet pregnancy with TRAP sequence, although there are several vascular anastomoses between an acardiac fetus and one fetus, the remaining 3rd fetus could also send blood indirectly via another vascular anastomoses. We hypothesize that the burden on the pump fetus of monochorionic triplet pregnancy with TRAP sequence would be different from that of monochorionic twin pregnancy with TRAP sequence. We report a case of monochorionic-triamniotic triplet pregnancy with TRAP sequence successfully treated with radiofrequency ablation, which did not develop polyhydramnios and heart failure although the estimated weight of the acardiac fetus increased twice as much as that of the direct pump fetus.

2. Case

A 38-year-old woman, gravida 4 para 1, was referred due to monochorionic-triamniotic triplet pregnancy at 10 weeks of gestation. We confirmed monochorionic-triamniotic triplet gestation, with absence of cardiac activity in one triplet. Reversed flow in the fetal umbilical cord was demonstrated on Doppler ultrasound examination. These findings were consistent with monochorionic-triamniotic gestation complicated with twin reversed arterial perfusion (TRAP) sequence. The acardiac fetus did not have an upper body.

Using Doppler ultrasound, the presence of anastomotic vessels was confirmed between triplets A (acardiac fetus) and

TABLE 1: Blood flow changes of the direct pump fetus and the indirect pump fetus around RFA.

	Direct pump fetus (fetus B)		Indirect pump fetus (fetus C)	
	Pre-intervention	Post-intervention	Pre-intervention	Post-intervention
UA-PI	1.25	1.19	0.97	0.95
MCA-PSV (cm/s)	24.3	22.2	21.5	23.4
DV-PI	0.42	0.48	0.37	0.45
UV-pulsation	no	no	no	no
MVP (cm)	4.3	4.5	3.8	4

UA-PI, pulsatility index of the umbilical artery; MCA-PSV, middle cerebral arterial peak systolic velocity; DV-PI, pulsatility index of the ductus venosus; UV-pulsation, pulsation of the umbilical vein; MVP, maximal vertical pocket.

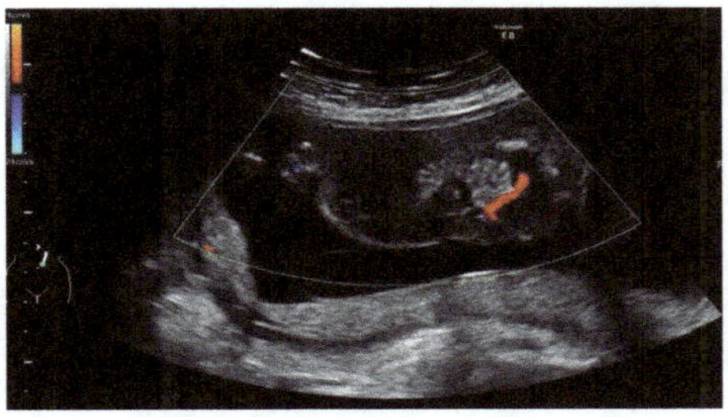

FIGURE 1: Ultrasonic color Doppler image of the acardiac fetus at 16 weeks of gestation. Blood flow is observed in the navel of the acardiac fetus, which is stuck to the anterior uterine wall. Complete cessation of blood flow in the acardiac fetus was successful with a single puncture.

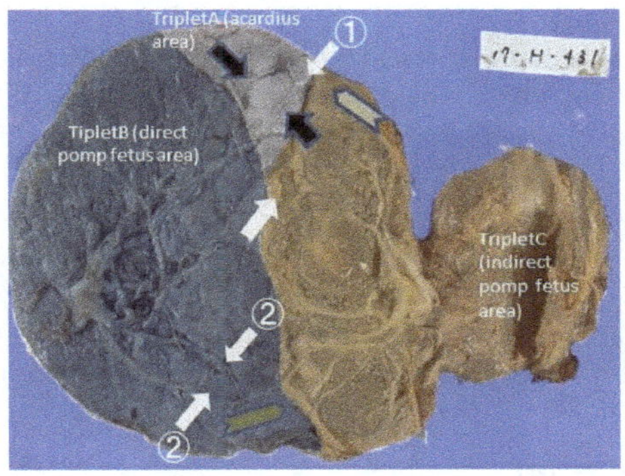

FIGURE 2: Photograph of the placental vascular surface. The black arrow indicates the anastomoses between the acardiac fetus and the direct pump fetus. The white arrow indicates the anastomoses between the direct pump fetus and the indirect pump fetus. ① is the anastomoses between the umbilical artery of the direct pump fetus and the umbilical artery of the indirect pump fetus. ② is the anastomoses between the umbilical vein of the direct pump fetus and the two umbilical veins of the indirect pump fetus. The gray arrow indicates the direction of blood flow in the vascular anastomoses.

B (direct pump fetus) but not between triplet A and triplet C (indirect pump fetus). The Doppler measurements of feeding vessel (umbilical artery) in the acardiac twin revealed pulse rate that was similar to FHR of twin B. The direct pump fetus could be distinguished from the indirect pump fetus by measuring FHR. The estimated fetal body weight (EFBW) of the acardiac fetus increased as pregnancy progressed. EFBW of an acardiac fetus can be obtained by the following equation: (grams) = (-1.66 × longest length [cm]) + (1.21 × longest length [cm]^2) [3]. At 14 weeks, body weight was 136 g for triplet A, 56 g for triplet B, and 59 g for triplet C. At 16 weeks, body weight was 227 g for triplet A, 109 g for triplet B, and 120 g for triplet C. In triplets *B* and *C*, we could not confirm polyhydramnios, absent umbilical artery end-diastolic velocity, umbilical venous pulsation, and absent or reverse blood flow in the ductus venosus.

We usually perform RFA when EFBW of an acardiac fetus is 0.7 times or more as much as that of a pump fetus, and heart failure and amniotic fluid excess are recognized. In the current case, weight of the acardiac fetus exceeded twice that of the pump fetus and weight of the acardiac fetus had increased further. We speculated that the pump fetus would develop heart failure with high probability in the future; thus, radiofrequency ablation (RFA) was performed at 18 weeks. The acardiac fetus was stuck to the anterior uterine wall and the other sac did not interfere with needle insertion (Figure 1). We used a 480 kHz radiofrequency generator and 20 cm-long, 17-gauge, internally cooled electrode with a 2 cm-long exposed metallic tip (Cool-tip RF system; Valleylab, Boulder, Co., USA). The patient had strong anxiety in a conscious state, so we performed surgery with general anesthesia. An electrode was transabdominally introduced and inserted into the fetal abdomen adjacent to the umbilical cord insertion area under continuous ultrasound guidance. Coagulation was initiated for 90 seconds, and complete blood flow cessation was successful in the acardiac fetus. In triplets B and C, preoperative and postoperative middle cerebral artery peak systolic velocities were the same and fetal anemia was not observed (Table 1).

During follow-up by weekly ultrasound, twin-to-twin transfusion syndrome, selective intrauterine growth restriction, and twin anemia–polycythemia sequence did not develop. At 37 weeks, a cesarean section was performed; two male newborn infants were delivered. Triplet B weighed 2,662 g, with Apgar scores of 8 and 9 at 1 and 5 minutes, respectively. Triplet C weighed 2,031 g, with Apgar scores of 8 and 9 at 1 and 5 minutes, respectively. Placental examination showed four vascular anastomoses between triplets B and C (Figure 2) and vascular anastomoses (i.e., umbilical artery and umbilical vein) between triplets A and B. The umbilical artery between

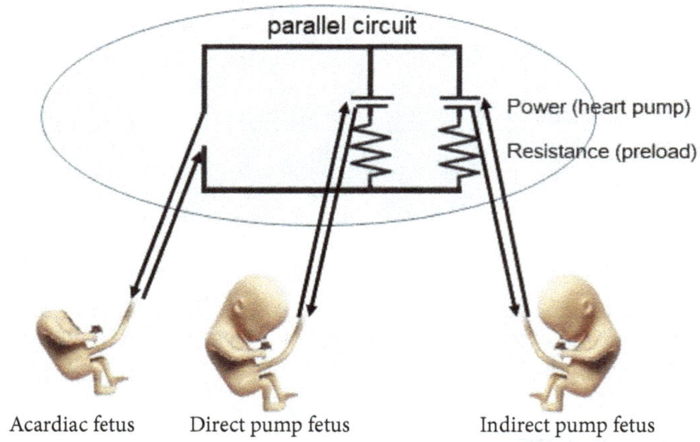

FIGURE 3: Schematic representation of the anastomosed blood vessels between triplets B and C. The anastomosed blood vessels comprised a parallel circuit, which provided blood flow to triplet A.

triplets A and B was anastomosed with a thin umbilical artery of triplet C. The umbilical vein between triplets A and B was anastomosed with two umbilical veins of triplet C. At 12 months, both children showed normal neurodevelopment.

3. Discussion

This is the first report on two liveborn infants delivered in term after successful RFA for monochorionic-triamniotic triplet pregnancy with TRAP sequence. There were two similar reports; however, the liveborn infants were preterm [4, 5]. In the current case, we succeeded in complete blood flow cessation with a single puncture on the acardiac fetus stuck to the anterior uterine wall.

The treatment methods of TRAP sequence are mainly RFA, bipolar cord coagulation, and intrafetal (or interstitial) laser coagulation. Recently, RFA and intrafetal (or interstitial) laser coagulation are mainly reported [6–8]. Laser surgery is generally selected at 14–16 weeks, and RFA is selected at 16–18 weeks because of fewer rate of premature labor [7]. Neonatal survival rate was comparable between the RFA and laser techniques (85% *vs* 82%, $P = 0.63$) [7]. In the current case, we decided intrauterine operation at 18 weeks, so we performed RFA.

Lee et al. [6] reported that there were no maternal deaths and no women required transfusions in patients treated for RFA. However, two women suffered thermal injuries at the site of the grounding pads. As a remedy, they changed to bigger grounding pads and had no further maternal thermal injuries. The cool-tip RF system we used this time comprised adopted pads which are bigger than the ground pads used at that time, and no complication was admitted.

Vascular anastomoses between triplets A and B were confirmed by Doppler ultrasound examination. Takahashi et al. reported that pump fetus identification was possible using dual-gate Doppler (ARIETTA 70) [5]. Here, we could distinguish the pump fetus from the indirect pump fetus based on the different baseline FHRs, which had relatively few fluctuations during gestation.

In monochorionic twin pregnancy with TRAP sequence, an acardiac fetus with an EFBW ≥0.7 times greater than that of the pump fetus is likely to develop heart failure [3]. Here, there was no abnormal blood flow or any sign of heart failure in triplet B (direct pump fetus), although the estimated weight of triplet A increased twice as much as that of triplet B. It can be inferred that triplet A was supplied with blood flow from triplet B and triplet C (indirect pump fetus) via another vascular anastomoses; this likely prevented triplet B from developing heart failure.

Without in utero treatment, the perinatal mortality rate for pump twins was approximately 55% [3]. Lewi et al. reported that intrauterine fetal death (IUFD) rate was the highest between the first and second trimester. It is also said that a poor prognostic factor of IUFD is a sudden increase in a pump fetus and accompanying heart failure [8]. In the current case, the direct pump fetus and the indirect pump fetus did not develop heart failure. However, the total weight of the direct pump fetus and the indirect pump fetus was almost the same as the acardiac fetus, and it was judged that the direct pump fetus and the indirect pump fetus are likely to develop heart failure in the future, and RFA was performed. It was possible to perform RFA before the onset of heart failure, leading to improvement in the prognosis of the both fetuses.

Argoti et al. [4] reported that blood flow to the acardiac fetus would be from direct pump and indirect pump fetuses via anastomosed blood vessels. However, the mechanism was not well understood. In their case, two live fetuses were simultaneously diagnosed with polyhydramnios; however, they did not develop heart failure. The fact that both direct pump and indirect pump fetuses simultaneously developed polyhydramnios indicated that the acardiac fetus was supplied with blood flow from both fetuses. Here, the umbilical artery between triplets A and B was anastomosed with a thin umbilical artery of triplet C. The umbilical vein between triplets A and B was anastomosed with two umbilical veins of triplet C. Figure 3 shows that the anastomosed blood vessels between triplets B and C comprised a parallel circuit, which provided blood flow to triplet A.

We hypothesized that increased preload has increased vascular resistance in triplet B. When vascular resistance of triplet B became higher than that of triplet C, blood flow from the acardiac fetus was probably diverted from triplet B to triplet C. In the previously reported cases, simultaneous polyhydramnios development in direct pump and indirect pump fetuses was probably because their preloads were equal. In an ideal parallel circuit, workloads of triplets B and C can be equal. However, there may have been other factors, such as placenta, blood flow, and preload, which differed between triplets B and C. Nevertheless, the burden on the pump fetus in monochorionic pregnancy with TRAP sequence can be lighter in triplet pregnancy than in twin pregnancy.

In the previous report [4], the capacity load of the direct pump fetus and the indirect pump fetus slowly progressed although the acardiac fetus rapidly increased. They succeeded in performing RFA before developing heart failure. From this and the previous cases, it appears that the progress of monochorionic-triamniotic triplet pregnancy with TRAP sequence is slow; it may be a disease in which it is possible to perform intrauterine therapy at the most appropriate timing before prognosis is poor. Therefore, monochorionic-triamniotic triplet pregnancy with TRAP sequence should be offered as an option of intrauterine therapy, such as RFA, to improve neonatal survival rate.

References

[1] D. L. Gillim and C. H. Hendricks, "Holoacardius: review of the literature and case report," *Obstetrics & Gynecology*, vol. 2, no. 6, pp. 647–653, 1953.

[2] Y. Imaizumi, "A comparative study of zygotic twinning and triplet rates in eight countries, 1972-1999," *Journal of Biosocial Science*, vol. 35, no. 2, pp. 287–302, 2003.

[3] T. R. Moore, S. Gale, and K. Benirschke, "Perinatal outcome of forty-nine pregnancies complicated by acardiac twinning," *American Journal of Obstetrics & Gynecology*, vol. 163, no. 3, pp. 907–912, 1990.

[4] P. S. Argoti, M. W. Bebbington, A. Johnson, and K. J. Moise Jr., "Indirect pump: unique presentation of a monochorionic-triamniotic triplet gestation complicated by TRAP sequence and successfully managed with radiofrequency ablation of the acardiac fetus," *Ultrasound in Obstetrics & Gynecology*, vol. 42, no. 1, pp. 115–117, 2013.

[5] Y. Takahashi, S. Iwagaki, R. Chiaki, K. Asai, M. Matsui, and I. Kawabata, "Ultrasonic identification of pump twin by dual-gate doppler in a monochorionic-triamniotic triplet twin reversed arterial perfusion sequence before preventative radiofrequency ablation: a case report," *Journal of Medical Ultrasonics*, vol. 45, no. 1, pp. 185–187, 2018.

[6] H. Lee, A. J. Wagner, E. Sy et al., "Efficacy of radiofrequency ablation for twin-reversed arterial perfusion sequence," *American Journal of Obstetrics & Gynecology*, vol. 196, e1, no. 5, p. 459, 2007.

[7] G. Pagani, F. D'Antonio, A. Khalil, A. Papageorghiou, A. Bhide, and B. Thilaganathan, "Intrafetal laser treatment for twin reversed arterial perfusion sequence: cohort study and meta-analysis," *Ultrasound in Obstetrics & Gynecology*, vol. 42, no. 1, pp. 6–14, 2013.

[8] H. Lee, M. Bebbington, and T. M. Crombleholme, "The north american fetal therapy network registry data on outcomes of radiofrequency ablation for twin-reversed arterial perfusion sequence," *Fetal Diagnosis and Therapy*, vol. 33, no. 4, pp. 224–229, 2013.

Uterine Tumor Resembling Ovarian Sex Cord Tumors Type II with Vaginal Vault Recurrence

Oriana Marrucci,[1] Paola Nicoletti,[1] Alessandro Mauriello,[2] Simone Facchetti,[2] Lodovico Patrizi,[1] Carlo Ticconi,[1] Francesco Sesti,[1] and Emilio Piccione[1]

[1]*Department of Surgical Sciences, Section of Gynecology and Obstetrics, University of Rome Tor Vergata, Italy*
[2]*Anatomic Pathology, Department of Experimental Medicine, University of Rome Tor Vergata, Italy*

Correspondence should be addressed to Oriana Marrucci; orianamarrucci@hotmail.it

Academic Editor: Maria Grazia Porpora

UTROSCTs (*Uterine Tumors Resembling Ovarian Sex Cord Tumors)* are rare neoplasms of unknown etiology usually occurring in middle-aged women. Less than 100 cases of UTROSCT have been reported so far. Although the typical behavior of UTROSCT is benign, metastatic and recurrent cases can occur. Here we describe an extremely rare case of vaginal vault recurrence of UTROSCT occurring 5 years after total hysterectomy with bilateral salpingo-oophorectomy. Though rare, UTROSCT should always be taken into account in the differential diagnosis of uterine masses initially considered leiomyomas.

1. Introduction

Uterine Tumors Resembling Ovarian Sex Cord Tumors (UTROSCTs) are rare neoplasms of unknown etiology [1]. They usually occur in middle-aged women. Most UTROSCTs behave as tumors of low malignant potential. Clinical characteristics are abnormal uterine bleeding and/or abdominal pain, along with an enlarged uterus or a palpable uterine mass without specific imaging finding [2]. Usually the diagnosis is incidental, following immunohistochemical and ultrastructural studies on the surgical specimen. UTROSCTs have a variable immunohistochemical profile with expression of sex cords, epithelial, and smooth muscle lineages markers. Hysterectomy with or without bilateral salpingo-oophorectomy is usually the treatment for UTROSCT. Here we report a rare case of vaginal vault recurrence (VVR) occurring 5 years after surgery in a woman who underwent hysterectomy with bilateral salpingo-oophorectomy for UTROSCT.

2. Case Presentation

In January 2013, a 54-year-old pluriparous woman was admitted to the Department of Obstetrics and Gynecology of Tor Vergata University Hospital (Rome) for recurrent postmenopausal abnormal uterine bleeding. At pelvic examination the uterine volume appeared increased by three times the standard volume.

Pelvic transvaginal ultrasound showed an intracavitary mass (80x73x74 mm) with heterogeneous echogenicity in which multiple anechoic areas with central and peripheral vascularization at power Doppler (RI 0.49) were present. The initial diagnosis was uterine leiomyoma. Other intramural leiomyomas, measuring 31x20x31 mm, 18x8 mm, and 9x6 mm, respectively, were identified. Ovaries appeared normal (see Figures 1(a) and 1(b)).

To exclude endometrial origin of bleeding, an office hysteroscopy was performed which was normal.

Laboratory blood tests showed no significant abnormalities. Total laparoscopic hysterectomy with bilateral salpingo-oophorectomy was performed. At gross pathologic examination, the uterus weighed 359 g and its dimensions were 8x3x4 cm. The uterine surface was deformed due to the presence of a grayish-yellow, polycyclic lesion measuring approximately 9 cm with a soft and fibrous consistency; the lesion also appeared poorly delineated with respect to the surrounding myometrium. On microscopic examination, it was composed of elements similar to the sex cords cells, with a trabecular and alveolar architectural pattern, and tubular elements. The

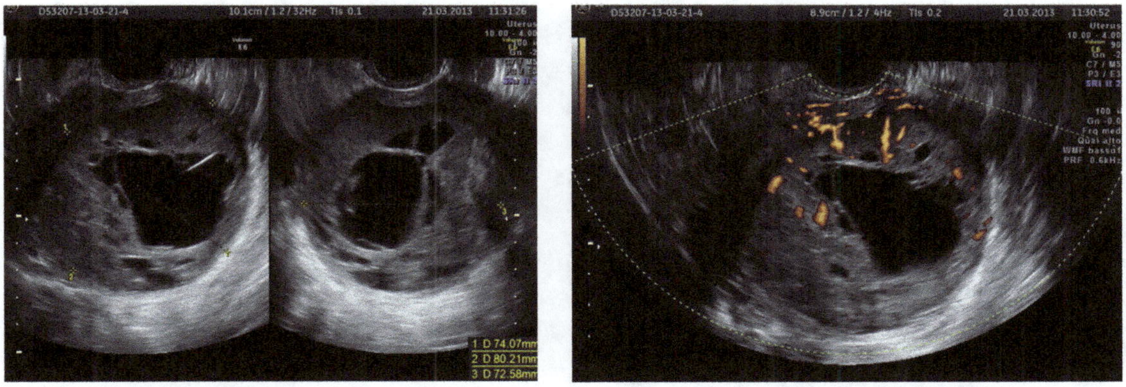

(a) (b)

FIGURE 1: (a) M-Mode findings: enlarged uterus with inhomogeneous echogenicity. (b) Power Doppler findings: multiple anechoic areas with central and peripheral vascularization.

cells showed an epithelioid appearance with irregular nuclei. The mitotic index was equal to 3 mitoses for 10 HPF assessed by means of Ki67 index, whereas proliferation index was 30%. Immunohistochemical profile showed the following: vimentin +, CD 56 +, CD 99 +, WT1 + / -, alpha actin -, desmin -, panCK -, EMA -, CD10 -, caldesmon -, S100 -, inhibin -, CroA -, and synaptophysin -. The diagnosis was uterine tumor with elements similar to the sex cords type II according to Blaustein's 2011 (UTROSCT, according to WHO) [3] (Figure 2).

The tubes and ovaries were histologically normal. At regular annual checks the patient remained asymptomatic with normal pelvic examination and ultrasound findings until December 2017 when a transvaginal ultrasound described the presence of a new solid lesion at level of the vaginal vault. The lesion was 45x19x20mm, highly vascularized (color score 4) and had a characteristic arboriform vascular pattern. It was adherent to the surrounding tissues but not to the bladder and bowel wall. These findings were confirmed by a CT scan of the abdomen and pelvis. A laparoscopy was performed with removal of the mass and partial infracolic omentectomy; multiple peritoneal biopsies were also taken (Figure 3(a)). Gross examination of the mass confirmed disease recurrence (Figure 3(b)).

At microscopic examination, the lesion showed elements similar to the sex cords cells, with trabecular and alveolar architecture, and tubular elements. The mitotic index was equal to 3 mitoses for 10 HPF assessed by means of Ki67 index, and proliferation index was 30%. Immunohistochemical profile showed the following: CD 56 +, CD 99 +/-, ER +, WT1 +, alpha actin -, panCK -, EMA -, CD10 -, S100 -, inhibin -, CroA -, calretinin-. The neoplasm was completely removed with free margins. It was compatible with the diagnosis of uterine tumor with elements similar to the sex cords type II according to Blaustein's 2011 (UTROSCT, according to WHO). The morphological and immunohistochemical characteristics were similar to those of the previous uterine neoplasm. No adjuvant therapy was administered according to the oncologic counselling. To date, the patient is asymptomatic, and pelvic examination and ultrasound are normal.

3. Discussion

To date, less than 100 cases of UTROSCT have been reported [4]. Although the typical behavior of UTROSCT is benign, metastatic and recurrent cases could occur [5]. To our knowledge, at present only 9 cases with extrauterine spread, distant metastatic disease, or recurrent disease have been reported [6].

UTROSCT is a rare and intriguing tumor. This neoplasm resembles an ovarian sex cord tumor. Even though several hypotheses have been raised to explain the histogenesis of UTROSCT—including its origin from sex cord cells, mesenchymal stem cells, and endometrial stromal tumors in which an excessive growth of sex cord cells occurs [7]—its pathogenesis is still unknown. In 1976, Clement and Scully [8] classified the neoplasm into two distinct subgroups based on clinical and histopathologic features. In the first group, the tumors showed a predominant endometrial stromal tumor-like differentiation and focal ovarian sex-cord-like areas (<50%) and were termed endometrial stromal tumors with sex-cord-like elements (ESTSCLE), whereas the neoplasms in the second group were composed predominantly of a sex-cord-like component accounting for 50% to 100% of the tumor, which was therefore called UTROSCT. UTROSCT has a high variability in the overall architecture of the tumor, as well as in its morphologic features and immunohistochemical characteristics. It shows a great variety of growth patterns, in which the cells are variably organized in sheets, cords, nests, trabeculae, and solid and hollow tubules. The neoplastic cells characteristically show low-grade atypia with round to oval nuclei, with regularly dispersed chromatin and small unnoticeable nucleoli. The cytoplasm is usually scarce and lightly eosinophilic [1]. A plethora of different immunohistochemical markers have been detected in UTROSCT. Some of these markers are (a) sex cord markers: α-Inhibin, calretinin, CD56, melan A, CD99, WT1, and MART-1; (b) epithelial markers: pancytokeratin, AE1/3, and epithelial membrane antigen; (c) myoid markers: α-smooth muscle actin, desmin, h-caldesmon, and histone-8 deacetylase; (d) neuroendocrine markers: estrogen receptors, progesterone

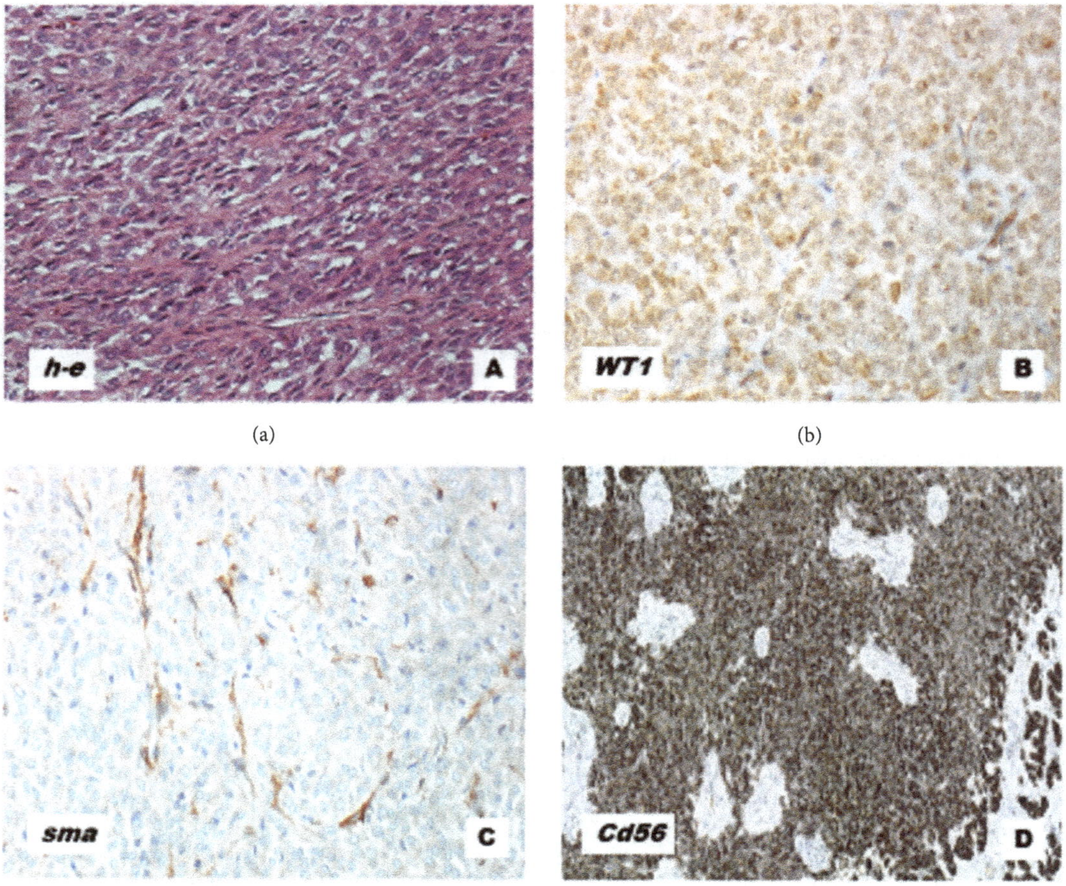

(a) (b) (c) (d)

FIGURE 2: Uterine tumor resembling an ovarian sex cord tumor. (a) Cords, nests, and trabeculae are seen, reminiscent of sex cord cells tumor of the ovary (H-E, 10x). (b) Positive stain for WT1 (10x). (c) Negative stain for smooth muscle actin (SMA, 10x). (d) Positive stain for CD56, a sex cord marker (10x).

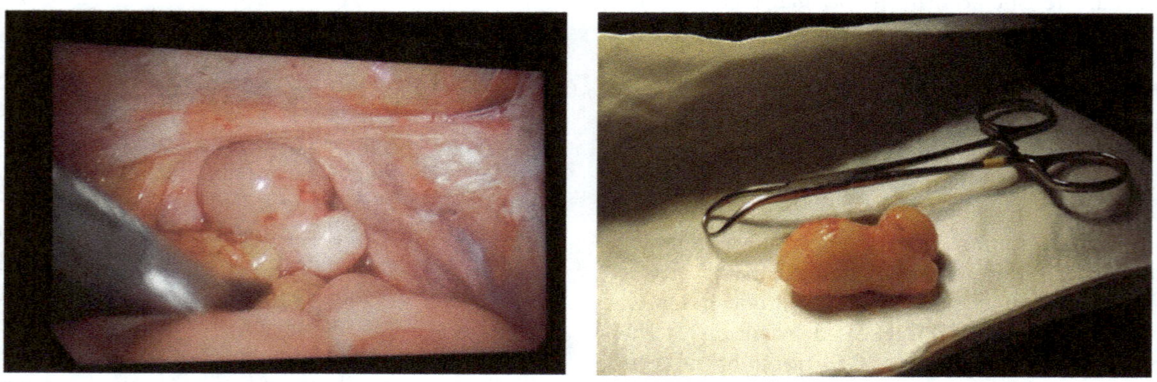

(a) (b)

FIGURE 3: (a) Laparoscopic appearance of the vaginal vault. (b) Macroscopic aspect of the excised mass.

receptors, androgen-receptors, and chromogranin; (e) miscellaneous markers: CD10, S100, CD117, and vimentin [1, 9]. These markers can be variably detected, often coexpressed, and, wherever expressed, can be expressed to a variable extent.

Immunoexpression for calretinin and at least for one of the other sex cord markers above reported is believed to be required to establish a diagnosis of UTROSCT [10]. Hysterectomy with or without bilateral salpingo-oophorectomy is the treatment of choice for UTROSCT [11]. At present, it is still impossible to predict aggressive disease. Traditional high-risk features of uterine cancer are of unclear value in UTROSCT. In UTROSCT lymphovascular space invasion and myometrial invasion have been reported in 4 out of 8 cases in which recurrence occurred [6]. These features have not been found in the present case, in which the initial clinical and US features suggested multiple uterine leiomyomas. Though very rare, UTROSCT should always be taken into account in the differential diagnosis of uterine masses initially considered leiomyomas. Although not specific, US and color Doppler findings could be helpful. There is no available information as to whether adjuvant therapy should be prescribed when VVR of UTROSCT occurs.

To our knowledge, the present case is the tenth one in which VVR of UTROSCT has been described. The possibility of VVR should be considered in the long-term follow-up of patients with UTROSCT, even if they are completely asymptomatic.

References

[1] D. Pradhan and S. K. Mohanty, "Uterine tumors resembling ovarian sex cord tumors," *Archives of Pathology & Laboratory Medicine*, vol. 137, no. 12, pp. 1832–1836, 2013.

[2] G. Giordano, M. Lombardi, F. Brigati, C. Mancini, and E. M. Silini, "Clinicopathologic features of 2 new cases of uterine tumors resembling ovarian sex cord tumors," *International Journal of Gynecological Pathology*, vol. 29, no. 5, pp. 459–467, 2010.

[3] C. J. Zaloudek, M. R. Hendrickson, and R. A. Soslow, "Mesenchymal tumors of the uterus," in *Blaustein's Pathology of the Female Genital Tract*, pp. 453–527, Springer, Boston, Mass, USA, 2011.

[4] S. M. Schraag, R. Caduff, K. J. Dedes, D. Fink, and A.-M. Schmidt, "Uterine tumors resembling ovarian sex cord tumors – treatment, recurrence, pregnancy and brief review," *Gynecologic Oncology Reports*, vol. 19, pp. 53–56, 2017.

[5] K. Biermann, L. C. Heukamp, R. Büttner, and H. Zhou, "Uterine tumor resembling an ovarian sex cord tumor associated with metastasis," *International Journal of Gynecological Pathology*, vol. 27, no. 1, pp. 58–60, 2008.

[6] M. L. Kuznicki, S. E. Robertson, A. Hakam, and M. M. Shahzad, "Metastatic uterine tumor resembling ovarian sex cord tumor: A case report and review of the literature," *Gynecologic Oncology Reports*, vol. 22, pp. 64–68, 2017.

[7] S. Croce, L. De Kock, T. Boshari et al., "Uterine tumor resembling ovarian sex cord tumor (UTROSCT) commonly exhibits positivity with sex cord markers FOXL2 and SF-1 but lacks FOXL2 and DICERI1 mutations," *International Journal of Gynecological Pathology*, vol. 35, no. 4, pp. 301–308, 2016.

[8] P. B. Clement and R. E. Scully, "Uterine tumors resembling ovarian sex-cord tumors: a clinicopathologic analysis of fourteen cases," *American Journal of Clinical Pathology*, vol. 66, no. 3, pp. 512–525, 1976.

[9] D. P. Hurrell and W. G. McCluggage, "Uterine tumour resembling ovarian sex cord tumour is an immunohistochemically polyphenotypic neoplasm which exhibits coexpression of epithelial, myoid and sex cord markers," *Journal of Clinical Pathology*, vol. 60, no. 10, pp. 1148–1154, 2007.

[10] A. A. Hashmi, N. Faridi, M. M. Edhi, and M. Khan, "Uterine tumor resembling ovarian sex cord tumor (UTROSCT), case report with literature review," *International Archives of Medicine*, vol. 47, pp. 1–4, 2014.

[11] R. Sadeh, Y. Segev, M. Schmidt, J. Schendler, T. Baruch, and O. Lavie, "Uterine tumors resembling ovarian sex cord tumors: case report of rare pathological and clinical entity," *Case Reports in Obstetrics and Gynecology*, vol. 2017, Article ID 2736710, 4 pages, 2017.

51

Development of Vaginal Pseudoaneurysm 3 Years after Cesarean Section Possibly Induced by Anticoagulant and Antiplatelet Therapies

Yui Kinjo, Tadatsugu Kinjo, Keiko Mekaru, Hayase Nitta, Hitoshi Masamoto, and Yoichi Aoki

Department of Obstetrics and Gynecology, Graduate School of Medicine, University of the Ryukyus, 207 Uehara Nishihara, Okinawa 903-0215, Japan

Correspondence should be addressed to Yoichi Aoki; yoichi@med.u-ryukyu.ac.jp

Academic Editor: Mehmet A. Osmanağaoğlu

Pseudoaneurysms generally develop when an arterial puncture site is inadequately sealed. We encountered a case of vaginal pseudoaneurysm that developed 3 years after cesarean section in a 35-year-old gravida 7 para 4 woman who was prescribed with anticoagulant and antiplatelet drugs after surgeries for ventricular septal defect and aortic valve replacement. Pelvic computed tomography scan revealed a large mass, which showed a dappled contrast filling on the arterial phase, located in the posterior vaginal wall. The vaginal pseudoaneurysm was completely occluded by embolization of the left vaginal artery. Anticoagulation and antiplatelet therapies can be potential causes of spontaneous pseudoaneurysm rupture. Extrauterine pseudoaneurysm has a long period of time between cesarean section and pseudoaneurysm discovery. Considering that pseudoaneurysm shows different clinical features for each patient, we should always consider pseudoaneurysm when we assess a patient with postpartum hemorrhage.

1. Introduction

Pseudoaneurysms (PAs) generally develop when an arterial puncture site is inadequately sealed. Uterine PA mainly shows postpartum vaginal bleeding after cesarean section (CS). Considering vascular wall vulnerability due to changes in hormonal and circulatory dynamics during pregnancy, PA can occur after not only invasive procedures, such as CS and dilatation and curettage (D&C), but also a normal vaginal delivery [1]. Typical cases of uterine PA exhibit vaginal bleeding 2 weeks to 1 month after CS [2, 3].

We encountered a case of vaginal PA that developed 3 years after CS in a patient who had been prescribed with anticoagulant and antiplatelet drugs until the PA rupture.

2. Case Report

A 35-year-old gravida 7 para 4 woman had histories of CS for four times and D and C for three times. The last CS was performed 3 years ago. Furthermore, surgeries for ventricular septal defect and aortic valve replacement were performed when she was 14 and 24 years old, respectively. Thereafter, anticoagulant and antiplatelet drugs (warfarin potassium at 2 mg/day and clopidogrel sulfate at 75 mg/day, respectively) had been prescribed until the PA rupture. Eventually, she complained of atypical vaginal bleeding for several days and then visited our department. Ultrasonography showed no abnormal findings in the uterus at that time. However, 3 days later, she experienced profuse vaginal bleeding and thereby was admitted to our hospital. Her blood pressure and pulse rate were 100/70 mmHg and 106 beats/min, respectively. Her laboratory results were as follows: white blood cell count, $3.7 \times 10^3/\mu l$; hemoglobin count, 6.2 g/dl; platelet level, 210 $\times 10^3/\mu l$; and prothrombin time-international normalized ratio, 1.95. However, second ultrasonography could not detect any uterine abnormality; therefore, contrast-enhanced computed tomography (CT) scan was performed. Pelvic CT scan

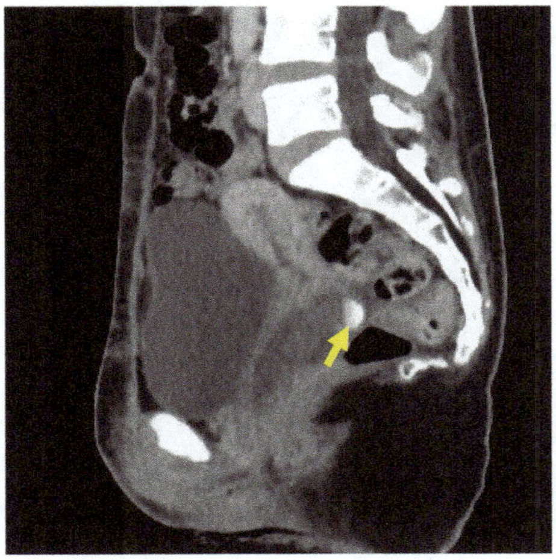

FIGURE 1: Pelvic computed tomography scan (sagittal view) reveals a large mass, which shows a dappled contrast filling on the arterial phase, located in the posterior vaginal wall (arrow).

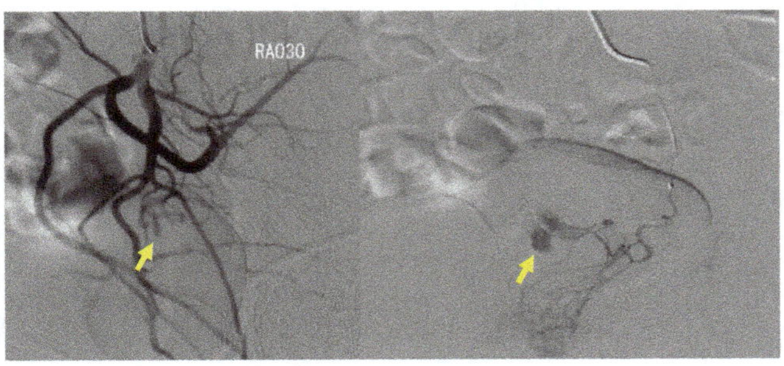

FIGURE 2: Pelvic angiography shows pseudoaneurysm formation in the left vaginal artery (arrows). (a) Angiography for the left internal iliac artery. (b) Selective angiography for the left vaginal artery.

revealed a large mass, which showed a dappled contrast filling on the arterial phase, located in the posterior vaginal wall (Figure 1). Thereafter, vascular radiologists performed emergency pelvic angiography, which revealed PA formation in the left vaginal artery (Figure 2). The PA was completely occluded by embolization of the left vaginal artery (Figure 3). Embolization procedures were performed with metallic coils and a gelatin sponge (Gelpart®; Nippon Kayaku, Tokyo, Japan), which measured 2 mm in diameter, via a microcatheter (Renegade® infusion catheter (2.5 Fr); Boston Scientific, Tokyo, Japan). Postembolization course was uneventful.

3. Discussion

A potential cause of spontaneous PA rupture in our case may be the use of anticoagulation and antiplatelet therapies after aortic valve replacement. Our patient had been prescribed with anticoagulant and antiplatelet drugs until the PA rupture. Several reports pointed out anticoagulation therapy as the possible cause of ruptured PA [4, 5]. According to a prospective study, failure of thrombosis was associated with considerably large PAs and the concomitant use of anticoagulation or antiplatelet agents [6]. Furthermore, late postpartum hemorrhage due to ruptured PA also occurs in patients with von Willebrand disease [7, 8]. In general, PAs are thrombosed spontaneously. Therefore, PA is formed as a result of repeated bleeding and thrombus due to abnormal hemostasis [4–8]. Hence, an underlying bleeding disorder or anticoagulation therapy should be considered in patients presenting with PA rupture-induced postpartum hemorrhage.

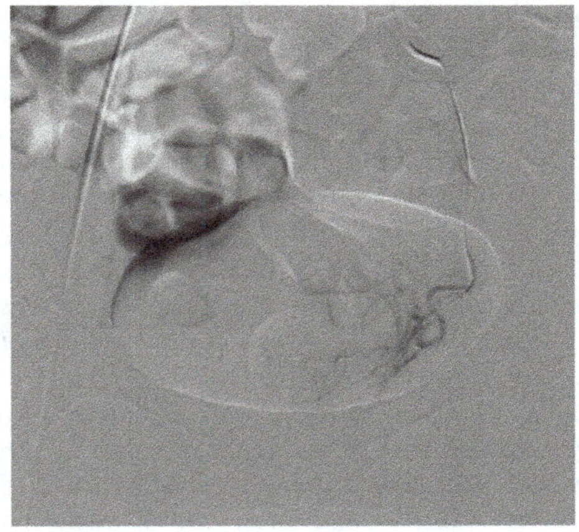

FIGURE 3: Complete occlusion of the left vaginal pseudoaneurysm by embolization of the left vaginal artery.

PA can occur after 3 years of CS. Toursarkissian et al. reported that spontaneous thrombosis of PA occurred in 88% of cases with small PAs at a mean of 23 days [9]. Isono et al. reviewed that the average time between preceding CS and PA is 14.5 days [2], whereas Baba et al. reported that it is at a median of 28 days and a maximum of 140 days [10]. Accordingly, a period of 3 years for PA to occur, as revealed in our case, is extremely rare. However, a large internal iliac pelvic PA combined with arteriovenous fistula appeared in a patient 20 years following an elective CS [11]; in another case, the time period between the CS and PA occurrence was approximately 10 years with no other potential causative factors [12]. Interestingly, Matsubara et al. speculated that extrauterine PA has a long period of time between CS and PA discovery [1].

The PA in our case developed from the vaginal artery and was located in the posterior vaginal wall, not in the uterus. Dohan et al. reported that seven out of 18 cases with PA after CS originated from the vaginal artery [3]. PA appearing in the internal iliac artery [11] or the Douglas pouch [12] and PA showing a pelvic mass [13] were also reported. Intrauterine PA undergoes morphological and functional dynamic changes in the uterus after CS, and it is easily damaged and ruptured. However, extrauterine PA does not suffer from such dynamic changes and is difficult to rupture; thus, time lag occurs between CS and extrauterine PA discovery [1].

In conclusion, anticoagulation and antiplatelet therapies can be potential causes of spontaneous PA rupture. Extrauterine PA has a long period of time between CS and PA discovery. Considering that PA shows different clinical features for each patient, we should always consider PA when we assess a patient with postpartum hemorrhage.

Acknowledgments

The authors would like to thank Enago (http://www.enago.jp/) for the English language review of this article.

References

[1] S. Matsubara, H. Takahashi, and Y. Baba, "Letter to 'Uterine artery pseudoaneurysm bleeding one decade after caesarean section: a case report': pseudoaneurysm anywhere and anytime," *The Journal of Obstetrics and Gynaecology Research*, vol. 43, no. 10, pp. 1660-1661, 2017.

[2] W. Isono, R. Tsutsumi, O. Wada-Hiraike et al., "Uterine Artery Pseudoaneurysm after Cesarean Section: Case Report and Literature Review," *Journal of Minimally Invasive Gynecology*, vol. 17, no. 6, pp. 687–691, 2010.

[3] A. Dohan, P. Soyer, A. Subhani et al., "Postpartum hemorrhage resulting from pelvic pseudoaneurysm: a retrospective analysis of 588 consecutive cases treated by arterial embolization," *Cardiovascular and Interventional Radiology*, vol. 36, no. 5, pp. 1247–1255, 2013.

[4] F. De Santis, G. Martini, T. Haglmüller, G. Mani, C. Conati, and G. Bonatti, "Anticoagulation therapy for postoperative deep vein thrombosis coupled with pulmonary embolism: a potential trigger for delayed popliteal artery injury presentation after total knee arthroplasty," *Phlebology*, vol. 28, no. 5, pp. 275–277, 2013.

[5] T. Horimatsu, K. Fujii, M. Shibuya et al., "Rupture of pseudoaneurysm of the superficial femoral artery over four years after self-expandable nitinol stent implantation," *Journal of Cardiology Cases*, vol. 12, no. 2, pp. 52–56, 2015.

[6] K. C. Kent, C. R. McArdle, B. Kennedy, D. S. Baim, E. Anninos, and J. J. Skillman, "A prospective study of the clinical outcome of femoral pseudoaneurysma and arteriovenous fistuals induced by arterial puncture," *Journal of Vascular Surgery*, vol. 17, no. 1, pp. 125–133, 1993.

[7] M. C. Salman, B. Cil, S. Esin, and O. Deren, "Late postpartum hemorrhage due to von Willebrand disease managed with uterine artery embolization," *Obstetrics and Gynecology*, vol. 111, 2 Part 2, pp. 573–575, 2008.

[8] M. Shimizu, E. Kondoh, M. Ueda, K. Kakui, K. Tatsumi, and I. Konishi, "Secondary postpartum hemorrhage due to uterine artery pseudoaneurysm rupture in von Willebrand disease," *The Journal of Obstetrics and Gynaecology Research*, vol. 37, no. 12, pp. 1887–1890, 2011.

[9] B. Toursarkissian, B. T. Allen, D. Petrinec et al., "Spontaneous closure of selected iatrogenic pseudoaneurysms and arteriovenous fistulae," *Journal of Vascular Surgery*, vol. 25, no. 5, pp. 803–809, 1997.

[10] Y. Baba, H. Takahashi, A. Ohkuchi et al., "Uterine artery pseudoaneurysm: its occurrence after non-traumatic events, and possibility of "without embolization" strategy," *European Journal of Obstetrics, Gynecology, and Reproductive Biology*, vol. 205, pp. 72–78, 2016.

[11] N. Papadakos, L. Wales, K. Hayes, A. M. Belli, I. Loftus, and S. Ray, "Post-traumatic pelvic pseudoaneurysm and arteriovenous fistula: combined endovascular and surgical approach," *European Journal of Vascular and Endovascular Surgery*, vol. 36, no. 2, pp. 164–166, 2008.

[12] L. Johannesson, J. Mason, and M. K. Oehler, "Uterine artery pseudoaneurysm bleeding one decade after caesarean section: a case report," *The Journal of Obstetrics and Gynaecology Research*, vol. 43, no. 5, pp. 939–942, 2017.

[13] T. Kuwata, S. Matsubara, Y. Kaneko, A. Izumi, M. Nakata, and M. Suzuki, "Asymptomatic uterine artery pseudoaneurysm after cesarean section," *The Journal of Obstetrics and Gynaecology Research*, vol. 36, no. 2, pp. 405–410, 2010.

52

Case of Ruptured Ectopic Pregnancy in the Uterosacral Ligament and Review of the Literature

Yasmin Abedin[1] and **Kanchi Chadha**[2]

[1]*Department of Obstetrics, Gynecology and Women's Health at Rutgers-New Jersey Medical School, Newark, New Jersey, USA*
[2]*Department of Obstetrics and Gynecology at Hackensack University Medical Center, Hackensack, New Jersey, USA*

Correspondence should be addressed to Yasmin Abedin; yabedin24@gmail.com

Academic Editor: Maria Grazia Porpora

Pregnancies that implant on the uterosacral ligament are rare. Here, we describe a case of ruptured ectopic pregnancy in the left uterosacral ligament in a patient with potential risk factors including possible endometriosis and recent hysteroscopic procedure. A 29-year-old female, para 0, presented to the emergency department with generalized abdominal pain. Pelvic examination was significant for fullness in the posterior cul-de-sac. Laboratory values were significant for beta-human chorionic gonadotropin (hCG) level of 6311 mIU/mL. Sonogram findings were significant for no intrauterine gestation, a $6.9 \times 4.6 \times 4.7$ cm^3 complex left adnexal mass, and moderate free fluid within the posterior cul-de-sac. The patient underwent laparoscopy, which revealed hemoperitoneum and unremarkable bilateral fallopian tubes and ovaries. An abnormal area was noted in the left uterosacral ligament. Tissue was bluntly removed and pathologically confirmed as chorionic villi within the left uterosacral ligament. After one week, her beta-hCG decreased to 784 mIU/mL. After two weeks, she was seen as an outpatient and was doing well without any symptoms. More information is required regarding these unique pregnancies to help understand the pathophysiology and determine the management.

1. Introduction

Pregnancies that implant on the uterosacral ligament are rare, and only a few other cases have been described in the literature. The incidence of these pregnancies ranges from 1 per 10,000 pregnancies to 1 per 30,000 pregnancies and approximately 1 per 100 ectopic pregnancies [1, 2]. These pregnancies present similar to tubal ectopic pregnancies and can be difficult to distinguish through ultrasonography; they can also be life threatening if not managed in a timely fashion. Here, we describe a case of ruptured ectopic pregnancy in the left uterosacral ligament in a patient with potential risk factors including possible endometriosis and recent hysteroscopic procedure. The pregnancy was managed with surgical intervention. Descriptions of such cases are needed in order to understand the pathophysiology of this disease and the best management guidelines. Moreover, we review other cases of ectopic pregnancies within the uterosacral ligament in order to gain insight into the risk factors and management of these pregnancies.

2. Case Presentation

This is a case of a 29-year-old female patient, para 0, who presented to the emergency department with worsening generalized abdominal pain. She had associated symptoms of fatigue and several episodes of diarrhea.

The patient's history was significant for infertility, for which she was undergoing evaluation at an outside institution. She had a hysterosalpingogram (HSG) about four months prior to presentation and three months prior to a hysteroscopy. Based on the HSG, there was suspicion for uterine polyps. One month prior to her presentation, she underwent a hysteroscopic procedure, which was uncomplicated. Two endometrial polyps were seen and removed, and bilateral tubal ostia were seen. She did not have a serum beta-human chori-

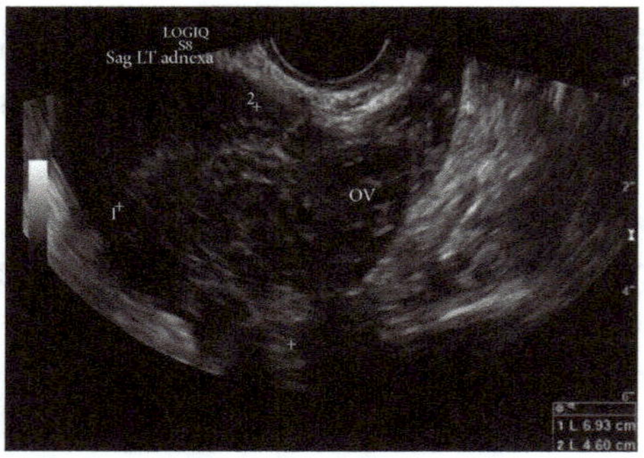

FIGURE 1: Transvaginal ultrasound image of left adnexa. OV depicts ovarian tissue. Complex left adnexal mass measuring $6.9 \times 4.6 \times 4.7\,\text{cm}^3$.

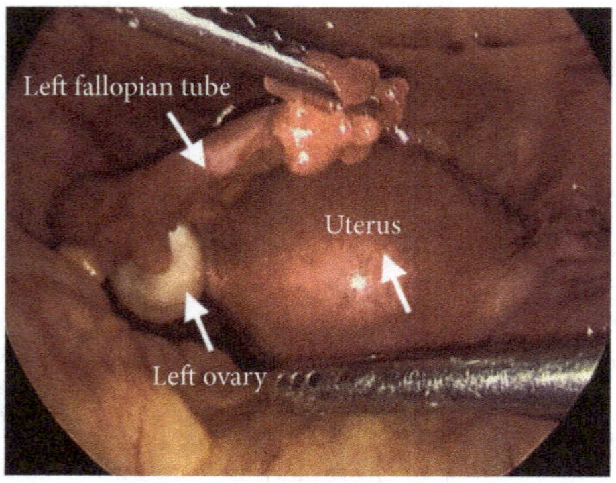

FIGURE 2: Laparoscopic image of unremarkable left fallopian tube and left ovary.

onic gonadotropin (hCG) test performed but urine beta-hCG was negative prior to the procedure. Her menstrual history was significant for irregular menses with intervals of 30-90 days. Her history otherwise was unremarkable.

On physical examination, the patient was pale and lethargic. She was tender on abdominal examination. Pelvic examination was significant for fullness in the right adnexa and posterior cul-de-sac. Laboratory values were significant for hemoglobin of 11.4 g/dL and beta-hCG level of 6311 mIU/mL. However, the patient was unaware of her pregnancy. Sonogram findings were significant for no intrauterine gestation, a $6.9 \times 4.6 \times 4.7\,\text{cm}^3$ complex left adnexal mass, and moderate free fluid within the posterior cul-de-sac and right upper quadrant (Figure 1). The adnexal mass appeared to be heterogeneous, and the image was certainly ambiguous since no discrete gestational sac, yolk sac, or fetal pole were seen. However, in the setting of a positive pregnancy test and acute abdominal findings, the adnexal mass was concerning for a ruptured ectopic pregnancy with hemoperitoneum.

The patient underwent a diagnostic laparoscopy for evaluation and management of the suspected ectopic pregnancy. On laparoscopy, hemoperitoneum of 1000 mL was visualized and evacuated. The uterus appeared to be unremarkable. The fimbriated end of the left fallopian tube was minimally erythematous, but no evidence of rupture or injury was noted and the left ovary was unremarkable (Figure 2). The right fallopian tube and ovary were also

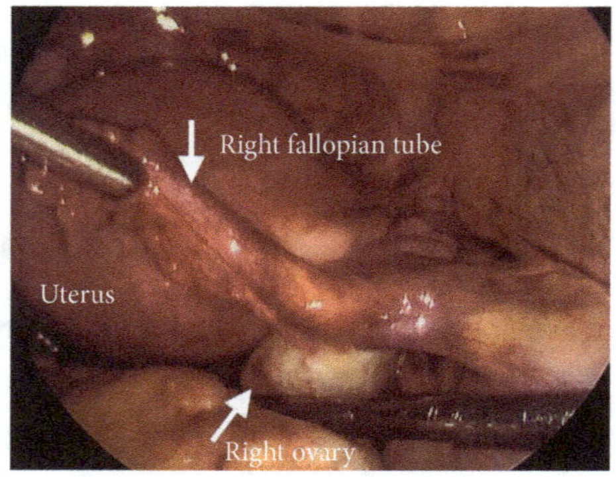

FIGURE 3: Laparoscopic image of unremarkable right fallopian tube and right ovary.

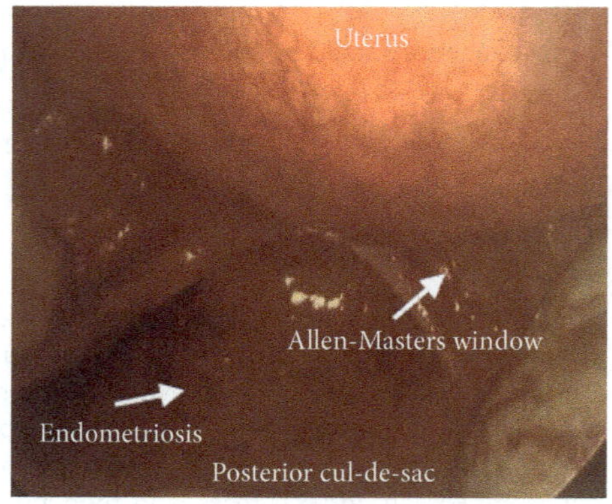

FIGURE 4: Laparoscopic image of posterior cul-de-sac, including endometriosis and Allen-Masters window.

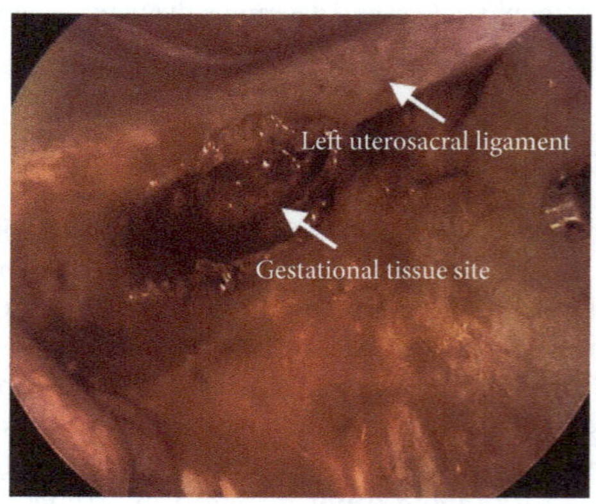

FIGURE 5: Laparoscopic image of left uterosacral ligament with the site of gestational tissue.

within normal limits (Figure 3). The posterior cul-de-sac appeared to have adhesions and several areas of endometriosis, including the Allen-Masters window (Figure 4). Upon closer examination, the left uterosacral ligament had a 2 cm defect with abnormal tissue with bleeding (Figure 5). The tissue was suspicious for an ectopic pregnancy; hence, it was removed bluntly from the peritoneum and sent to pathology for assessment. Thereafter, this area of the left uterosacral ligament was copiously irrigated and suctioned. Persistent oozing of blood was observed, and

TABLE 1: Summary of prior cases with an ectopic pregnancy within the uterosacral ligament.

Authors	Shin et al. [4]	Lo and Lau [5]	Lo and Lau [5]	Gundabattula and Pochiraju [6]	Cheung and Rosenthal [7]	Dasari and Devi [8]	Present case
Age (years)	28	33	32	30	24	22	29
Gravidity and parity	G2P0010	G1P0	G4P2	G3P1011	Not reported	G2P1	G1P0
Serum beta-HcG (mIU/mL)	Not reported	Not reported	Not reported	5699 to 81 after one week	1654	Not reported	6311 to 3807 after procedure to 784 after 1 week
Risk factors	None	Endometriosis	None	None	None	Intrauterine device	Endometriosis and recent hysteroscopic procedure
Management	Surgical removal via laparotomy	Surgical removal via laparoscopy converted to laparotomy	Surgical removal via laparoscopy	Surgical removal via laparoscopy followed by parenteral methotrexate 50 mg/m^2	Surgical removal via laparoscopy	Surgical removal via laparotomy	Surgical removal via laparoscopy

SURGIFLO hemostatic matrix with thrombin was used to achieve excellent hemostasis.

At the end of the case, there was no identifiable pregnancy within the fallopian tubes or peritoneal cavity. The patient was extubated and had tolerated the procedure well. On postoperative day one, the patient did well and the repeat beta-hCG was 3807 mIU/mL.

Pathology results on postoperative day 2 revealed that the first specimen was a blood clot and that the second specimen was chorionic villi within the left uterosacral ligament. After one week, the patient's beta-hCG had decreased to 784 mIU/mL. After two weeks, the patient was seen as an outpatient and was doing well without complaints.

3. Discussion

Primary peritoneal pregnancy is a rare gynecologic morbidity. The incidence has been variable depending on the literature, ranging from 1 per 10,000 pregnancies to 1 per 30,000 pregnancies and approximately 1 per 100 ectopic pregnancies [1, 2]. The risks to the patient are similar as that of a ruptured tubal pregnancy; however, identification preoperatively is not trivial [2]. According to Studdiford, a primary peritoneal pregnancy needs to meet the following criteria: both fallopian tubes and ovaries appear to be normal without evidence of rupture or injury, absence of uteroperitoneal fistula, and the presence of a pregnancy related exclusively to the peritoneal surface and early enough to eliminate the possibility of secondary implantation [3]. We believe that our case met these criteria after laparoscopy was done and after pathology results confirmed chorionic villi within the peritoneum. However, the initial diagnosis was assumed to be a ruptured tubal ectopic pregnancy given the patient's presentation and unclear sonographic findings (Figure 1). The sonogram was ambiguous since no distinct gestational sac, yolk sac, or fetal pole were seen. However, an adnexal mass in the setting of a positive pregnancy test and acute abdominal findings was concerning for a ruptured ectopic pregnancy. Primary peritoneal pregnancies can have dire consequences, such as intraperitoneal hemorrhage with need for transfusion and even death. It is important for gynecologic surgeons to realize that the sonogram cannot always correctly diagnose a peritoneal pregnancy. There should also be a high index of suspicion for either ruptured tubal or abdominal pregnancy when a patient has a hemoperitoneum in the setting of a positive pregnancy test, and emergent laparoscopy is key to reduce morbidity. Furthermore, when an ectopic pregnancy is suspected and laparoscopy is initiated, it is imperative to perform a thorough pelvic and abdominal survey in order to locate the pregnancy implantation site.

There is a paucity of information regarding primary peritoneal pregnancies implanting in the uterosacral ligament, mostly because it is a rare entity. There have been few case reports on this topic (Table 1) [4–8].

Shin et al. described a 28-year-old G2P0010 patient with a ruptured ectopic pregnancy within the uterosacral ligament that was surgically removed via laparotomy. This patient did not have any apparent risk factors [4]. Lo and Lau described two cases; the first case was a 33-year-old female G1P0 with a history of pelvic endometriosis who had a ruptured ectopic pregnancy within the uterosacral ligament [5]. She was surgically managed with laparoscopy, which was converted to laparotomy [5]. The second case was a 32-year-old G4P2 with similar presentation, without any risk factors, managed with laparoscopic excision of abnormal tissue [5]. Gundabattula and Pochiraju described a 30-year-old G3P1011 with no significant risk factors with a ruptured ectopic pregnancy within the uterosacral ligament, which was managed with laparoscopy and one dose of parenteral methotrexate 50 mg/m^2. There was a significant decline in her beta-hCG levels after one week (5699 mIU/mL to 81 mIU/mL) [6]. Cheung and Rosenthal discussed a 24-year-old female patient with similar presentation and no risk factors, managed with laparoscopy only [7]. Finally, Dasari and Devi reported a 22-year-old female G2P1 with a ruptured uterosacral ligament pregnancy, which was managed with laparotomy. An intrauterine device (IUD) was listed as a possible risk factor [8]. See Table 1.

The majority of these cases did not document any risk factor; however, pelvic endometriosis and IUD were listed as potential risk factors for having a primary peritoneal pregnancy within the uterosacral ligament. Our case did not have any of these documented risk factors prior to her procedure. She did not have any prior sonographic images depicting endometriosis and did not undergo laparoscopy previously. Based on our assessment during the laparoscopic procedure, it was evident that she did have endometriosis in the posterior cul-de-sac (Figure 4), which could have been a contributing risk factor to the peritoneal pregnancy within the left uterosacral ligament.

The pathophysiology of pregnancies that implant on the uterosacral ligament involves sperm that accumulates in the posterior cul-de-sac and ovum that also lies in the same region due to the physiologic flow of peritoneal fluid [9, 10]. Interestingly, hysteroscopy has not previously been described as a potential or definite risk factor for uterosacral ligament ectopic pregnancies, and it is remarkable that our case underwent this procedure just one month prior to presentation. It is possible that the hysteroscopic fluid could have assisted with patency of the fallopian tubes to allow for the sperm and ovum to meet in the peritoneum and implant in the uterosacral ligament, which can be considered a risk factor. On the contrary, one must also consider whether or not the hysteroscopic fluid could have facilitated the movement of an early tubal pregnancy into the peritoneum. However, the patient's urine beta-hCG was negative prior to her hysteroscopic procedure, so pregnancy was unlikely at that time. Also, as mentioned previously, we believe our case meets Studdiford's criteria and was a primary peritoneal pregnancy.

Management of pregnancies in the uterosacral ligament will vary depending on the patient's condition, gestational age, size of ectopic, and surgeon's experience. The use of surgery via laparoscopy [5–7] and laparotomy [4, 5, 8] has been described as above. Administration of methotrexate and/or intracardiac potassium chloride has also been described in the past for treatment of abdominal pregnancies [6, 10–13]. Not all of the prior reported cases of pregnancies in the uterosacral ligament trended beta-hCG levels [6]. This should be considered a crucial part of management, especially if the location of pregnancy or diagnosis of intra-abdominal pregnancy cannot be confirmed immediately. In our case, we successfully used laparoscopy and blunt removal of the gestational tissue from the uterosacral ligament and also followed beta-hCG values.

4. Conclusion

In summary, we reported a case of a ruptured ectopic pregnancy that implanted in the left uterosacral ligament. The patient was treated with surgical removal of gestational tissue, and she was followed postoperatively. Primary peritoneal pregnancies are rare, and pregnancies in the uterosacral ligament occur even more infrequently. Cases of such pregnancies should be reported in order for clinicians to understand the pathophysiology and determine the best management practices. Providers should have a high index of suspicion and be vigilant in performing laparoscopy/laparotomy in the setting of a positive pregnancy test and hemoperitoneum. It is imperative to perform a thorough pelvic and abdominal survey during surgery and obtain tissue for pathological analysis in order to determine a diagnosis.

References

[1] H. K. Atrash, A. Friede, and C. J. Hogue, "Abdominal pregnancy in the United States: frequency and maternal mortality," *Obstetrics and Gynecology*, vol. 69, 3, Part 1, pp. 333–337, 1987.

[2] F. G. Hailu, G. T. Yihunie, A. A. Essa, and W. . Tsega, "Advanced abdominal pregnancy, with live fetus and severe preeclampsia, case report," *BMC Pregnancy and Childbirth*, vol. 17, no. 1, p. 243, 2017.

[3] W. E. Studdiford, "Primary peritoneal pregnancy," *American Journal of Obstetrics and Gynecology*, vol. 44, no. 3, pp. 487–491, 1942.

[4] J. S. Shin, Y. J. Moon, S. R. Kim, K. T. Kim, H. Moon, and Y. Y. Hwang, "Primary peritoneal pregnancy implanted on the uterosacral ligament: a case report," *Journal of Korean Medical Science*, vol. 15, no. 3, pp. 359–362, 2000.

[5] K. W.-K. Lo and T.-K. Lau, "Ectopic pregnancy in uterosacral ligament," *The Journal of Obstetrics and Gynaecology Research*, vol. 23, no. 5, pp. 415–419, 1997.

[6] S. R. Gundabattula and M. Pochiraju, "Primary abdominal pregnancy in the uterosacral ligament with haemoperitoneum: a near miss," *Journal of Clinical and Diagnostic Research*, vol. 8, no. 5, pp. OD08–OD09, 2014.

[7] V. Y. T. Cheung and D. M. Rosenthal, "Abdominal pregnancy," *Journal of Minimally Invasive Gynecology*, vol. 12, no. 1, p. 9, 2005.

[8] P. Dasari and S. Devi, "Primary peritoneal pregnancy: a case report," *The Journal of Obstetrics and Gynaecology Research*, vol. 26, no. 1, pp. 45–47, 2000.

[9] D. Cavanagh, "Primary peritoneal pregnancy," *American Journal of Obstetrics and Gynecology*, vol. 76, no. 3, pp. 523–532, 1958.

[10] N. Agarwal and F. Odejinmi, "Early abdominal ectopic pregnancy: challenges, update and review of current management," *The Obstetrician & Gynaecologist Gynaecologist*, vol. 16, no. 3, pp. 193–198, 2014.

[11] L. Cobellis, L. Stradella, and E. M. Messalli, "Contribution to the choice of therapy in abdominal pregnancy," *Panminerva Medica*, vol. 42, no. 2, pp. 159–161, 2000.

[12] P. M. Anderson, E. K. Opfer, J. M. Busch, and E. F. Magann, "An early abdominal wall ectopic pregnancy successfully treated with ultrasound guided intralesional methotrexate: a

case report," *Obstetrics and Gynecology International*, vol. 2009, Article ID 247452, 3 pages, 2009.

[13] D. Deka, A. Bahadur, A. Singh, and N. Malhotra, "Successful management of heterotopic pregnancy after fetal reduction using potassium chloride and methotrexate," *Journal of Human Reproductive Sciences*, vol. 5, no. 1, pp. 57–60, 2012.

53

Intrauterine Transfusion Complicated by Umbilical Artery Thrombosis

Roopali V. Donepudi and Kenneth J. Moise Jr.

Department of Obstetrics, Gynecology and Reproductive Medicine, Division of Maternal-Fetal Medicine, UT Health-School of Medicine at Houston, The Fetal Center, Children's Memorial Hermann Hospital, Houston, TX, USA

Correspondence should be addressed to Roopali V. Donepudi; roopalivdonepudi@gmail.com

Academic Editor: Giovanni Monni

Background. Fetal anemia results from several conditions; however intrauterine transfusion (IUT) remains the treatment for severe cases. The complications of this procedure are rare and yet can result in preterm delivery or fetal death. *Case.* 31 y/o G3P2002 with Rh alloimmunization underwent IUT from 19 to 35 weeks. Umbilical artery thrombosis was noted after her 5th IUT. Further transfusions were performed without any complications and she delivered a full term male infant with APGARS of 8 and 9 at 1 and 5 minutes, respectively. *Conclusion.* The complication of umbilical artery thrombosis is unusual and the optimal management is unclear. We report such a case and propose that the presence of Hyrtl's anastomosis near the placental cord insertion may explain the reassuring fetal status throughout the pregnancy.

1. Introduction

The incidence of fetal anemia secondary to Rhesus alloimmunization has decreased since the implementation of Rh immunoglobulin prophylaxis in Rh-negative women. However, intrauterine transfusion (IUT) continues to be the standard treatment for fetal anemia. Typically this is undertaken by accessing the umbilical vein near the placental cord insertion. The procedure is not without complications including preterm premature rupture of membranes (PPROM), preterm labor (PTL), preterm birth (PTB), infection, and cord complications including cord hematoma, bleeding, and fetal bradycardia [1]. We report a case of umbilical artery thrombosis after intrauterine transfusion with delivery at term without any further complications. We obtained consent for publication by the patient.

2. Case Presentation

The patient was a 31 y/o Gravida 3 Para 2 who presented to our center at 19-week gestation. She had two prior uncomplicated full term vaginal deliveries and received Rh immunoglobulin during and after each of her previous pregnancies. She has no significant past medical or surgical history.

During this pregnancy, her first trimester studies revealed an anti-D titer of 2048. The fetal status was noted to be RHD positive on amniocentesis.

On her initial evaluation at 19-week gestation at our center, the middle cerebral artery (MCA) Doppler revealed a peak systolic velocity (PSV) of 2.37 MoM. There was mild ascites and cardiomegaly.

After counseling the patient underwent the first in a series of combined intravascular/intraperitoneal intrauterine transfusions (see Table 1). The ascites and cardiomegaly resolved after the second transfusion.

The fourth transfusion was complicated by an episode of transient bradycardia with spontaneous recovery after removal of the procedure needle from the umbilical vein. On a preoperative ultrasound prior to her sixth procedure, thrombosis of one of the umbilical arteries was noted (see Figure 1). A review of earlier ultrasounds indicated two patent umbilical arteries although visualization of the cord was not specifically undertaken postoperatively after the fourth procedure or before and after the fifth procedure. Based on the reassuring status of the fetus, a decision was made to

TABLE 1: Intraoperative fetal transfusion data.

Gestational Age (weeks)	Initial Hct (%)	Final Hct (%)	IVT volume (mL)	IPT volume (mL)	Complication
19.1	6	24	8	5	None
19.6	22.4	37.6	10	10	None
21.6	30.5	40.9	12	20	None
25	27.8	30.1	15	Postponed	Fetal bradycardia
25.1				50	None
28.1	29.2	45.7	50	80	None
31.6	28.6	Unable to obtain final Hct due to dislodged needle.	70	115	2VC noted pre-op.
35	26	40.7	100	150	None

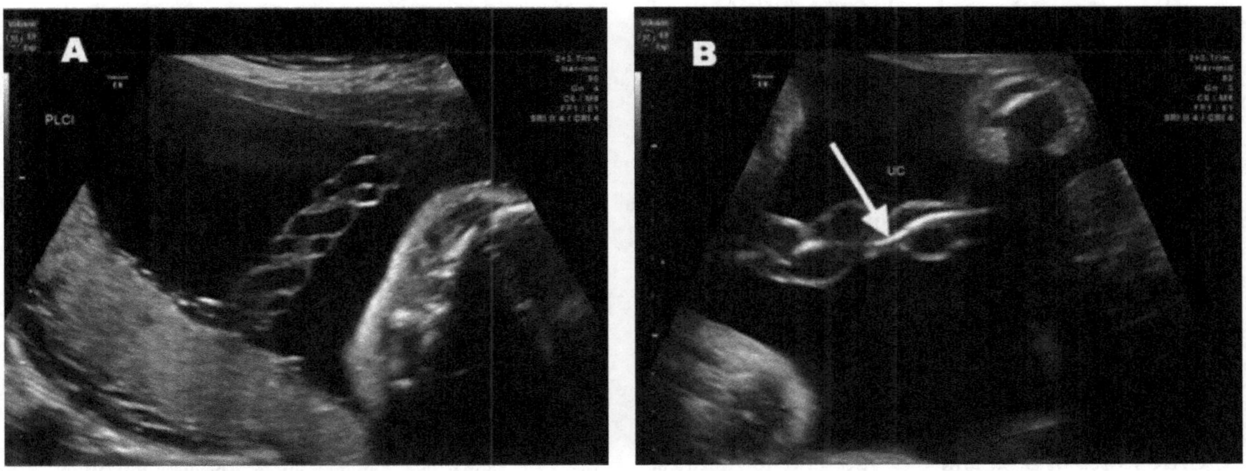

(a) (b)

FIGURE 1: (a) Three-vessel cord with two patent umbilical arteries was noted on initial evaluation. (b) Thrombosed umbilical artery (arrow) is seen in this segment of the cord.

continue serial intrauterine transfusions. Antenatal testing was initiated with weekly biophysical profiles and daily kick counts.

In addition to fetal anemia, this pregnancy was complicated by diet controlled gestational diabetes and mild polyhydramnios with an AFI of 29. The estimated fetal weight at 35 weeks ultrasound was 3193gms (87th %ile). She underwent a cesarean section at 37 weeks, delivering a 3480-gram male fetus in vertex presentation with APGARS of 8 and 9 at 1 and 5 minutes, respectively. After delivery the umbilical cord was examined and a 3-vessel cord with an intraluminal hematoma in one umbilical artery was confirmed. The hematocrit was 37% after birth. The total bilirubin was 9.9mg/dL and the direct bilirubin was 2.6 mg/dL. As per our neonatal protocols weekly hematocrit levels were monitored which remained above 30%; hence no transfusions were needed during this period.

3. Discussion

In pregnancies complicated by Rh alloimmunization for the first time fetal status should be confirmed by cell free DNA or fetal RHD gene testing on amniocentesis in cases of paternal heterozygosity or unknown status. These cases are managed conservatively initially by following serial antibody titers that should ideally be done in the same laboratory since variations in titers among laboratories commonly occurs. Once critical titers are exceeded MCA Dopplers should be performed to identify fetuses that are anemic. Serial titers are no longer monitored after reaching this critical titer. When the MCA PSV is > 1.5 MoM [2] for gestational age, a fetal blood sampling and intrauterine transfusion is done when anemia is confirmed. This procedure is performed between 18 and 35 weeks, as cases <18 weeks are limited by the small size of the vessels, thereby increasing the complications. We perform a combination of intravascular, in the umbilical vein, and intraperitoneal transfusions as this provides a more stable hematocrit and increases the duration between transfusions thereby reducing total number of procedures [3]. The technical aspects of performing an IUT have been previously described by the coauthor (KJM) [4]. Serial MCA Dopplers have been reported to be unreliable following an IUT especially after 2 transfusions. Therefore, we do not use these Dopplers to determine the timing of subsequent transfusions. The second, third, and subsequent IUTs are performed at 7-, 14-, and 21-day intervals, respectively, based on the expected drop in the hemoglobin level each day [4, 5]. The procedure-related loss after IUT has been reported to be 2% [6]; however there is limited information on the incidence of umbilical artery thrombosis and further management if this occurs.

We report a case of severe fetal anemia secondary to Rh alloimmunization requiring multiple intrauterine transfusions starting at 19 weeks. The bradycardia noted during the fourth transfusion may have been secondary to umbilical arterial puncture. We suspect that the thrombosis of the umbilical artery may be secondary to this inadvertent puncture while attempting to insert the needle in to the umbilical vein for the IUT. Although her treatment course was complicated by thrombosis of one of the umbilical arteries, subsequent transfusions were successful resulting in a term delivery.

Smith et al. [7] described a similar case. After two intravascular transfusions, a single umbilical artery was seen on ultrasound. They attempted another transfusion 4 weeks later, which was complicated by fetal bradycardia with the need for discontinuation of the procedure. Several weeks later, during an intravascular transfusion, the fetus developed refractory bradycardia and the infant was delivered by emergent cesarean section. The infant weighed 1920gms and had APGAR scores of 4, 2, and 6 at 1, 5, and 10 minutes, respectively. On pathology, coagulative necrosis and luminal thrombosis of one of the umbilical arteries were noted.

We believe that the presence of Hyrtl anastomosis explains the favorable outcome in our case. Joseph Hyrtl first described this anastomosis in 1870 as a communication between the umbilical arteries near the placental surface. This anastomosis is seen in 95% of all placentas [8]. It is believed to play a role in equalizing the blood pressure between the different parts of the placenta supplied by the umbilical arteries [9] and was thought to be protective in cases of compression or occlusion of one artery. This is particularly important late in pregnancy during uterine contractions when compression of one umbilical artery is well tolerated.

Gordon et al. [10] performed a quantitative analysis of the hemodynamic characteristics of the flow through this anastomosis. They demonstrated the importance of the presence of Hyrtl's anastomosis for the regulation of blood flow in discordant arteries. The anastomosis resulted in a redistribution of flow from the unaffected artery to the affected artery and equilibration of pressure gradients in the arteries to improve placental perfusion.

One of the most common umbilical cord anomalies is the presence of a single umbilical artery (SUA) that can be detected early by ultrasound. In cases of isolated SUA, fetal growth restriction and increased perinatal mortality has been reported [11]. Suess et al. [12] found an increase in the size of this isolated umbilical artery with gestational age, which may be an adaptive mechanism to enhance the placental perfusion. Hyrtl anastomosis is absent in these cases of SUA. The absence of the Hyrtl anastomoses near the placental cord insertion and failure of the arterial dilatation are likely responsible for the poor placental perfusion and complications like growth restriction and perinatal mortality. When the umbilical cord has two umbilical arteries, initially the loss of one vessel can be compensated for by the Hyrtl anastomosis. Adequate perfusion of the placenta may still be possible in these cases.

In conclusion, we suggest that while the detection of thrombosis of one of the umbilical arteries following IUT deserves a cautious approach, continuing the pregnancy and future transfusions may be a reasonable option especially in the case of prematurity and reassuring fetal status.

References

[1] I. T. M. Lindenburg, I. L. Van Kamp, and D. Oepkes, "Intrauterine blood transfusion: current indications and associated risks," *Fetal Diagnosis and Therapy*, vol. 36, pp. 263–271, 2014.

[2] R. Zimmermann, P. Durig, R. J. Carpenter Jr., and G. Mari, "Longitudinal measurement of peak systolic velocity in the fetal middle cerebral artery for monitoring pregnancies complicated by red cell alloimmunisation: a prospective multicentre trial with intention-to-treat," *BJOG: An International Journal of Obstetrics & Gynaecology*, vol. 109, pp. 746–752, 2002.

[3] K. J. Moise, R. J. Carpenter, B. Kirshon, R. L. Deter, J. D. Sala, and L. E. Cano, "Comparison of four types of intrauterine transfusion: effect on fetal hematocrit," *Fetal Diagnosis and Therapy*, vol. 4, pp. 126–137, 1989.

[4] K. J. Moise Jr, "Management of rhesus alloimmunization in pregnancy," *Obstetrics & Gynecology*, vol. 112, pp. 164–176, 2008.

[5] M. Scheier, E. Hernandez-Andrade, E. B. Fonseca, and K. H. Nicolaides, "Prediction of severe fetal anemia in red blood cell alloimmunization after previous intrauterine transfusions," *American Journal of Obstetrics & Gynecology*, vol. 195, pp. 1550–1556, 2006.

[6] K. J. Moise Jr., "Management of rhesus alloimmunization in pregnancy," *Obstetrics & Gynecology*, vol. 100, pp. 600–611, 2002.

[7] J. F. Smith Jr., K. D. Warner, M. Bergmann, and M. J. Pushchak, "Umbilical artery regression: a rare complication of intravascular fetal transfusion," *Obstetrics & Gynecology*, vol. 93, pp. 828-829, 1999.

[8] K. Benirschke and S. L. Pekarske, "Placental pathology casebook. extensive calcification of the umbilical cord and placenta," *Journal of perinatology: official journal of the California Perinatal Association*, vol. 15, pp. 81–83, 1995.

[9] L. Raio, F. Ghezzi, E. Di Naro et al., "In-utero characterization of the blood flow in the Hytrl anastomosis," *Placenta*, vol. 22, pp. 597–601, 2001.

[10] Z. Gordon, O. Eytan, A. J. Jaffa, and D. Elad, "Hemodynamic analysis of hyrtl anastomosis in human placenta," *American Journal of Physiology-Regulatory, Integrative and Comparative Physiology*, vol. 292, pp. R977–R982, 2007.

[11] S. Burshtein, A. Levy, G. Holcberg, A. Zlotnik, and E. Sheiner, "Is single umbilical artery an independent risk factor for perinatal mortality?" *Archives of Gynecology and Obstetrics*, vol. 283, pp. 191–194, 2011.

[12] G. Suess, L. Raio, A. Kuhn, E. Di Naro, and D. Surbek, "Arterial-adaptive dilatation and doppler velocimetry in normal fetuses with a single umbilical artery," *Ultraschall in der Medizin*, vol. 30, pp. 485–489, 2009.

54

Hidradenitis Suppurativa Recurrence in a Caesarean Scar

K. M. Darch, T. L. Holland, and L. J. Spelman

Veracity Clinical Research, Suite 18 Level 1 250 Ipswich Rd., Woolloongabba QLD 4102, Australia

Correspondence should be addressed to K. M. Darch; darchkatherine@gmail.com

Academic Editor: Mehmet A. Osmana ao lu

Hidradenitis suppurativa (HS), also known as acne inversa, is a chronic, relapsing inflammatory skin condition characterised by the presence of painful nodules, abscesses, and sinus tracts or scarring. Affecting up to 4% of the population, it is not uncommon and is seen predominantly in females at a ratio of 3 : 1. HS carries a substantial burden for those who suffer from it, from the significant psychosocial impact, to the cost of the multitude of topical and systemic treatments which often do not successfully control its symptoms. In this case report, we discuss a 33-year-old female known to our clinic, who presented with a recurrence of her HS in a caesarean scar, with otherwise silent disease. From our review of the literature, this appears to be only the second case of recurrence of HS in a caesarean scar reported to date. With a predilection for females of reproductive ages, involvement of sensitive areas, and an average of greater than seven years from onset of symptoms until diagnosis, the ability to recognise HS and ensure referral for specialist management is essential for all who are regularly involved in the management of this patient group.

1. Introduction

Affecting up to 4% of the population, HS is a common, chronic and debilitating disease, seen more commonly in females with a ratio of 3 : 1 [1]. It may occur at any time from the age of puberty, with only 2% of cases occurring before the age of 11 [2]. The exact aetiology of HS and its resultant painful nodules, abscesses, sinus tracts, and scarring remain unknown; however, recent evidence points to the dysregulation of skin immunity around hair follicles in affected regions [1]. Its sequelae, painful nodules, abscesses, and sinus tracts, are thought to be the result of inflammation of the hair follicle and resultant hyperkeratosis which leads to follicular occlusion and subsequent rupture of the follicle, with the release of the contents of the follicle perpetuating the inflammatory response of the surrounding dermis [1]. Studies have revealed elevated levels of IL-1b, TNF, IL-10, and IL-17 in the lesional skin of those with HS and have shown abnormalities in antimicrobial peptides and Toll-like-receptor signalling [1, 3].

The longstanding theory that HS is the result of infection of the apocrine sweat glands is no longer supported, with studies revealing that cultures taken from discharging lesions of HS most commonly show either no growth or growth of normal skin flora [1], though the secondary infection of sinus tracts and abscesses is possible. HS is known to beassociated with a number of other conditions including inflammatory bowel disease, depression and other psychiatric conditions, and the metabolic syndrome [1], highlighting the importance of a multidisciplinary approach to its management.

2. Case

This is the case of a 33-year-old female known to our clinic for management of HS, successfully managed with Humira (adalimumab) 40 mg injections weekly. She became pregnant with her first child and continued Humira until the end of the second trimester. She gave birth via emergency caesarean at 39 weeks to a healthy 3.59 kg male following induction of labor, failure to progress, and foetal bradycardias. Her HS remained silent throughout the pregnancy and after the birth, until approximately one week later when three painful nodules appeared in her left axilla. She self-recommenced Humira at this time, after ceasing breast feeding, and these nodules settled. Approximately two months later, she noted the appearance of small nodules and inflammatory tracts around her caesarean scar. These were initially thought to represent a fungal infection and were treated with an over-the-counter antifungal cream with limited efficacy. She was subsequently treated with topical antimicrobial preparation containing gramicidin, neomycin sulfate, nystatin, and triamcinolone acetonide, followed by oral amoxycillin and clavulanic acid, and potassium permanganate soaks to the area, all of which provided minimal improvement. Our patient reported excellent compliance with all wound care instructions at the time of delivery and noted significant distress at being told that her symptoms were the result of insufficient wound care and recurrent infection of the area.

She was seen in our clinic one month after the onset of symptoms. We noted the presence of a number of small, well-defined HS lesions, with nodules and discharging sinus tracts around the caesarean scar. Her disease elsewhere remained silent, and her compliance with Humira was excellent. She was subsequently diagnosed with a recurrence of HS in her caesarean scar, providing her with a sense of relief following the multiple previous presentations and reviews.

Her HS lesions involving her caesarean site responded well to treatment with doxycycline 100 mg daily and Prontosan Wound Gel and Wash (polyaminopropyl biguanide (polihexanide), betaine surfactant) in addition to Humira, with discharging sinus tracts persisting until review six months after the onset of symptoms, and complete resolution by review at one year.

3. Discussion

Our extensive search of the literature reveals only one other case of a recurrence of HS in a caesarean scar. This recently published report describes the case of a 34-year-old female with Hurley Stage II HS since the age of 18. The appearance of nodules and discharging fistulae were noted approximately five months following her second caesarean section, with the appearance of similar nodules also noted following her first caesarean section. Unlike our patient, she was also noted to have active disease in bilateral axillae. She was treated with doxycycline 100 mg twice a day, and topical treatment with both the antiseptic octenidine and a clindamycin/benzoyl peroxide gel [4]. There has been one other case report published which describes wound dehiscence following caesarean section in a female with HS, with multiple other comorbidities including obesity, gestational diabetes, and current smoker. The case report described that wound dehiscence was common following excision of HS lesions and as a result suggested that HS was the cause for the patient's postoperative complications [5].

The potential for HS to show Koebnerisation, or the predilection for areas of injury or trauma to otherwise "normal" skin, has been discussed in the literature previously. A case series that detailed 14 patients with HS lesions in locations not typical for the disease has described the presence of lesions, including nodules, abscesses, cysts, and in one patient a draining sunus tract, at the level of the waistband [6]. Seven of these patients had lesions excised, with histopathology results supporting the diagnosis of HS in all cases. All of the participants were obese, and all had a history of HS elsewhere. From this, the authors hypothesised that these HS lesions were the result of Koebnerisation following "traumatisation from external factors." They provide the details of another two studies, both describing female participants who were also obese and had a history of HS, in whom HS lesions were found to be present in line with where the edge of their bra sits [7, 8] and suggest that this may also be the result of Koebnerisation.

Further to this, Boer et al. investigated the potential for mechanical stressors to cause Koebnerisation of HS [9]. They suggested that the biomechanical stressors on inverse and concave skin areas are different to that in other areas, and that these constant mechanical forces are enhanced in obese patients and could be the reason for HS's predilection for these areas. They also note that mechanical stress on the skin induces a proinflammatory environment, epidermal hyperplasia, and hyperkeratosis and cited other associated conditions such as acne mechanica, which develops in areas exposed to mechanical stressors.

3.1. Management of HS. Successful management of HS remains a significant clinical challenge. The average time from onset of HS symptoms to diagnosis is 7.2 years [10]. This delay perpetuates the distress experienced by those who suffer from HS and is thought to result from of a lack of familiarity of clinicians with the condition, the frequent misdiagnosis of the inflammatory lesions of HS as recurrent boils or folliculitis which understandably fail to respond to conventional antimicrobial therapies [11] and the resultant reluctance of patients to continue to present to healthcare providers. Education, advocacy, referral, and early diagnosis are essential for adequate management of this population of patients. It has been suggested that in conjunction with medical therapies, all patients must receive adequate counselling and support for known comorbidities, including adequate analgesia, support to lose weight and for smoking cessation, treatment of superinfection, and proper education regarding management of active lesions [2].

Given the population most commonly affected by HS, knowledge of best management of the disease in women who are considering pregnancy, who are pregnant, and who are breast feeding is essential. Most women experience no change in their HS during pregnancy, with 20% reporting improvement while pregnant, and 8% experiencing worsening of their disease [12]. An article by Perng et al. [12] published in 2017 provides a summary of the treatment options available for women during pregnancy. They discuss the use of topical antibiotics, with clindamycin (1%), metronidazole (0.75%), and erythromycin (2%) classified as FDA pregnancy category B drugs. Though often considered to be first-line treatment in the non-pregnant population, the use of oral tetracyclines is contraindicated during pregnancy, and they are not recommended for use in lactation. The combination of oral clindamycin and rifampicin may provide significant benefit for patients with moderate-to-severe HS, and with clindamycin listed as pregnancy category B, and rifampicin as pregnancy category C, a short course of this combination therapy may be considered in pregnant patients where the benefit of treatment outweighs any potential risks, and where there are no other contraindications to their use or drug-drug interactions.

Biologic agents such as adalimumab and infliximab are considered to be category B drugs in pregnancy; however, the evidence to support their use in pregnancy is controversial [12, 13]. Given the high molecular weight of adalimumab, it is likely to require active transport to cross the placenta [14]. For this reason, it is suggested that biologic agents such as adalimumab should be ceased prior to the third trimester of pregnancy when active transport of maternal IgG occurs in order to limit potential foetal exposure [12, 14]. Evidence for their use in breastfeeding is also limited.

3.2. Psychological Impact of HS. HS has been said to cause "tremendous psychological stress" for those who suffer from it [15]. The psychosocial impact of HS may be mediated by a number of factors. The pain and discharge from draining sinuses and abscesses may significantly impair a patient's ability to work, exercise, and socialise. The physical appearance of the lesions and their predilection for sensitive areas often cause significant shame and embarrassment for those who suffer from them, which again has an impact on their ability to work and socialise and on their relationships. HS remains a significant challenge to successfully manage, and the expense of multiple topical and systemic treatments also carries a significant impact.

Studies have shown that depression is diagnosed at a higher rate (5.9%) in those with HS when compared to the rate in matched controls (3.5%), and at a higher rate in females who suffer from the condition [12]. "Anxiety" was similarly diagnosed at a higher rate in those with HS (3.9%) when compared to matched controls (2.4%) [12], and the study discussed a nonstatistically significant increase in the rate of diagnosis of other psychiatric conditions such as schizophrenia and bipolar disorder in those who suffered from HS compared to matched controls.

For our patient, the fact that she felt that she was not listened to and that she was told it was not possible for her HS to recur in a caesarean scar added significantly to her distress.

4. Conclusions

In this case report, we have discussed the recurrence of HS in a caesarean scar of a patient with otherwise silent disease. This appears to be only the second case of this that has been reported in the literature to date, with a similar case recently published. We have discussed the significant burden that HS and misdiagnosis of the condition have on those who suffer from it. Patient education, early referral, and a multidisciplinary team approach to management may greatly assist to ease this disease burden and may have significantly improved the experience of our patient.

Given that HS is more likely to affect women and can be seen from the age of puberty, a knowledge of the management of HS during pregnancy and breast feeding forms an essential part of the holistic management of the HS patient. We hope that this case may serve as a reminder of the significant distress that HS can cause, that it may present in atypical sites, and the difference that holistic management can make.

Consent

Informed consent was obtained from the subject of this case report prior to preparation of this manuscript.

References

[1] C. Vinkel and S. F. Thomsen, "Hidradenitis suppurativa: causes, features, and current treatments," *The Journal of Clinical and Aesthetic Dermatology*, vol. 11, no. 10, pp. 17–23, 2018.

[2] W. Gulliver, C. C. Zouboulis, E. Prens, and G. B. Jemec, "Evidence-based approach to the treatment of hidradenitis suppurativa/acne inversa, based on the European guidelines for hidradenitis suppurativa," *Reviews in Endocrine & Metabolic Disorders*, vol. 17, no. 3, pp. 343–351, 2016.

[3] G. Kelly and E. P. Prens, "Inflammatory mechanisms in hidradenitis suppurativa," *Dermatologic Clinics*, vol. 34, no. 1, pp. 51–58, 2016.

[4] E. Agiasofitou, T. Kanni, E. Platsidaki et al., "Development of new lesions of hidradenitis suppurativa on a caesarean section scar: a manifestation of the Koebner phenomenon?," *Skin Appendage Disorders*, vol. 6, pp. 1–3, 2020.

[5] M. Fernando and M. J. Schultz, "Recurrent wound dehiscence and small bowel herniation following caesarean section in a woman with hidradenitis suppurativa," *Journal of Surgical Case Reports*, vol. 2014, no. 5, pp. 5-6, 2014.

[6] J. Boer, "Should hidradenitis suppurativa be included in dermatoses showing Koebnerization? Is it friction or fiction?," *Dermatology*, vol. 233, no. 1, pp. 47–52, 2017.

[7] J. Boer, "Resolution of hidradenitis suppurativa after weight loss by dietary measures, especially on frictional locations," *Journal of the European Academy of Dermatology and Venereology*, vol. 30, no. 5, pp. 895-896, 2016.

[8] J. Boer and D. Mihajlovic, "Boils at frictional locations in a patient with hidradenitis suppurativa," *Acta Dermatovenerologica Croatica*, vol. 24, no. 4, pp. 303-304, 2016.

[9] J. Boer, M. Nazary, and P. T. Riis, "The role of mechanical stress in hidradenitis suppurativa," *Dermatologic Clinics*, vol. 34, no. 1, pp. 37–43, 2016.

[10] A. B. Kimball, M. M. Okun, D. A. Williams et al., "Two phase 3 trials of adalimumab for hidradenitis suppurativa," *The New England Journal of Medicine*, vol. 375, no. 5, pp. 422–434, 2016.

[11] H. Van der Zee, J. Laman, J. Boer, and E. Prens, "Hidradenitis suppurativa: viewpoint on clinical phenotyping, pathogenesis and novel treatments," *Experimental Dermatology*, vol. 21, no. 10, pp. 735–739, 2012.

[12] P. Perng, J. G. Zambella, and G. A. Okoye, "Management of hidradenitis suppurativa in pregnancy," *Journal of the American Academy of Dermatology*, vol. 76, no. 5, pp. 979–989, 2017.

[13] M. L. Porter, S. J. Lockwood, and A. B. Kimball, "Update on biologic safety for patients with psoriasis during pregnancy," *International Journal of Women's Dermatology*, vol. 3, no. 1, pp. 21–25, 2017.

[14] C. D. Chambers, D. L. Johnson, R. Xu et al., "Birth outcomes in women who have taken adalimumab in pregnancy: a prospec-

tive cohort study," *PLOS ONE*, vol. 14, no. 10, article e0228603, p. e0223603, 2019.

[15] E. Shavit, J. Dreiher, T. Freud, S. Halevy, S. Vinker, and A. D. Cohen, "Psychiatric comorbidities in 3207 patients with hidradenitis suppurativa," *Journal of the European Academy of Dermatology and Venereology*, vol. 29, no. 2, pp. 371–376, 2015.

Permissions

All chapters in this book were first published by Hindawi Publishing Corporation; hereby published with permission under the Creative Commons Attribution License or equivalent. Every chapter published in this book has been scrutinized by our experts. Their significance has been extensively debated. The topics covered herein carry significant findings which will fuel the growth of the discipline. They may even be implemented as practical applications or may be referred to as a beginning point for another development.

The contributors of this book come from diverse backgrounds, making this book a truly international effort. This book will bring forth new frontiers with its revolutionizing research information and detailed analysis of the nascent developments around the world.

We would like to thank all the contributing authors for lending their expertise to make the book truly unique. They have played a crucial role in the development of this book. Without their invaluable contributions this book wouldn't have been possible. They have made vital efforts to compile up to date information on the varied aspects of this subject to make this book a valuable addition to the collection of many professionals and students.

This book was conceptualized with the vision of imparting up-to-date information and advanced data in this field. To ensure the same, a matchless editorial board was set up. Every individual on the board went through rigorous rounds of assessment to prove their worth. After which they invested a large part of their time researching and compiling the most relevant data for our readers.

The editorial board has been involved in producing this book since its inception. They have spent rigorous hours researching and exploring the diverse topics which have resulted in the successful publishing of this book. They have passed on their knowledge of decades through this book. To expedite this challenging task, the publisher supported the team at every step. A small team of assistant editors was also appointed to further simplify the editing procedure and attain best results for the readers.

Apart from the editorial board, the designing team has also invested a significant amount of their time in understanding the subject and creating the most relevant covers. They scrutinized every image to scout for the most suitable representation of the subject and create an appropriate cover for the book.

The publishing team has been an ardent support to the editorial, designing and production team. Their endless efforts to recruit the best for this project, has resulted in the accomplishment of this book. They are a veteran in the field of academics and their pool of knowledge is as vast as their experience in printing. Their expertise and guidance has proved useful at every step. Their uncompromising quality standards have made this book an exceptional effort. Their encouragement from time to time has been an inspiration for everyone.

The publisher and the editorial board hope that this book will prove to be a valuable piece of knowledge for researchers, students, practitioners and scholars across the globe.

List of Contributors

Saki Yamamoto, Tomohiro Kikuchi, Hiroyuki Fujii, Yuko Otake, Mitsuru Matsuki, Masashi Endo and Harushi Mori
1Department of Radiology, Jichi Medical University School of Medicine, Tochigi, Japan

Risa Narumi and Hiroyuki Fujiwara
Department of Obstetrics and Gynecology, Jichi Medical University School of Medicine, Tochigi, Japan

Lily Criscione, Kristen Elmezzi and Saioa Torrealday
Walter Reed National Military Medical Center, 8901 Rockville Pike, Bethesda, MD 20889, USA

Barton C. Staat and Kimberly Hickey
Uniformed Services University, 4301 Jones Bridge Rd., Bethesda, MD 20814, USA

Dereje Tegene, Sultan Nesha, Befikadu Gizaw and Tadele Befikadu
Department of Obstetrics and Gynecology, Adama Hospital Medical College, Adama, Ethiopia

Mansooreh Haghiri, Sedigheh Borna, Sedigheh Hantoushzadeh and Maasoumeh Saleh
Maternal, Fetal and Neonatal Research Center, Vali-e-Asr Hospital, Tehran University of Medical Sciences, Tehran, Iran

Kamran Hessami
Department of Obstetrics and Gynecology, Baylor College of Medicine, Houston, TX, USA
Maternal-Fetal Medicine Research Center, Shiraz University of Medical Sciences, Shiraz, Iran

Ali Sharifi
Department of Surgery, Beesat Hospital, Hamadan University of Medical Sciences, Tehran, Iran

Seyed Mohsen Ahmadi Tafti
Department of Surgery, Tehran University of Medical Sciences, Tehran, Iran

Mahrooz Malek
Department of Radiology, Vali-e-Asr Hospital, Tehran University of Medical Sciences, Tehran, Iran

Nasim Pourdamghan
Department of Obstetrics and Gynecology, Kerman University of Medical Sciences, Tehran, Iran, Kerman, Iran

Abolfazl Shirdel Abdolmaleki
School of Medicine, Shiraz University of Medical Sciences, Shiraz, Iran

Luke William Nelson and Elliot MacKenzie
Dunedin Public Hospital, 201 Great King Street, Dunedin 9010, New Zealand

Yusuke Sagae, Masumi Sunada and Akihito Horie
Department of Gynecology and Obstetrics, Kyoto University, Kyoto, Japan

Daisuke Katsura, Shunichiro Tsuji, Kaori Hayashi, Kazutaka Yamada, Shinsuke Tokoro, Kounosuke Suzuki, Fuminori Kimura and Takashi Murakami
Department of Obstetrics and Gynecology, Shiga University of Medical Science Hospital, Setatsukinowa-cho, Otsu, Shiga 520-2192, Japan

Suzuko Moritani
Department of Diagnostic Pathology, Shiga University of Medical Science Hospital, Setatsukinowa-cho, Otsu, Shiga 520-2192, Japan

Osamah Hasan
Midwestern University Chicago College of Osteopathic Medicine, 555 31st St, Downers Grove, IL 60515, USA

Grant S. Johnson and James J. Siegert
Franciscan Health, 20201 South Crawford Avenue, Olympia Fields, IL 60461, USA

Francisco Garcini
Silver Cross Hospital, 1890 Silver Cross Boulevard, Suite 210, New Lenox, IL 60451, USA

Thai T. Nguyen
Advanced Urology Associates, 1541 Riverboat Center Drive, Joliet, IL 60431, USA

Mohamed Rishard, Prabhodana Ranaweera and Athula Kaluarachchi
Department of Obstetrics and Gynecology, Faculty of Medicine, University of Colombo 25, Kynsey Road, Colombo 08, Sri Lanka
De Soysa Hospital for Women Kynsey Road, Colombo 08, Sri Lanka

Tushani Ranawaka
Department of Obstetrics and Gynecology, Faculty of Medicine, University of Colombo 25, Kynsey Road, Colombo 08, Sri Lanka

Suren Perera, Kushan Jayasinghe, Amila Rubasinghe, Sanjaya Athapaththu, Malindu Edirisinghe, Priyankara Jayawardana and Zacky Haniffa
De Soysa Hospital for Women Kynsey Road, Colombo 08, Sri Lanka

Ali Azadi
University of Arizona, College of Medicine, 475 N 5th St, Phoenix, AZ 85004, USA
Star Urogynecology, 14155 N 83rd Ave, Suite 138, Peoria, AZ 85381, USA

Alexandra Wolfe
OMS-IV Midwestern University, 19555 N 59th Ave, Glendale, AZ 85308, USA

Greg J. Marchand
The Marchand Institute for Minimally Invasive Surgery, 10238 E Hampton Ave, Suite 212, Mesa, AZ 85209, USA

Kwaku Asah-Opoku
Department of Obstetrics and Gynecology, University of Ghana School of Medicine and Dentistry (UGSMD), Korle-Bu, Accra, Ghana
Korle-Bu Teaching Hospital, Department of Obstetrics and Gynaecology, Korle-Bu, Accra, Ghana
Department of Obstetrics and Gynaecology, University Medical Centre Utrecht, Utrecht University, Utrecht, Netherlands
Julius Global Health, Julius Centre for Health Sciences and Primary Care, University Medical Centre Utrecht, Utrecht University, Utrecht, Netherlands

Nana Essuman Oduro, Alim Swarray-Deen, Isaac Osei Koranteng and Rita Catherine Senker
Korle-Bu Teaching Hospital, Department of Obstetrics and Gynaecology, Korle-Bu, Accra, Ghana

Kareem Mumuni and Kobinah Nkyekyer
Department of Obstetrics and Gynecology, University of Ghana School of Medicine and Dentistry (UGSMD), Korle-Bu, Accra, Ghana
Korle-Bu Teaching Hospital, Department of Obstetrics and Gynaecology, Korle-Bu, Accra, Ghana

Marcus Rijken
Department of Obstetrics and Gynaecology, University Medical Centre Utrecht, Utrecht University, Utrecht, Netherlands
Julius Global Health, Julius Centre for Health Sciences and Primary Care, University Medical Centre Utrecht, Utrecht University, Utrecht, Netherlands

F. Richard Ervin
South Carolina Department of Health and Environmental Control, South Carolina, USA

Tadatsugu Kinjo, Keiko Mekaru, Miyuki Nakada, Sugiko Oishi, Chiaki Urasoe, Kozue Akamine, Hayase Nitta, Hitoshi Masamoto and Yoichi Aoki
Department of Obstetrics and Gynecology, Graduate School of Medicine, University of the Ryukyus, 207 Uehara Nishihara, Okinawa 903-0215, Japan

Oriel Nissim and Deeksha Jandhyala
Medical University of South Carolina, Charleston, South Carolina, USA

Susan E. Dorman
Medical University of South Carolina, Charleston, South Carolina, USA
South Carolina Department of Health and Environmental Control, South Carolina, USA

Kyohei Yamaguchi, Hiroaki Tanaka, Fumi H. Furuhashi, Kayo Tanaka, Eiji Kondo and Tomoaki Ikeda
Department of Obstetrics and Gynecology, Mie University, Mie, Japan

Drishti Madhok and Erik Gunderson
Bundaberg Base Hospital, 271 Bourbong St Bundaberg, QLD 4670, Australia

Vinayak Smith
Department of Obstetrics and Gynaecology, Monash University, 252 Clayton Road, 3168 VIC, Australia

Atsushi Yoshida, Asumi Okumura, Masahiro Nakao and Ryo Suzuki
Department of Obstetrics and Gynecology, Sakakibara Heart Institute, Fuchu, Tokyo, Japan

Ali Hosiani
Department of Obstetrics & Gynaecology, Blacktown Hospital, Blacktown, New South Wales, Australia

James Brown and Indika T. Alahakoon
Department of Maternal Foetal Medicine, Westmead Hospital, Westmead, New South Wales, Australia

Stephanie L. Pierce and Rodney K. Edwards
Department of Obstetrics and Gynecology, College of Medicine, University of Oklahoma Health Sciences Center, Oklahoma City, OK, USA

Dena R. Shibib
Department of Pathology, College of Medicine, University of Oklahoma Health Sciences Center, Oklahoma City, OK, USA
Department of Pathology, Oklahoma City VA Health Care System, Oklahoma City, OK, USA

Denise Robison
OU Medicine Microbiology Laboratory, Oklahoma City, OK, USA

Sofia Jovina Domingues
Centro Hospitalar de Setúbal, Setúbal, Portugal

Luísa Pinto
Centro Hospitalar e Universitário Lisboa Norte, Lisbon, Portugal

Shravya Govindappagari
Department of Obstetrics and Gynecology, Division of Maternal-Fetal Medicine, Cedars-Sinai Medical Center, Los Angeles, CA, USA

Michelle Nguyen
Department of Obstetrics and Gynecology, Adventist Health White Memorial, Los Angeles, CA, USA

Megha Gupta
Department of Obstetrics and Gynecology, Division of Maternal-Fetal Medicine, University of Texas Health Science Center at Houston, Houston, TX, USA

Ramy M. Hanna
Department of Medicine, Division of Nephrology, UCLA David Geffen School of Medicine, Los Angeles, CA, USA

Richard M. Burwick
Department of Obstetrics and Gynecology, UCLA David Geffen School of Medicine, Los Angeles, CA, USA

Department of Obstetrics and Gynecology, Division of Maternal-Fetal Medicine, Cedars-Sinai Medical Center, Los Angeles, CA, USA

Angela Vidal and Carolin Dhakal
Department of Obstetrics and Gynecology, Lucerne Cantonal Hospital, Switzerland

Dani Zoorob, Kristrun Kristinsdottir and Thomas Klein
University of Toledo, Department of Obstetrics and Gynecology Academic Offices, 2142 N. Cove Blvd., Toledo, OH 43606, USA

Sonyoung Seo-Patel
ProMedica Health System, Women's Services, 2142 N. Cove Blvd., Toledo, OH 43606, USA

Yumika Takaki, Atsushi Daimon, Misa Nunode, Tomohito Tanaka, Daisuke Fujita and Masahide Ohmichi
Department of Obstetrics and Gynecology, Osaka Medical and Pharmaceutical University, 2-7 Daigaku-Machi, Takatsuki, Osaka 569-8686, Japan

Archana Ayyar, Rachel D. Seaman and Mary C. Tolcher
Department of Obstetrics and Gynecology, Baylor College of Medicine, Houston, Texas, USA

Kalpalatha Guntupalli
Department of Medicine, Pulmonary and Critical Care, Baylor College of Medicine, Houston, Texas, USA

Ubong Akpan, Chinyere Akpanika and Saturday Etuk
Department of Obstetrics and Gynaecology, University of Calabar, Calabar, Nigeria

Victor Nwagbara
Department of General Surgery, University of Calabar, Calabar, Nigeria

Udeme Asibong
Department of Family Medicine, University of Calabar, Calabar, Nigeria

Manisha Chhetry
Department of Obstetrics and Gynecology, BP Koirala Institute of Health Science, Nepal

Aruna Pokharel and Amar Nath Chaudhary
Department of Obstetrics and Gynecology, Nobel Medical College and Teaching Hospital, Nepal

Kathy Mostajeran, Hillary Boswell and Ziad Haidar
Gulf Coast Educational Consortium/HCA Houston Healthcare West, 12141 Richmond Ave. Houston, TX 77082, USA

Anastasia A. Salame, Mohammad J. Jaffal, Marco A. Mouanness, Amal R. Nasser Eddin and Labib M. Ghulmiyyah
American University of Beirut Medical Center, Beirut, Lebanon

Mariam Ayyash, Nicolina Smith and Madhurima Keerthy
Department of Obstetrics and Gynecology, Henry Ford Health System, Detroit, Michigan, USA

Ashina Singh
Department of Gastroenterology and Hepatology, Henry Ford Health System, Detroit, Michigan, USA

Majid Shaman
Division of Maternal and Fetal Medicine, Department of Obstetrics and Gynecology, Henry Ford Health System, Detroit, Michigan, USA

Narges Montazeri and Mohammad Hassan Darabi
Maternal-Fetal Medicine Research Center, Shiraz University of Medical Sciences, Shiraz, Iran

Ramin Shekouhi and Maryam Sohooli
Colorectal Research Center, Department of Surgery, Shiraz University of Medical Sciences, Shiraz, Iran

Tahereh Shamsi and Fateme Bagheri
School of Medicine, Shiraz University of Medical Sciences, Shiraz, Iran

Mohammad Amin Shahrbaf
Faculty of Medicine, Shahid Beheshti University of Medical Sciences, Tehran, Iran

Kurabachew Mengistu
Department of Anesthesiology, College of Medicine and Health Sciences, Hawassa University, Hawassa, Ethiopia

Tufa Bobe and Gashaw Tilahun
Department of Obstetrics and Gynaecology, College of Medicine and Health Sciences, Madda Wallabu University, Robe, Ethiopia

Kibru Kifle
Department of Obstetrics and Gynaecology, College of Medicine and Health Sciences, Hawassa University, Hawassa, Ethiopia

Dereje Geleta
School of Public and Environmental Health, College of Medicine and Health Sciences, Hawassa University, Hawassa, Ethiopia

Joan Tymon-Rosario
Department of Obstetrics & Gynecology and Women's Health, Albert Einstein College of Medicine, Montefiore Medical Center, Bronx, NY, USA

Jessica M. Atrio
Department of Obstetrics & Gynecology and Women's Health, Albert Einstein College of Medicine, Montefiore Medical Center, Bronx, NY, USA
Division of Family Planning, Department of Obstetrics & Gynecology and Women's Health, Bronx, NY, USA

Hyun Ah Yoon
Department of Pathology, Albert Einstein College of Medicine, Montefiore Medical Center, Bronx, NY, USA

David Erlichman
Department of Radiology, Albert Einstein College of Medicine, Montefiore Medical Center, Bronx, NY, USA

Veronica Lerner
Department of Obstetrics & Gynecology and Women's Health, Albert Einstein College of Medicine, Montefiore Medical Center, Bronx, NY, USA
Division of Minimally Invasive Surgery, Department of Obstetrics & Gynecology and Women's Health, Bronx, NY, USA

Junsuke Muraoka, Teruo Otsuka, Aya Yamauchi and Kiminari Terao
Department of Obstetrics and Gynecology, Perinatal Medicine, Miyazaki Prefectural Nobeoka Hospital, 2-1-10 Shinkoji, Nobeoka, Miyazaki 882-0835, Japan

Lauryn C. Gabby
Department of Obstetrics, Gynecology, & Reproductive Sciences, University of California, San Diego, California, USA

Katherine E. McDaniel, Brian J. Gordon and Laila A. Al-Marayati
Department of Obstetrics and Gynecology, University of Southern California, Los Angeles, California, USA

Josephine Eva Gathura, Amro Elfeky, Rodney McLaren Jr., David Herzog and Richard Grazi
Department of Obstetrics and Gynecology, Maimonides Medical Center, Brooklyn, New York, USA

D. Ricard-Gauthier and D. E. Huber
Department of Gynecology and Obstetrics, Valais Hospital, Sion, Switzerland

M.-A. Panchard
Department of Underwater and Hyperbare, University Hospital of Geneva, Switzerland

Boban Gjakov and Mateja Vukmanič Pohar
Department of Gynecology and Obstetrics, Brežice General Hospital, Černelčeva cesta 15, 8250, Brežice, Slovenia

Darja Kopač
Division of Obstetrics and Gynecology, University Medical Center Ljubljana, Šlajmerjeva 3, 1000 Ljubljana, Slovenia

Miha Lučovnik
Division of Obstetrics and Gynecology, University Medical Center Ljubljana, Šlajmerjeva 3, 1000 Ljubljana, Slovenia
Medical Faculty, University of Ljubljana, Vrazov trg 2, 1000 Ljubljana, Slovenia

David M. B. Rosen, Sarah Choi, Mujahid Bukhari, Gregory M. Cario and Danny Chou
Sydney Women's Endosurgery Centre (SWEC), Sydney, Australia

Dave R. Listijono
Sydney Women's Endosurgery Centre (SWEC), Sydney, Australia
IVF Australia, Sydney, Australia

Angeliki Rouvali, Panagiotis Vlastarakos, Sofoklis Stavros, Maria Giourga, Kalliopi Pappa, Alexandros Rodolakis and Ekaterini Domali
1st Department of Obstetrics and Gynaecology, Alexandra Hospital, National and Kapodistrian University of Athens, Athens, Greece

Angeliki Gerede
Department of Obstetrics and Gynecology Democritus, University of Thrace Alexandroupolis, Greece

Joshua M. Samuel, Fatima Ali, Jonathan Faro and Jonathan D. Baum
Department of Obstetrics and Gynecology, Jersey Shore Medical Center, Neptune, NJ 07754, USA

Yuri Suminaga, Yoshitsugu Chigusa, Haruko Okamoto, Yosuke Kawamura, Mana Taki, Masaki Mandai and Haruta Mogami
Department of Gynecology and Obstetrics, Kyoto University, 54 Shogoin Kawahara-cho, Sakyo-ku, Kyoto 606-8507, Japan

Tadakazu Kondo
Department of Hematology and Oncology, Kyoto University, 54 Shogoin Kawahara-cho, Sakyo-ku, Kyoto 606-8507, Japan

Allison Eubanks, Katherine Dengler and Daniel Gruber
Department of Urogynecology in Obstetrics & Gynecology, Walter Reed National Military Medical Center, Bethesda, MD, USA

Yuichiro Sato and Murasaki Aman
Department of Diagnostic Pathology, Faculty of Medicine, Miyazaki University Hospital, University of Miyazaki, 5200 Kihara, Kiyotake, Miyazaki 889-1692, Japan

Tomoko Yamaguchi, Jyunsuke Muraoka and Hajime Taniguchi
Department of Obstetrics and Gynecology, Miyazaki Prefectural Nichinan Hospital, 1-9-5, Kiyama, Nichinan, Miyazaki 887-0013, Japan

Atsushi Kisanuki
Department of Diagnostic Pathology, Miyazaki Prefectural Nichinan Hospital, 1-9-5, Kiyama, Nichinan, Miyazaki 887-0013, Japan

Kazunari Maekawa, Atushi Yamashita and Yujiro Asada
Department of Pathology, Faculty of Medicine, University of Miyazaki, 5200 Kihara, Kiyotake, Miyazaki 889-1692, Japan

Yuki Kodama and Hiroshi Sameshima
Department of Obstetrics and Gynecology, Faculty of Medicine, University of Miyazaki, 5200 Kihara, Kiyotake, Miyazaki 889-1692, Japan

Maria Grazia Piccioni, Martina Derme, Laura Salerno, Elisa Morrocchi, Francesco Pecorini, Maria Grazia Porpora and Roberto Brunelli
Department of Gynecological, Obstetrical and Urological Sciences, University of Rome "Sapienza", Viale del Policlinico, 155, 00161 Rome, Italy

Sheeba Marwah, Reenu Kanwar, Shahida Naghma and Anjali Dabral
Department of Obstetrics and Gynaecology, New Delhi 110029, India
VMMC and Safdarjung Hospital, New Delhi 110029, India

Nitesh Gupta
VMMC and Safdarjung Hospital, New Delhi 110029, India
Department of Pulmonary, Critical and Sleep Medicine, New Delhi 110029, India

Andréanne Durivage, Geneviève Le Templier, Annabelle Cumyn and Nadine Sauvé
Department of General Internal Medicine, Faculty of Medicine, University of Sherbrooke, Quebec, Canada

Shuusaku Kobori
Department of Maternal and Fetal Medicine, Miyagi Children's Hospital, Miyagi 989-3126, Japan

Yuichiro Takahashi
Department of Fetal and Maternal Medicine, Nagara Medical Center, Gifu, Japan

Shusaku Kobori, Masatake Toshimitsu, Shinichi Nagaoka and Jun Murotsuki
Department of Maternal and Fetal Medicine, Miyagi Children's Hospital, Sendai, Miyagi 989-3126, Japan

Oriana Marrucci, Paola Nicoletti, Lodovico Patrizi, Carlo Ticconi, Francesco Sesti and Emilio Piccione
Department of Surgical Sciences, Section of Gynecology and Obstetrics, University of Rome Tor Vergata, Italy

Alessandro Mauriello and Simone Facchetti
Anatomic Pathology, Department of Experimental Medicine, University of Rome Tor Vergata, Italy

Yui Kinjo
Department of Obstetrics and Gynecology, Graduate School of Medicine, University of the Ryukyus, 207 Uehara Nishihara, Okinawa 903-0215, Japan

Yasmin Abedin
Department of Obstetrics, Gynecology and Women's Health at Rutgers-New Jersey Medical School, Newark, New Jersey, USA

Kanchi Chadha
Department of Obstetrics and Gynecology at Hackensack University Medical Center, Hackensack, New Jersey, USA

Roopali V. Donepudi and Kenneth J. Moise Jr.
Department of Obstetrics, Gynecology and Reproductive Medicine, Division of Maternal-Fetal Medicine, UT Health-School of Medicine at Houston, The Fetal Center, Children's Memorial Hermann Hospital, Houston, TX, USA

K. M. Darch, T. L. Holland and L. J. Spelman
Veracity Clinical Research, Suite 18 Level 1 250 Ipswich Rd., Woolloongabba QLD 4102, Australia

Index

www.ingramcontent.com/pod-product-compliance
Lightning Source LLC
LaVergne TN
LVHW082151200926
848484LV00008B/2139
* 9 7 9 8 8 8 7 4 0 6 4 8 0 *